Preparation and Revision for the DRCOG

Commissioning Editor: Ellen Green
Project Development Manager: Siân Jarman
Project Manager: Nancy Arnott
Designer: Erik Bigland
Illustrator: David Gardner

THIRD EDITION

Preparation and Revision for the
DRCOG

Janice Rymer
MD FRCOG FRANZCOG ILTM
Senior Lecturer/Consultant in Obstetrics and
Gynaecology, Guy's, King's and St Thomas' School of Medicine,
Guy's and St Thomas' Hospital Trust, London

Gregory Davis
MD FRCOG FRANZCOG
Staff Specialist/Conjoint Senior Lecturer,
Department of Obstetrics and Gynaecology,
St George Hospital, University of New South Wales

Adam Rodin
BSc FRCOG
Consultant in Obstetrics and Gynaecology,
Barnet and Chase Farm Hospitals NHS Trust

Michael Chapman
MD FRCOG FRANZCOG
Professor of Obstetrics and Gynaecology,
St George Hospital, University of New South Wales

CHURCHILL
LIVINGSTONE

EDINBURGH LONDON NEW YORK PHILADELPHIA ST LOUIS SYDNEY TORONTO 2003

CHURCHILL LIVINGSTONE
An imprint of Elsevier Limited

First edition 1990
Second edition 1998
Third edition 2003
   Reprinted 2007, 2008, 2009

ISBN: 978-0-443-07224-6

British Library Cataloguing in Publication Data
A catalogue record for this book is available from the British Library.

Library of Congress Cataloging in Publication Data
A catalog record for this book is available from the Library of Congress.

Note
Medical knowledge is constantly changing. As new information becomes
available, changes in treatment, procedures, equipment and the use of drugs
become necessary. The editors, contributors and the publishers have, as far as
it is possible, taken care to ensure that the information given in this text is
accurate and up to date. However, readers are strongly advised to confirm that
the information, especially with regard to drug usage, complies with the latest
legislation and standards of practice.

Working together to grow
libraries in developing countries

www.elsevier.com | www.bookaid.org | www.sabre.org

ELSEVIER   BOOK AID International   Sabre Foundation

your source for books,
journals and multimedia
in the health sciences

www.elsevierhealth.com

The
publisher's
policy is to use
paper manufactured
from sustainable forests

Printed in China

Preface

The Diploma of the Royal College of Obstetricians and Gynaecologists is an examination to establish that a medical practitioner is adequately prepared to undertake obstetrics and gynaecology in a general practice setting. This book aims to provide basic knowledge of the syllabus and to assist the candidate to pass the examination. We begin by describing the structure of the examination in detail and devote a chapter to each section. In these chapters advice on preparation is given and example questions are provided for practice. We emphasize in the text that the place to learn obstetrics and gynaecology is on the wards, in clinics and in the operating theatre. Discussion with colleagues and background reading is essential in obstetrics and gynaecology as there are many areas of controversy.

In covering the syllabus we have aimed for a 'common-sense' approach without dealing with minutiae. We have highlighted controversial areas and acknowledged that other views exist.

Each chapter commences with a section outlining the 'expectations of the examiners' to provide guidance for the candidate to concentrate on the core of the subject. The coverage is not definitive and should be augmented with other texts, as described in 'Suggested reading'.

We thank our eight contributors for providing their specialist expertise and acknowledge Christine Watson who wrote the chapters on 'Family Planning' and 'Psychosexual Counselling' for our first two editions. As this is the third edition assistance has been needed with updating certain chapters and we are particularly grateful to Philippa Kyle, Jennifer Higham and Elizabeth Owen for their help with fetal medicine, menstrual disorders, and recurrent miscarriage. We are also grateful to Roger Jackson from the Royal College of Obstetricians and Gynaecologists who has given us advice about the examination. In addition, we are indebted to Tracy Alderton, who has diligently typed the manuscript and coped with the never-ending alterations.

Every conception needs a father, and this book has had Dr Joe Rosenthal (general practitioner) who has painstakingly read and criticized every chapter. He has provided us with excellent consumer critique and we are eternally grateful.

It is our hope that this book will provide the medical practitioner with many of the necessary skills for passing examinations in obstetrics and gynaecology, and also a basic knowledge of the subject. We envisage that it will not only appeal to DRCOG candidates, medical students and MRCOG candidates but also have a place in the surgery of the general practitioner as a ready reference book for common problems.

London 2003   J.R.

Contributors

Barry Auld MRCOG
Consultant in Obstetrics and
Gynaeology, Conquest Hospital,
St Leonards-on-Sea

Simon Barton BSc MD FRCOG FRCP (Edin)
Consultant Physician and Clinical
Director, Department of
HIV/Genitourinary Medicine,
St Stephen's Centre, Chelsea and
Westminster Hospital, London

Michael Chapman MD FRCOG FRANZCOG
Professor of Obstetrics and Gynaecology,
University of New South Wales,
St George Hospital, Sydney

Gregory Davis MD FRCOG FRANZCOG
Staff Specialist/Conjoint Senior Lecturer,
Department of Obstetrics and
Gynaecology, St George Hospital,
New South Wales, Australia

Ann Duthie MD MRCP FRCPCH
Consultant in Paediatrics, Whipps Cross
Hospital, London

Antony Hollingworth PhD FRCS MRCOG
MBA
Consultant in Obstetrics and
Gynaecology, Whipps Cross Hospital,
London

Marie McDonald RGN, RM, ADM,
MBA (Health)
Midwifery Consultant, London

Helen Massil MRCOG MFFP
Consultant in Reproductive Health,
Department of Reproductive Health,
Community Health, St Giles, London

Ian Page FRCOG
Consultant in Obstetrics and
Gynaecology, Whangarei Base Hospital,
New Zealand

Valerie Price MBChB MFFP
Senior Medical Officer in Reproductive
Health, St Giles, Community Health
South London

Adam Rodin BSc MRCOG
Consultant in Obstetrics and
Gynaecology, Wellhouse NHS Trust,
London

Jonathan Rosenthal BSc MSc MBBCH
MRCGP DRCOG DFFP
Senior Lecturer in General Practice,
Department of Primary Care and
Population Sciences, Royal Free Hospital
School of Medicine, London

Janice Rymer MD MRCOG FRANZCOG ILTM
Senior Lecturer/Consultant in Obstetrics
and Gynaecology, Guy's, King's and
St Thomas' School of Medicine, Guy's
and St Thomas' Hospital Trust, London

Contents

CONTENTS

Section I

The examination

Station 1

For Examiner's Use Only

Correct   No Mark

Total

What common gynaecological procedure has been
carried out in the laparoscopic picture illustrated?

For Exam important facts that your patient should be
aware of about the procedure and which you should discuss
with her.

Name the sutures and fontanelles that are marked on the
specimen. Numbers 1-6.

No Mark

1 General information

Janice Rymer

DIPLOMA OF THE ROYAL COLLEGE OF OBSTETRICIANS AND GYNAECOLOGISTS (DRCOG)

The College awards a Diploma to registered medical practitioners who have appropriate postgraduate training and who satisfy the examiners. The Diploma is intended to recognize a general practitioner's interest in obstetrics and gynaecology and is not a specialist qualification.

The Royal College of Obstetricians and Gynaecologists (RCOG) produces a booklet entitled *Diploma Examination Regulations* which can be obtained from the Head of the Examination Department. The address is given at the end of this chapter.

You should obtain a copy of the Diploma Examination Regulations at the time of commencing your training.

Eligibility
The regulations state that:

1. The candidate must be *fully* registered as a medical practitioner in the register maintained by the General Medical Council or the Medical Council of Ireland.
2. The candidate must have held a recognized appointment for 6 consecutive months. (Recognized appointments are limited to the United Kingdom and Republic of Ireland.) It is not essential that this appointment is completed by the time of the examination, but evidence of having completed this training is required from successful candidates who wish to register as a Diplomate of this College.

If you want advice on your eligibility, contact the Diploma Secretary in the Examination Department.

Sample certificate
A sample certificate is shown in Figure 1.1.

SAMPLE CERTIFICATE

RECOGNISED APPOINTMENT FOR THE DIPLOMA EXAMINATION (DRCOG)

TO: The Examination Office
       RCOG

This is to confirm that Dr ***
has completed/is expected to complete to my satisfaction a six
month **combined** appointment at the above hospital, recognised for
the purposes of the diploma examination (DRCOG). The post
commenced on */*/** and terminated/will terminate on */*/**.

I further confirm that Dr ***
is clinically competent to attempt the Diploma examination.

Signed... FRCOG/MRCOG

Date.................................... Hospital...

Fig. 1.1   A sample appointment certificate.

The College can refuse an application and does not have to give the reason
for refusal.

If you withdraw your application after the closing date or fail to appear, then
you will forfeit the examination fee.

DATES OF THE EXAMINATION

The examination is held in April and October. The closing date for applications should be obtained from the College. Late applications are not accepted.
The Multiple Choice Question (MCQ) paper and Objective Structured Clinical
Examination (OSCE) are taken on the same day and you will be assigned to
a centre chosen by the College. The entry fee (in sterling) must be sent with

the application; the fee is subject to annual review. Details of the entry fee are available from the Head of the Examination Department.

EXAMINATION FORMAT

The examination is conducted in two parts:

1. *An MCQ paper of 2 hours' duration.*
2. *An OSCE*—this examination consists of 22 stations, each station lasting 6 minutes (a total of approximately 2 hours and 15 minutes).

You may not attempt the Diploma examination more than five times.

SUBJECT MATTER

The syllabus includes the following topics:

Obstetrics
1. Routine procedures in modern antenatal care
2. Epidemiology of maternal and perinatal morbidity and mortality
3. Complications of early pregnancy
4. Shared care and specialist referral
5. Prepregnancy counselling
6. Prenatal diagnosis
7. Methods of education for pregnancy, childbirth and the newborn
8. The importance of social and emotional factors in childbearing
9. Antenatal and intrapartum infections
10. The roles of health care team members
11. The common conditions for which antenatal admission is required
12. The onset of labour
13. Normal labour
14. Pain relief in labour
15. Induction of labour
16. Physiology of uterine activity and oxytocic drugs
17. Fetal heart rate monitoring and acid–base studies
18. Abnormal labour
19. Abnormal presentations
20. Operative deliveries
21. Resuscitation of a shocked patient
22. Breech deliveries
23. Multiple pregnancies
24. Shoulder dystocia
25. The third stage of labour
26. Episiotomies

27. Breast-feeding
28. Puerperal infections
29. Puerperal disorders, both physical and psychological
30. Physiology of the normal puerperium
31. Maternal immunization with anti-D
32. Rubella vaccinations
33. Home deliveries
34. Indications for the flying squad.

Neonatal medicine
1. Examination of the newborn
2. Resuscitation of the newborn
3. Common diseases in the newborn infant
4. Normal development of the newborn
5. Congenital abnormalities in the newborn.

Gynaecology
1. Health education and preventive medicine
2. Gynaecological history
3. Gynaecological examination
4. Appropriate gynaecological investigations
5. Congenital abnormalities of the female genital tract
6. Psychosexual problems
7. Infertility
8. Abortions (miscarriages)
9. Menstrual disorders
10. Benign lesions of the genital tract
11. Gynaecological malignancies
12. Menopause
13. Urinary tract disorders and genital prolapse
14. Vaginal discharge
15. Sexually transmitted diseases
16. Family planning
17. Medical records and clinical audit
18. Communication skills.

RESULTS

Each candidate receives a written result stating whether a pass or fail has been attained. The results are also posted on a board in the College and are available on the RCOG website.

Successful candidates are required to pay a registration fee and provide a certificate confirming satisfactory completion of 6 months' recognized DRCOG training before being granted the Diploma of the Royal College of

Obstetricians and Gynaecologists. The amount of the current registration fee is available from the Head of the Examination Department.

WHEN YOU PASS

Once you have passed and received your Diploma certificate, you are entitled to use the letters DRCOG after your name. The College has a 'Register of Diplomates', and you will receive details of College meetings, functions and events. The College also has limited accommodation which is available to Diplomates visiting London. Duplicate certificates cannot be provided in the event of loss or damage.

ADDRESSES

United Kingdom
Head of Examination Department
Royal College of Obstetricians and Gynaecologists
27 Sussex Place
Regent's Park
London
NW1 4RG
(Telephone: 44 (0)20 7772 6200
Fax: 44 (0)20 7723 0575
Website: www.rcog.org.uk)

Australia and New Zealand
The Royal Australian and New Zealand College of Obstetricians and Gynaecologists also has a Diploma examination and its regulations can be obtained from:
Examination Secretary
Royal Australian and New Zealand College of Obstetricians and
Gynaecologists
254 Albert Street
East Melbourne
Victoria 3002
Australia
(Telephone: 61 (0)3 9417 1699
Fax: 61 (0)3 9419 0672
Website: www.ranzcog.edu.au)

2

Preparing for the examination

Janice Rymer

The Diploma examination is intended for general practitioners who have an interest in obstetrics and gynaecology. It is not a specialist qualification. The examiners will expect a 'common-sense' approach to problems, and management aimed at safe medical practice. To emphasize this we open each chapter in our syllabus section with 'Expectations of the examiners' to stress what important knowledge is to be acquired. It is very easy to waste time on minutiae when studying for such a broadly based examination as the DRCOG.

The following points are outlined to assist your preparation:

1. The best preparation for the DRCOG is a Senior House Officer (SHO) post on a busy obstetric and gynaecological rotation with teaching from senior staff. Time spent on wards and in clinics is invaluable as the examination is so 'practically' orientated.
2. Ideally, reading should commence before the post starts, and the syllabus in this book provides a good basic knowledge. Thereafter consistent reading around subjects and conditions as they present on the wards will provide the substance of your learning. This is superior to reading a book from cover to cover.
3. It is advisable to plan a reading programme using the College guidelines for the DRCOG syllabus.
4. In all sections of the DRCOG the examiners will ask questions relevant to current practice. They are often particularly interested in current issues that appear in the lay as well as the medical press. Therefore it is wise to keep up to date, and this is best achieved by reading the following journals:
   a. *British Journal of Obstetrics and Gynaecology*
   b. *British Medical Journal*
   c. *British Journal of General Practice*
   d. *The Lancet*
   e. *The Diplomate*
   f. Review articles in the *British Journal of Hospital Medicine, Practical Therapeutics* and *Hospital Update*.
5. Journal clubs are a painless way of learning, and discussion around the topics is very valuable.

6. Each unit should have organized teaching sessions, and these are very worthwhile, especially if senior colleagues are present.
7. Revision courses for the DRCOG are good for consolidating knowledge and for practising skills in OSCEs, especially if you have not been exposed to this format of examination previously. These are usually advertised at your hospital or in the *British Medical Journal*. It is important to realize that these courses do not cover the whole syllabus, but are valuable for identifying deficiencies in your knowledge and allowing controversial areas to be discussed. When you only learn obstetrics and gynaecology in one unit it is easy to miss the fact that certain areas of management are controversial.
8. Senior colleagues have experience and a lot to teach. Listen to them!

In 1993 the RCOG published a document entitled 'Report of the DRCOG Working Party'. The working party defined three basic aims of training which are worthwhile keeping in mind during your preparation for the examination:

1. To ensure that doctors completing a defined programme of training have acquired knowledge, clinical skills and attitudes to enable them to undertake the practice of obstetrics and gynaecology within the setting of primary health care
2. To encourage the philosophy of updating knowledge and skills by means of further training or study
3. To facilitate the integration of primary and secondary health care in relation to obstetrics and gynaecology.

3   The written paper

Janice Rymer

GENERAL INFORMATION

The written paper consists of a multiple choice question (MCQ) paper lasting 120 minutes. The paper consists of 60 five-part MCQs in book form.

MULTIPLE CHOICE QUESTIONS

A key word or introductory statement (the stem) is followed by five words or statements (parts) which relate to the stem. The candidate must decide whether each of the five parts is true or false. For each statement correctly answered true or false one mark is given and for an incorrect answer no mark is awarded.

The most important advice is to read the stem very carefully. Once you have done this, read it again. You are allowed to write on the question booklet so you can mark your answers on it and put a question mark beside those of which you are unsure. You are advised to guess if you have no idea whether the statements are true or false, as there is no negative marking.

The first response to a question is more often correct than a later response, so it is unwise to alter the initial answers.

Remember to leave yourself time to complete the answer sheet.

Figure 3.1 is an example of a computer answer sheet.

Examples of multiple choice questions follow below.

Obstetrics

1. *In pregnancy:*
   A. the plasma volume increases more in singleton than in multiple pregnancies
   B. the blood pressure falls in the second trimester
   C. oxygen consumption rises
   D. the glomeruler filtration rate (GFR) decreases
   E. the fasting blood sugar levels rise.

Royal College of Obstetricians and Gynaecologists
Diploma Examination (DRCOG)

SURNAME (FAMILY NAME)		CANDIDATE NUMBER			

SURNAME
(FAMILY NAME) — *JOHNSON*

OTHER
NAME(S) — *PETER ALAN*

Please us HB pencil. Rub out all errors thoroughly   T = True
Mark lozenges like ▬ NOT like ✓ ✗ ⊖   F = False

CANDIDATE NUMBER

1	2	7	5
0 ▭	0 ▭	0 ▭	0 ▭
1 ▬	1 ▭	1 ▭	1 ▭
2 ▭	2 ▬	2 ▭	2 ▭
3 ▭	3 ▭	3 ▭	3 ▭
4 ▭	4 ▭	4 ▭	4 ▭
5 ▭	5 ▭	5 ▭	5 ▬
6 ▭	6 ▭	6 ▭	6 ▭
7 ▭	7 ▭	7 ▬	7 ▭
8 ▭	8 ▭	8 ▭	8 ▭
9 ▭	9 ▭	9 ▭	9 ▭

IMPORTANT NOTES
1. When you have finished, check that you have NOT left any blanks.
2. Erasures should be left clean, with no smudges where possible. (The document reading machine will accept the darkest response for each item.)

	A	B	C	D	E		A	B	C	D	E
1	T/F	T/F	T/F	T/F	T/F	16	T/F	T/F	T/F	T/F	T/F
2	T/F	T/F	T/F	T/F	T/F	17	T/F	T/F	T/F	T/F	T/F
3	T/F	T/F	T/F	T/F	T/F	18	T/F	T/F	T/F	T/F	T/F
4	T/F	T/F	T/F	T/F	T/F	19	T/F	T/F	T/F	T/F	T/F
5	T/F	T/F	T/F	T/F	T/F	20	T/F	T/F	T/F	T/F	T/F
6	T/F	T/F	T/F	T/F	T/F	21	T/F	T/F	T/F	T/F	T/F
7	T/F	T/F	T/F	T/F	T/F	22	T/F	T/F	T/F	T/F	T/F
8	T/F	T/F	T/F	T/F	T/F	23	T/F	T/F	T/F	T/F	T/F
9	T/F	T/F	T/F	T/F	T/F	24	T/F	T/F	T/F	T/F	T/F
10	T/F	T/F	T/F	T/F	T/F	25	T/F	T/F	T/F	T/F	T/F
11	T/F	T/F	T/F	T/F	T/F	26	T/F	T/F	T/F	T/F	T/F
12	T/F	T/F	T/F	T/F	T/F	27	T/F	T/F	T/F	T/F	T/F
13	T/F	T/F	T/F	T/F	T/F	28	T/F	T/F	T/F	T/F	T/F
14	T/F	T/F	T/F	T/F	T/F	29	T/F	T/F	T/F	T/F	T/F
15	T/F	T/F	T/F	T/F	T/F	30	T/F	T/F	T/F	T/F	T/F

CHECK THAT YOU HAVE ANSWERED EVERY ITEM TRUE OR FALSE

Fig. 3.1   An example of a computer answer sheet. You must mark either the T or the F lozenge for each question, using an HB pencil.

2. *A raised maternal serum α-fetoprotein (AFP) may be associated with:*
   A. normal pregnancy
   B. trisomy 21
   C. threatened abortion
   D. twins
   E. anencephaly.

3. *Rhesus isoimmunization:*
   A. does not occur during the first pregnancy
   B. is no longer a problem in the UK since the introduction of anti-D prophylaxis
   C. may cause fetal ascites in a severely affected case
   D. may lead to Chadwick's sign being detected on ultrasound in early pregnancy
   E. 50 μg of anti-D following a first trimester abortion is sufficient.

4. *The following antenatal complications are more common in multiple than singleton pregnancies:*
   A. premature labour
   B. placenta praevia
   C. congenital abnormalities
   D. polyhydramnios
   E. pre-eclampsia.

5. *Relating to diabetes and pregnancy:*
   A. polyhydramnios complicates 60% of pregnancies in established diabetics
   B. pre-eclampsia is more common in diabetic pregnancies
   C. a type 1 diabetes patient with retinopathy should be advised to avoid pregnancy
   D. the glycosylated haemoglobin level gives an indication of diabetic control over the preceding weeks
   E. congenital abnormality is now the most important contributor to perinatal morbidity and mortality.

6. *A 20-year-old primigravida at 34 weeks presents to the antenatal clinic with a blood pressure of 150/95 mmHg and proteinuria of 4 g/24 hours:*
   A. she should be told to rest in bed at home with daily visits from the community midwife
   B. a serum urate of 0.45 mmol/l is consistent with severe disease
   C. she may have thrombocytopenia
   D. delivery should always be by lower segment caesarean section (LSCS)
   E. if she has oedema, the disease will be more severe.

7. *Preterm delivery:*
   A. preterm delivery accounts for 75% of all perinatal deaths
   B. genital infection is not a risk factor
   C. previous preterm labour is not a risk factor
   D. by identifying at-risk patients (by risk screening) the incidence of preterm delivery can be reduced
   E. tocolytic drugs delay delivery by a minimum of 1 week.

8. *The following are associated with a breech presentation:*
   A. placenta praevia
   B. multiple pregnancy
   C. an incidence of 3% at term
   D. Potter's syndrome
   E. Tay–Sachs disease.

9. *Non-stressed antepartum cardiotocography (CTG) performed at 36 weeks:*
   A. can be interpreted using the same criteria as for a pregnancy at 26 weeks
   B. if the rate is 110/minute, delivery should be undertaken as soon as possible
   C. deceleration in response to movement is a normal finding
   D. may show uterine activity
   E. if there is reduced variability for 20 minutes, the fetus may be sleeping.

10. *The following are appropriate indications for chorionic villus sampling (CVS):*
    A. a woman aged 39 with a confirmed 12 weeks' gestation
    B. a woman aged 45 with a confirmed 8 weeks' gestation
    C. a woman who is known to be a translocation carrier
    D. a woman whose son has Niemann–Pick disease
    E. a woman aged 30 whose husband is aged 45.

11. *The following statements relating to vaccination in pregnancy are correct:*
    A. rabies vaccine is safe for use in pregnancy
    B. poliomyelitis vaccination is contraindicated in pregnancy
    C. inadvertent administration of rubella vaccination in pregnancy is an indication for termination
    D. tetanus vaccination carries no risk of intrauterine fetal infection
    E. human varicella zoster immunoglobulin should be given to the term newborn of a mother who has shown evidence of varicella zoster infection in the second trimester.

12. *The following features in a patient's history should alert the obstetrician to the possibility of systemic lupus erythematosus (SLE):*
    A. early onset severe pre-eclampsia
    B. second trimester intrauterine death
    C. early severe intrauterine growth retardation
    D. photosensitive skin rashes
    E. recurrent first trimester abortions.

13. *When a pregnant woman develops hepatitis B:*
    A. the course of acute hepatitis B is unaffected by pregnancy
    B. demonstration of hepatitis B e antigen in the mother's serum makes congenital infection unlikely
    C. caesarean delivery is indicated to reduce the risk of viral infection in the newborn
    D. most cases can be managed as outpatients
    E. transmission from mother to baby is commoner amongst Asian than Caucasian patients.

14. *The following statements about oral iron prophylaxis during pregnancy are correct:*
    A. diarrhoea and constipation can occur
    B. if prophylaxis is not given, iron deficiency will develop
    C. non-compliance of the mother occurs in less than 10% of cases
    D. maternal iron prophylaxis is recognized to reduce the incidence of infant iron deficiency anaemia
    E. oral maternal iron prophylaxis is associated with an increase in MCV.

15. *The following statements about severe pre-eclampsia are correct:*
    A. disseminated intravascular coagulation (DIC) is a recognized underlying cause
    B. epidural anaesthesia is contraindicated if the platelet count is < 100
    C. plasma volume is reduced
    D. diuretics are helpful in management
    E. the serum urate concentration is typically elevated.

16. *A patient at 38 weeks is found to have a uterine size of 32 weeks. The following ultrasound observations are suggestive of intrauterine growth retardation:*
    A. oligohydramnios
    B. an abdominal circumference on the 50th percentile for 32 weeks
    C. an anterior placenta
    D. a biparietal diameter (BPD) on the 50th percentile for 38 weeks
    E. fetal tachycardia.

17. *Regarding labour:*
    A. induction of labour is not associated with an increased caesarean section rate
    B. prolonged labour in a multiparous woman is likely to be due to inefficient uterine action
    C. Kjelland's forceps are associated with an increased incidence of neonatal cerebral irritability
    D. the average length of the second stage in a nulliparous patient is 60 minutes
    E. the minimum acceptable rate of cervical dilatation in the active phase of labour is 1 cm/hour.

18. *Puerperal psychosis:*
    A. occurs in about 1 in 1000 mothers
    B. is characteristically manic in type
    C. usually only results in a 2–3 weeks' hospital stay
    D. is not recurrent in future pregnancies
    E. is best treated by separation of the mother and the baby because of the risk of infanticide.

19. *Regarding forceps deliveries:*
    A. Wrigley's forceps have a cephalic curve but no pelvic curve
    B. incorrect application of the forceps can result in cranial nerve palsies
    C. if the station of the head is –1 it is acceptable to use Kjelland's forceps
    D. a pudendal block can be used
    E. the patient does not need to be catheterized.

20. *Postpartum haemorrhage:*
    A. a previous postpartum haemorrhage is a risk factor for a subsequent postpartum haemorrhage
    B. can be prophylactically treated with an intravenous oxytocic with the delivery of the anterior shoulder followed by an intravenous infusion over 3 hours
    C. is defined as a blood loss of 500 ml within the first 12 hours

D. can occur with morbid adherence of the placenta

    E. is the main cause of maternal deaths in the latest triennial report.

Statistics

21. *In the Confidential Enquiry into Maternal Deaths (England and Wales) for the period 1994–1996:*

    A. hypertensive disease was the commonest cause of direct maternal death

    B. the death rate from ectopic pregnancy had fallen

    C. there was a maternal death rate of 12.2 per 100 000 total maternities (direct and indirect deaths)

    D. the risk of maternal death in black women was higher than in Caucasian women

    E. death in association with abortion was not included in the true maternal mortality rate.

22. *Concerning the 1994–1996 Maternal Mortality Report:*

    A. the last report was published 5 years previously

    B. anaesthetic causes still claim the most lives

    C. direct mortality is lowest in women having their second baby

    D. genital sepsis remains a major cause of maternal death

    E. the major cause of the 134 indirect deaths was epilepsy.

23. *Concerning perinatal mortality in Britain:*

    A. the perinatal mortality rate includes stillbirths and first-week neonatal deaths

    B. the three major causes are low birth weight, malformation and asphyxia

    C. the perinatal death rate decreases with increasing parity

    D. the lowest rate occurs in social class III

    E. if an infant is born before 24 weeks' gestation and shows signs of life, but then dies within the first 24 hours, it is not included as a perinatal death.

Neonatal medicine

24. *Babies of diabetic mothers have an increased risk of:*

    A. respiratory distress syndrome

    B. intrauterine growth retardation (IUGR)

    C. macrosomia

    D. anaemia

    E. hyperbilirubinaemia.

25. *In herpes neonatorum:*

    A. the majority of mothers have a history of herpes genitalis

    B. the herpes simplex virus (HSV) is frequently recovered from the amniotic fluid of infected infants

    C. type I HSV is usually involved

    D. the presence of maternal antibodies is protective

    E. maternal viraemia is characteristically the cause.

26. *The following statements about neonatal resuscitation are correct:*
    A. an apnoeic baby at birth with a heart rate of less than 80 beats/minute should be intubated
    B. in a baby who has been exposed to meconium inhalation it is important to visualize the cords
    C. drying and warming the baby together with simple stimulation normally correct terminal apnoea
    D. the effects of pethidine given to the mother late in labour may be corrected during resuscitation of the newborn by the administration of naloxone (0.01 mg/kg) via an umbilical vein
    E. a diaphragmatic hernia is a recognized cause of a newborn failing to respond to resuscitation including intermittent positive pressure ventilation.

27. *Congenital cytomegalovirus (CMV) is:*
    A. present in up to 20% of babies
    B. usual if the mother has a primary infection
    C. rare if the mother is immune prior to pregnancy
    D. usually symptomatic if the virus is recovered from the neonate at birth
    E. characteristically associated with significant neurological impairment following a primary maternal infection.

28. *Recognized complications of preterm birth include:*
    A. poor temperature control in the newborn
    B. transient tachypnoea of the newborn
    C. jaundice
    D. meconium aspiration syndrome
    E. apnoeic attacks.

29. *The normal infant delivered at term has:*
    A. a head circumference of 40 cm
    B. an impalpable liver
    C. a plasma glucose above 1.7 mmol/l
    D. brown adipose tissue
    E. no adult haemoglobin.

30. *Regarding fetal circulation:*
    A. the ductus venosus carries blood to the inferior vena cava from the umbilical artery
    B. the ductus arteriosus carries blood from the pulmonary artery to the aorta
    C. the foramen ovale permits blood to pass from the right to the left ventricle
    D. the ductus arteriosus is contractile
    E. the umbilical vein becomes the ligamentum teres of the adult.

Gynaecology

31. *During a normal menstrual cycle:*
    A. the proliferative phase of the endometrium follows ovulation

B. the plasma progesterone concentration rises following ovulation
    C. the average menstrual blood loss is 200 ml
    D. ovulation is dependent upon an intact hypothalamic pituitary portal circulation
    E. the blood loss is normally fluid because of the presence of fibrinolysins.

32. *The climacteric is usually associated with:*
    A. a reduction in the level of follicle stimulating hormone (FSH)
    B. a reduction in circulating oestrogens
    C. an elevated serum 5-hydroxytryptamine level
    D. hyperprolactinaemia
    E. a reduction in the serum cholesterol concentration.

33. *The following statements about colposcopy are correct:*
    A. mild dyskaryosis on a smear should not be referred for colposcopy, but the smear should be repeated annually until a more significant change is detectable
    B. severe dyskaryosis on a smear always indicates cervical intraepithelial neoplasia (CIN) 3
    C. an 'incomplete' colposcopic assessment can safely be followed by laser ablation providing a biopsy has confirmed CIN
    D. a mosaic pattern suggests intraepithelial dysplasia
    E. during prepuberty the transformation zone is more likely to be in the endocervical canal.

34. *The following statements concerning endometrial cancer are correct:*
    A. the risk of developing endometrial cancer is increased in diabetics
    B. postcoital bleeding is the classic symptom
    C. a dilatation and curettage is not required if the colposcopic assessment is normal
    D. the incidence is decreased in nulliparous women
    E. the incidence is increased in women who receive unopposed oestrogen therapy.

35. *Regarding ectopic pregnancies:*
    A. 95% occur in the fallopian tube
    B. pelvic inflammatory disease (PID) is the most important aetiological factor
    C. ultrasound should always be performed prior to referral to hospital
    D. bleeding is usually the first symptom
    E. if the urine pregnancy test is negative the diagnosis is ruled out.

36. *The following investigations should be performed routinely on a woman who presents with symptoms of urinary urgency:*
    A. barium enema
    B. mid-stream urine (MSU)
    C. urodynamics
    D. abdominal X-ray
    E. pelvic examination.

37. *Concerning infertility:*
    A. Artificial insemination—husband (AIH) has been proven to increase the 'take home baby rate' in couples who have unexplained infertility
    B. clomifene can be given to induce ovulation in anovulatory women
    C. if the postcoital test is normal, then a semen sample is not needed
    D. Gamete intrafallopian transfer (GIFT) is used in women who have tubal disease
    E. stress can cause anovulation.

38. *Concerning carcinoma of the cervix:*
    A. the peak age is 50–59 years
    B. it is the commonest malignant tumour of the genital tract
    C. early spread occurs via the venous system
    D. a microinvasive lesion has invaded the stroma to a depth of 3 mm and the lymphatics are involved
    E. it is more common in women who smoke.

39. *Polycystic ovarian syndrome:*
    A. clinical features include hirsutism, anorexia and dysfunctional bleeding
    B. can be treated with clomifene
    C. LH levels are usually raised
    D. women who have this disorder are at increased risk of endometrial cancer
    E. wedge resection of the ovaries is a common successful form of treatment.

40. *Therapeutic abortion:*
    A. mortality and morbidity increase with increasing gestational age
    B. uterine perforation requires immediate laparotomy
    C. secondary infertility is a recognized late complication of first trimester abortion
    D. the mortality rate of legal abortion is less than 1 per 1 000 000 maternities
    E. prostaglandins in an asthmatic can cause acute bronchospasm.

41. *Endometriosis:*
    A. can be treated with the CO_2 laser
    B. can be treated with danazol to create a 'pseudo-pregnancy'
    C. can cause Asherman syndrome
    D. can cause dyspareunia
    E. if severe can cause infertility.

42. *Hirsutism:*
    A. polycystic ovarian syndrome and idiopathic hirsutism account for over 90% of cases
    B. is a side-effect of danazol
    C. is a side-effect of spironolactone
    D. shaving increases hair growth
    E. LH, FSH and testosterone levels should be measured.

43. *Contraindications to oestrogen replacement therapy for postmenopausal women include:*
    A. cervical carcinoma
    B. past history of breast cancer
    C. past history of deep venous thrombosis (DVT)
    D. diabetes
    E. past history of endometrial cancer.

44. *Infertility:*
    A. the incidence of unexplained infertility in infertile couples is about 10–15%
    B. there is a decline in fecundity with age
    C. if the husband is identified as having 'poor' sperm, then investigations in the partner can be abandoned
    D. azoospermia is associated with small testes and a low FSH level
    E. GIFT can be used in women with unexplained infertility.

45. *Genital prolapse:*
    A. can be caused by vaginal delivery
    B. vaginal narrowing can occur after colporrhaphy
    C. vaginal hysterectomies have less postoperative morbidity than abdominal hysterectomies if prophylactic antibiotics are used
    D. cannot occur in a nulliparous woman
    E. can become worse after the climacteric.

46. *Hydatidiform mole:*
    A. can produce ovarian enlargement and breathlessness
    B. can present with pre-eclampsia before 20 weeks
    C. when complete is totally maternally derived
    D. if partial, has more chance of being followed by choriocarcinoma than a complete mole
    E. can be treated by hysterectomy in the older woman.

47. *The vagina:*
    A. the anterior wall is longer than the posterior wall
    B. the normal epithelium contains mucus-secreting glands
    C. is related in its lower third to the bladder base
    D. the pH is acidic during the reproductive phase of life
    E. ovarian function can be assessed by the cytology of vaginal wall smears.

48. *A 25-year-old nulliparous woman is referred from her general practitioner with an abnormal smear:*
    A. a smear should always be repeated before referral
    B. menstruation is the best time to perform colposcopy as the transformation zone is easily seen
    C. ideally, ectocervical cells should be seen on the smear
    D. colposcopic assessment may be incomplete
    E. at colposcopy bizarre vessel branching suggests CIN.

49. *Ovarian cancer:*
    A. 30% have metastases beyond the pelvis at the initial diagnosis
    B. can be properly staged using a Pfannenstiel incision

C. the mortality rate has significantly changed over the past 20 years

    D. laparoscopy is acceptable as a 'second-look' operation

    E. can present with vague symptoms of dyspepsia, tiredness and abdominal distension.

50. *Dysfunctional uterine bleeding:*
    A. is a diagnosis of exclusion
    B. a dilatation and curettage is therapeutic
    C. the endometrial curettings are abnormal
    D. danazol can be used as treatment
    E. laser ablation of the endometrium is acceptable treatment.

Sexually transmitted infections

51. *Trichomonas vaginalis:*
    A. can be diagnosed by colposcopy
    B. causes clue cells on microscopy
    C. on a wet mount, preparation may reveal motile flagellated protozoa
    D. can be treated with metronidazole
    E. classically produces a thick white discharge.

52. *Regarding AIDS:*
    A. vertical transmission appears to occur in 30% of infants delivered to HIV-infected women
    B. transmission of HIV to the fetus has been proven to occur in the first trimester
    C. is caused by a retrovirus
    D. nosocomial exposure is an important mode of spread
    E. the diagnosis of HIV in children is difficult due to passive acquisition of maternal HIV antibodies.

53. *Hepatitis B infection in a pregnant woman:*
    A. carries a 1.8% chance of mortality
    B. is associated with congenital abnormalities
    C. infection in a pregnant woman carries a 60% increase in preterm delivery
    D. in the third trimester the risk of vertical transmission is 20%
    E. newborns of HbsAg-positive mothers should have hepatitis B immunoglobulin at birth.

54. *The lesions of syphilis include:*
    A. perivascular inflammation
    B. cranial nerve lesions
    C. aortic aneurysm
    D. vulval ulceration
    E. condylomata acuminata.

Family planning

55. *The combined oral contraceptive pill is protective against:*
    A. ovarian cancer
    B. endometrial cancer

C. cervical cancer
D. ectopic pregnancy
E. pelvic inflammatory disease.
56. *Regarding intrauterine devices (IUDs):*
    A. menorrhagia is an absolute contraindication
    B. encrustation of a copper device is associated with failure
    C. actinomycosis may be seen with prolonged use of IUDs
    D. they are contraindicated in women who have had a caesarean section
    E. IUDs inserted within 5 days of unprotected intercourse can act as post-coital contraception.
57. *Sterilization:*
    A. the failure rate is 1–5 per 1000 procedures (in females)
    B. vasectomy is safer than female sterilization
    C. in males is deemed successful if two postoperative seminal specimens are 'sperm-free'
    D. postoperatively, menstrual loss should decrease
    E. the failure rate is increased if performed at the time of abortion.
58. *Regarding the combined oral contraceptive pill:*
    A. it should not be prescribed to women over the age of 37 years
    B. if diarrhoea occurs, the pill may not be absorbed
    C. in higher doses it can be used as the morning after pill
    D. it is associated with an increased incidence of pulmonary embolism
    E. it should not be prescribed in diabetic women.

ANSWERS TO MULTIPLE CHOICE QUESTIONS

The correct answers are given below.

Obstetrics
1. B.C.
2. A.C.D.E.
3. C.E. Rhesus isoimmunization has dramatically decreased in incidence but has by no means disappeared. Chadwick's sign is a clinical sign of early pregnancy.
4. A.B.C.D.E. This question emphasizes the fact that nearly all antenatal complications are more common in multiple pregnancies.
5. B.D.E. Polyhydramnios complicates 25% of pregnancies in established diabetics. Diabetic retinopathy, diabetic vascular disease and neuropathy are not adversely affected by pregnancy.
6. B.C.
7. A. There is no evidence that identification of risk factors reduces the incidence of preterm delivery. Tocolysis has not been shown to reduce perinatal morbidity or mortality.
8. A.B.C.D.

9. D.E. At 26 weeks the variability may be reduced. If there are no other adverse features, a fetal heart rate of 110/minute is normal. Decelerations in response to movements are an ominous sign. Fetuses do have sleep cycles of 20 minutes, so a CTG must be continued for longer than 20 minutes to see if it becomes reactive.
10. A.C.D. CVS is not normally performed at less than 11 weeks due to a possible risk of limb defects.
11. A.D. If vaccination is required in pregnancy, live vaccines should be avoided. Passive immunization is available with antirabies human immunoglobulin. The Salk inactivated virus is used for poliomyelitis vaccination in pregnancy.
12. A.B.C.D.E.
13. D.E. Acute maternal infection with hepatitis B virus may result in congenital hepatitis and the risk depends on the trimester in which maternal infection occurs, being highest at term.
14. A.E.
15. B.C.E. Severe pre-eclampsia can result in DIC. As the plasma volume is reduced in these women, diuretics are contraindicated.
16. A.B.
17. C.E. In the active phase of the first stage of labour the cervix dilates at up to 3 cm and 6 cm/hour in primigravidae and multigravidae respectively. (The minimum acceptable rate is 1 cm/hour.) The average length of the second stage in primigravidae is 40 minutes, and in multigravidae, 20 minutes.
18. A.
19. B.D.
20. A.B.D. A postpartum haemorrhage is defined as a blood loss of ≥ 500 ml within the first 24 hours after delivery. Hypertensive diseases of pregnancy were the main cause of maternal deaths in the latest triennial report.

Statistics
21. B.C.D. For the period 1994–1996, the leading direct cause of death was thromboembolism.
22. C.D. The report on confidential enquiries into maternal deaths in England and Wales is drawn up every 3 years. The major cause of indirect deaths was cardiac disease (39), then epilepsy (19) and then psychiatric causes (9).
23. A.B. The perinatal mortality rate is the number of stillbirths and first-week deaths occurring from 24 completed weeks of pregnancy to 7 days after birth per 1000 total births, but if an infant is born before 24 weeks' gestation and shows signs of life, but then dies within 7 days, it is to be included as a perinatal death.

Neonatal medicine
24. A.B.C.E. Severe diabetics are at risk of IUGR.
25. A.

26. A.B.D.E.
27. A. CMV is the most common viral infection during pregnancy. By the time an infant is born with the stigmata of congenital CMV infection, damage has occurred in utero and therapy at birth is not effective. There are currently no therapies or immunization practices.
28. A.B.C.E. The passage of meconium is rare in preterm infants and, if it occurs, listeriosis should be considered.
29. C.D.
30. B.D.E.

Gynaecology

31. B.D.E. The average menstrual blood loss is about 40 ml.
32. B. FSH and luteinizing hormone (LH) levels rise, and oestradiol levels fall.
33. D.E.
34. A.E. Intermenstrual bleeding is the classic symptom of endometrial carcinoma and postcoital bleeding is suggestive of cervical carcinoma. A post-menopausal woman who has bleeding should be referred for endometrial biopsy.
35. A.B.
36. B.C.E.
37. B.E.
38. A.E. Cervical cancer is second to ovarian as the commonest malignant tumour of the genital tract. The incidence of cervical cancer has fallen but the peak age is still 50–59 years, and the incidence has doubled in women under 40 years. The lymphatics are not involved in a microinvasive lesion.
39. B.C.D.
40. A.C.E. If uterine perforation occurs during the procedure, a laparoscopy should be performed and the completion of the evacuation performed while another operator is watching through the laparoscope. Laparotomy is carried out if the uterine tear is actively bleeding.
41. A.D.E. Danazol creates a 'pseudo-menopause'.
42. A.B.E. Spironolactone is used in the treatment of hirsutism.
43. B.E.
44. A.B.E. It is common in cases of 'infertility' to have 'subfertility' in both partners. Men with azoospermia have small testes and high FSH levels.
45. A.B.C.E.
46. A.B.E. Complete hydatidiform moles are totally paternally derived.
47. D.E.
48. D.E. A smear showing severely dyskaryotic cells demands colposcopic referral and a smear showing malignant cells demands urgent referral.
49. D.E. 75% of women with ovarian carcinoma have stage III or stage IV disease at time of presentation. A vertical incision is essential for correct staging. Laparotomy is usually performed, but laparoscopy is acceptable and this is done at 1 year postoperation.
50. A.D.E. A dilatation and curettage is a diagnostic procedure.

Sexually transmitted infections

51. A.C.D. *Trichomonas* is easily diagnosed by colposcopy and typical Y-shaped vessels are seen. Clue cells are usually associated with *Gardnerella vaginalis*. The classic discharge of *Trichomonas* is usually profuse, offensive and greenish-yellow.
52. B.C.E. Vertical transmission occurs in approximately 15%.
53. A.E. Hepatitis infection in pregnancy is associated with a 20% increase in preterm delivery. In the third trimester the risk of vertical transmission is 66%; it is less than 10% if the virus is acquired earlier.
54. A.B.C.D.

Family planning

55. A.B.D.E.
56. B.C.E. Beware of questions that say 'absolute'.
57. A.B.C.E.
58. B.C.D.

4   Objective structured clinical examination

Janice Rymer

Objective structured clinical examinations (OSCEs) are well established as a method of student assessment and are gradually being introduced into post-graduate assessment. In 1994 the RCOG commenced OSCEs for the Diploma examination. Major weaknesses were identified with the previous form of assessment, namely clinicals and vivas. OSCEs have been developed because they are valid, reliable, have high fidelity and are a feasible method of assessment.

The examination consists of a circuit of 22 stations, of which 20 are marked. At each station the candidate has to perform a task and these stations may test knowledge, skills, communication or problem-solving ability. Depending on the type of station there may be a role-player, a patient, a photograph or a clinical scenario. The stations are laid out in a clockwise direction numbered 1 to 22 and on your entrance card are the station number and circuit number at which you start. The invigilator will instruct you as to when to proceed to your station number. When you sit down it is important that you check that you are at the right station and there will be an answer book on the desk with your name and candidate number on it. Again, you need to check that these are correct and, if not, alert one of the invigilators. In the answer books it is imperative that you only write within the boxes and you must use the pencil provided.

At each station you will have 6 minutes and then a bell will sound. When this occurs you move in a clockwise direction to the next station. There will be two rest stations within the OSCE. You can use the time at these stations for a rest and to check your answer sheet.

KNOWLEDGE OR FACTUAL STATION

These stations purely assess your knowledge regarding certain subjects. The material provided may be a photograph, results of investigations or a clinical scenario. The answer sheets are designed so that you only write within the boxes—only one answer within one box. The columns on the right-hand side are for the examiners only, so do not write within them as they are optically read and erroneous marks may mean incorrect marking. The following are examples:

Station 1

For Examiner's Use Only	
Correct	No Mark
Total	

1. What common gynaecological procedure has been carried out in the laparoscopic picture illustrated?

> < > <

2. Give three important facts about the procedure that your patient should be aware of and which you should discuss with her.

> < > <
> < > <
> < > <

3. What is the usual failure rate of the procedure?

> < > <

4. Is the procedure shown in the photograph an appropriate procedure to carry out in the week following delivery?

> < > <

5. State a reason.

> < > <

6. Name the metal structures used for this procedure.

> < > <

7. If the patient had had her LMP 6 weeks prior to the procedure, what investigation would you perform?

> < > <

8. What medium has been used to distend the abdomen?

> < > <

Station 2

For Examiner's Use Only	
Correct	No Mark
Total	

Name the sutures and fontanelles that are marked on this specimen. Numbers 1–6

1.   > <   > <
2.   > <   > <
3.   > <   > <
4.   > <   > <
5.   > <   > <
6.   > <   > <

Define denominator

7.   > <   > <

What is the denominator of the following presentations: vertex, breech, face?

8.   > <   > <
9.   > <   > <
10.   > <   > <

CLINICAL SKILLS STATION

As with the pre-existing clinicals you may be asked to examine a patient.

(You may be asked to examine a pregnant patient, although this is unlikely due to the feasibility of having pregnant patients within an OSCE circuit. It would be more likely to be a plastic model or a role-player. Your instructions as to what to examine will be quite clear.)

The following are guidelines for examination:

General examination

Observe the patient's facies, demeanour and nutritional state. Ask yourself, 'does the patient look well?' A pregnant patient should have 'the bloom of pregnancy' due to vasodilatation and increased blood volume. Start by looking at the patient's hands. The blood pressure can then be taken, in the seated semiprone or lateral position. Check the conjunctivae for evidence of anaemia. If the patient is hypertensive, remember to examine the optic fundi but do not spend too much time on this aspect. Look for thyroid enlargement, and inspect and palpate the patient's breasts. The heart and lungs should be auscultated. Sacral oedema and pretibial oedema should be tested for. The legs should be inspected for varicosities, and the reflexes must be tested.

Abdominal examination

As with every medical examination, remember: inspection, palpation, percussion and auscultation.

Inspection

Observe for striae gravidarum. Is the swelling symmetrical? Are fetal movements seen? Are there any scars present? (Look particularly for a laparoscopy scar.)

Palpation

Firstly, palpate the upper margin of the uterine fundus and measure the symphysiofundal height with a tape measure. Then feel for the presenting part and determine whether it is engaged or not. (The examiner may ask you to express this in fifths palpable above the brim.) Then palpate the uterus to determine which side the fetal back is on. If you are unable to determine the presentation, don't panic, as in some cases this may be difficult.

Percussion

This is seldom necessary.

Auscultation

You must listen for the fetal heart in the appropriate place. (You may be asked to demonstrate the fetal heart with the sonicaid.)

Vaginal examination

In the context of an OSCE, this would be more likely with a pelvic model and you may be asked to pass a speculum, take a cervical smear or swab and then do a bimanual examination. Marks could be given for technique and dexterity. In this situation it would be appropriate to talk to the model as if it was a live patient.

The following is an example of a clinical skills station relating to an obstetric patient.

Prior to a skills or communication station you may have a rest station where information will be given to you for the actual communication station. This will give you time to prepare. The marking system will not be given to you, but a sample marking system is given here.

Station 3—Rest station

At the next station you will meet Mrs R. T. She is a 34-year-old primigravida and is currently at 37 weeks' gestation. You need to check her BP, examine her abdomen and check for oedema.

Station 4

Marks awarded for: **Marks**

Examiner to mark

1. Introducing yourself   1
2. Taking BP correctly (positioning etc.) and obtaining the correct BP   1
3. Observing abdomen and detecting scar   1
4. Measuring symphysiofundal height   1
5. Assessing presentation   1
6. Determining engagement of head   1
7. Determining lie   1
8. Testing for oedema adequately   1

Role-player to mark

1. Rapport   1
2. Not hurting patient during examination   1

COMMUNICATION STATION

Remember that at these stations communication is being assessed and knowledge is often secondary. The purpose of these stations is to assess your ability to communicate with the patients, so you must always treat the patients as individuals and be considerate. You want to convey to the examiner that you are a kind, compassionate and discerning clinician. As soon as you arrive at this station introduce yourself to the patient or role-player. Remember that some patients are excellent historians and some are not. The role-player may have been briefed not to communicate well and therefore the station is assessing your skill to extract information. If there is a role-player at the station, she will have been briefed to give the same scenario to each candidate. Remember the role-player or patient may well be awarding some marks.

The following is an example of a communication station and of how the marking may be awarded. In this case the information is given to you at the rest station preceding the station where the patient/role-player is.

Station 5—Rest station

At the next station you will be seeing a patient. Please read the following scenario to prepare yourself:

> Mrs Trihard is a 27-year-old woman who has been trying to become pregnant for 2 years. This is the first time she has come to see you (you are her general practitioner). Please take a relevant history from her and explain to her that you wish to arrange for a day 21 progesterone and semen analysis.

Remember you will only have 6 minutes.

Role-player information (information not given to candidate)

You have been trying for a pregnancy for 2 years. You are rather embarrassed about the subject but it is very important to you and your husband is not very helpful. You have been taking your temperature for 18 months and you are finding it all very stressful. You are having intercourse twice a week but it is all becoming rather forced, especially at the appropriate time. You have regular periods and have no history of pelvic infection. It does worry you that your husband may be having an affair with his secretary.

Your answer sheet will be blank apart from the marking columns, but the allocation of marks is shown here for your information.

Station 6

Please hand this sheet to the examiner

	For Examiner's Use Only	
	Correct	No Mark
	Total	
Candidate introducing him/herself	> <	> <
Making patient feel comfortable	> <	> <
Extracting appropriate information	> <	> <
Listening to patient	> <	> <
Explaining the serum progesterone test	> <	> <
Explaining the semen analysis	> <	> <
Checking if patient has any questions	> <	> <
Future plan of management	> <	> <
Role-player to mark confidence of candidate	> <	> <
Role-player to mark rapport	> <	> <

SUMMARY

An OSCE ensures that each candidate is exposed to the same examination questions and environment. Therefore the marking is very rigid and standardized.

Station 1—Answers   Marks

1. Laparoscopic sterilization with clips   1
2. Failure rate
   Relative irreversibility
   That it may require an open operation
   Anaesthesia
   Ectopic risk
   Postoperative regret   3
3. 1:200–1:500   1
4. No   1
5. Tubes too thick, therefore higher failure rate   1
6. Filschie clips   1
7. Pregnancy test   1
8. CO_2 1

Station 2—Answers   Marks

1. Frontal suture
2. Anterior fontanelle (bregma)
3. Coronal suture
4. Sagittal suture
5. Posterior fontanelle
6. Lambdoidal suture   6
7. The denominator is a defined point of the presenting part
   and is used to describe the fetal position   1
8. Cephalic—occiput
9. Breech—sacrum
10. Face—mentum   3

SECTION II

The syllabus

A. GYNAECOLOGY

B. OBSTETRICS

C. MISCELLANEOUS SUBJECTS

5

The menstrual cycle

Gregory Davis

Expectations of the examiners

A basic knowledge of the menstrual cycle is essential to the understanding of most gynaecological disorders and hormonal methods of contraception. Examiners will not expect a detailed knowledge of the endocrinology of the menstrual cycle but could ask about the basic principles.

HYPOTHALAMUS–PITUITARY–OVARY AXIS

In the fifth month of intrauterine life, primordial follicles in the ovary of the female fetus reach their maximum number (approximately 6–7 million per ovary). From then on, follicles continue to grow and become atretic until the menopause. This process occurs independently of gonadotrophin stimulation and under all physiological circumstances including ovulation, pregnancy and periods of anovulation. As most women ovulate 400–500 times in their life, it is the fate of the vast majority of these follicles to become atretic.

Full development of a follicle does not occur until the onset of puberty. At puberty, changes in the hypothalamus result in the pulsed secretion of gonadotrophin releasing hormone (GnRH) from the hypothalamus. This causes a similar pulsed release of the gonadotrophins, follicle stimulating hormone (FSH) and luteinizing hormone (LH), from the anterior pituitary. Thereafter, FSH and LH are secreted in pulses every 70–220 minutes depending on the phase of the cycle. This pattern of release is modulated by feedback on the hypothalamus and pituitary by oestrogen and the peptides produced by the follicle—inhibin, activin and follistatin.

Follicular phase

At the beginning of each cycle, FSH stimulates further growth in follicles that have reached a stage in their development at which they are responsive to FSH. In normal cycles, the development of one follicle outstrips the others (dominant follicle). The production of inhibitory factors by the dominant follicle and the falling levels of FSH in the mid-follicular phase lead to atresia in the remaining follicles (see Fig. 5.1). As the dominant follicle grows, oestrogen production within the follicle increases dramatically and rising levels of oestradiol are seen in the peripheral blood. LH promotes the conversion of cholesterol to androgens in the theca cells. These androgens are converted to oestradiol by the action of aromatase.

Ovulation

The rising levels of oestradiol in the peripheral circulation trigger the LH surge from the pituitary. Ovulation occurs 36 hours after the initial rise in LH. The mid-cycle surge of LH (and to a lesser extent FSH) stimulates the completion of meiosis in the oocyte and the production of progesterone and prostaglandins in the follicle. Progesterone enhances the activity of proteolytic enzymes that are responsible, with prostaglandins, for digestion and rupture of the follicular wall. The mid-cycle rise in FSH is responsible for freeing the oocyte from its attachments to the surrounding granulosa cells so that it can be released. The follicular phase varies but is usually 14 days or longer.

Luteal phase

With the release of the ovum, the follicle shrinks and the granulosa cells produce a yellow pigment, lutein, that gives the corpus luteum its name. The corpus luteum produces all three classes of sex steroids: androgens, oestrogens and progestins, but it is the production of progesterone that distinguishes the

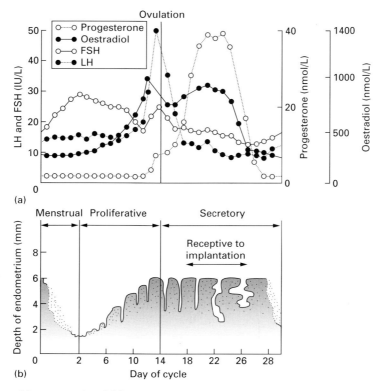

Fig. 5.1 (a) Hormonal and (b) endometrial changes during the menstrual cycle.

luteal from the follicular phase. The massive secretion of progesterone is important in preparing the endometrium for implantation and also suppresses the growth of new follicles past a certain stage. The life span of the corpus luteum is 9–11 days, after which it regresses and steroid levels fall unless pregnancy intervenes. Human chorionic gonadotrophin (HCG) from the implanting pregnancy maintains the production of steroids from the corpus luteum until the 9th or 10th week of gestation, by which time placental steroidogenesis is well established. As the menopause approaches, the follicles become more and more resistant to stimulation. The pituitary responds to the low oestradiol concentration by increasing the amount of FSH, released. Finally, despite high concentrations of FSH, there are no further responsive follicles and amenorrhoea (the menopause) ensues.

ENDOMETRIAL CYCLE

Proliferative phase

This corresponds to the follicular phase in the ovary. The most obvious response to oestradiol in the endometrium is cell division (hence the name 'proliferative phase'). Mitosis occurs in both stromal and epithelial cells, leading to growth of the glands and thickening of the endometrium from 0.5 mm in the menstrual phase to 3.5–5 mm in height at the end of the proliferative phase.

Secretory phase

With the rise in progesterone from the corpus luteum, mitotic activity in the endometrium and growth cease. Microscopically, the first sign of the effect of progesterone is the appearance of vacuoles at the base of the epithelial cells lining the glands. The nuclei are displaced towards the gland lumen and mitotic activity ceases. The glands continue to grow and the spiral arterioles become progressively more coiled and tortuous. The glandular cells, presumably full of secretory products, bulge into the glands and the glands become dilated with secreted material.

The stroma becomes oedematous in the mid-secretory phase and stromal cells undergo decidualization. They change from thin fibroblast-like cells to the large polyhedral cells seen in true decidua in pregnancy.

Menstrual phase

Falling levels of oestradiol and progesterone at the end of the secretory phase cause cyclical constriction and dilatation of the spiral arterioles in the endometrium. These spasms are successively more intense and prolonged, leading to generalized vasoconstriction, ischaemia and cell disintegration with release of lysosomal enzymes. Neutrophil leukocytes infiltrate the endometrium and breakdown continues until rising concentrations of oestradiol in the subsequent menstrual cycle initiate healing.

LOWER GENITAL TRACT CHANGES

Cervix

Cervical changes during the menstrual cycle are of major importance in fertility. Their use to predict ovulation has largely been superseded in the treatment of infertility by more objective measures but they are still used by many women to avoid pregnancy.

The cervical mucus becomes more profuse and less viscous as oestradiol rises in the follicular phase. Immediately prior to ovulation (2–3 days) when oestradiol peaks, the mucus demonstrates the capacity to be drawn out into a long thread without losing its continuity (spinnbarkeit). On scanning electron microscopy this change is evident as an increase in the pore size of the honeycomb-like appearance of the mucus. This facilitates sperm migration through the cervix. Under the influence of exogenous progesterone the pore size is decreased in the luteal phase and the mucus is more viscous.

The changes in cervical mucus can also be observed by drying the mucus on a microscopy slide. As ovulation approaches, the dried mucus assumes the appearance of a fern frond (ferning). The cervical os is more open around the time of ovulation, which facilitates sperm transport.

Vagina

Vaginal secretions are increased in response to oestradiol but the most striking change in the vagina is in the morphology of the vaginal epithelium. Oestradiol stimulates the growth and maturation of superficial cells in the stratified squamous epithelium of the vagina. Therefore, in smears taken from women just prior to ovulation superficial cells are dominant, while more intermediate cells are seen in smears early in the cycle or later in the cycle in the presence of progesterone.

'PHYSIOLOGICAL' TREATMENTS IN GYNAECOLOGY

Infertility

Steroids

Progesterone supplementation to support the luteal phase of the cycle is controversial. It is used on the basis that it helps prepare the endometrium adequately, thereby increasing the chances of successful implantation and reducing subsequent miscarriage. Its use in women with recurrent miscarriages has not been shown to be effective and it is likely that the low levels of progesterone seen in these women reflect the fact that the pregnancies are already failing rather than any inherent progesterone deficiency.

In women with premature menopause wishing to conceive, sequential therapy with oestrogen followed by oestrogen and progesterone (mimicking a natural cycle) is used to prepare the endometrium for the implantation of donor eggs that have been fertilized with either the partner's or a donor's semen.

Clomifene (clomiphene)

Clomifene (clomiphene) acts principally as an anti-oestrogen. It binds for weeks to oestrogen receptors in the pituitary but does not activate them, and downregulates receptor production. This blocks the binding of oestradiol, preventing feedback inhibition of FSH secretion. The pituitary secretes more FSH, increasing the stimulation of ovarian follicles. A side-effect of this is to increase the chance of multiple ovulation and consequent multiple pregnancy. Clomifene should only be used for women with ovulatory disorders and will not induce ovulation in premature ovarian failure.

FSH/LH

An alternative method of inducing ovulation is to bypass the pituitary completely and to give FSH. Previously, FSH and LH purified from the urine of menopausal women (human menopausal gonadotrophins, HMG) were used but have now been superseded by recombinant FSH. In anovulatory infertility, when clomifene (clomiphene) has failed, low doses of FSH are used over several weeks. For superovulation, either in combination with intrauterine insemination (IUI) or prior to in vitro fertilization (IVF), larger doses are used over a shorter period of time. In this regimen, the pituitary may also be bypassed by giving HCG to mimic the LH surge and induce ovulation. LH and HCG are structurally similar but HCG is used as it is cheaper, large quantities being extracted from the urine of pregnant women. In IVF treatment cycles injections of HCG are continued through the luteal phase to maintain the corpus luteum until pregnancy or the next period supervenes.

GnRH analogues (agonists)

More recently, synthetic GnRH analogues that have a longer half-life than natural GnRH have been used to abolish a woman's endogenous cycle. These act by initially causing an outpouring of LH and FSH but then downregulation of GnRH receptors in the pituitary and desensitization of gonadotroph cells. This leads to very low levels of LH and FSH and, consequently, oestrogen.

Increasing use of this hypo-oestrogenic state has been seen in treatments in gynaecology. It is widely employed in assisted reproduction where an artificial cycle is imposed using FSH and HCG. Improved pregnancy rates have been reported using this method. Three-month courses of these agents are employed for shrinking fibroids prior to surgery and 6-month courses are used in the treatment of endometriosis. They are employed less commonly in other hormone-dependent conditions such as menorrhagia, premenstrual syndrome, and breast and prostatic carcinoma.

GnRH antagonists

Although GnRH antagonists are theoretically more appropriate for clinical use than the agonists, side-effects have hindered their use until recently. Antagonists have similar effects to the agonists but work more quickly. Whereas agonists take several weeks to attain their maximal effect and a similar time for the effects to wear off, the antagonists work in days rather than weeks. As these agents are developed we will see their increasing use in clinical situations where agonists are currently used.

Contraception

Contraceptive pills

The two major contraceptive actions of the combined oral contraceptive pill are to prevent ovulation and to make the cervical mucus resistant to sperm transport. Ovulation is prevented because the constantly elevated levels of oestrogen and progesterone inhibit gonadotrophin secretion, preventing follicle development and the LH surge. The change in the cervical mucus is an action of progesterone and is the main contraceptive action of the progestin-only pill.

Depot progestins

Long-acting progestin preparations are used as contraceptives and to control menorrhagia. They induce the cervical mucus changes described above and the continuous negative feedback on the pituitary inhibits the LH surge, thereby preventing ovulation (unlike the progestin-only pill). The constant suppression of the endometrium leads to reduced menstruation and, eventually, amenorrhoea in two-thirds of women who use these preparations long-term. Three-monthly intramuscular injections of depot medroxyprogesterone acetate (Depo-Provera) have been widely used for many years.

Abnormal bleeding

Anovulatory bleeding

This is a common cause of irregular bleeding, particularly at the extremes of a woman's reproductive life, and is associated with PCOS. Failure to ovulate leads to prolonged endometrial stimulation and irregular, incomplete shedding of the endometrium. It is treated by replacing the absent cycle regulator, i.e. the corpus luteum, with exogenous progesterone for 10–14 days to achieve endometrial maturation and subsequent shedding after progesterone is withdrawn. Alternatively, the woman's endogenous hormone production can be suppressed and artificially replaced using the combined oral contraceptive pill or, in older women, hormone replacement therapy (see Ch. 14).

Menorrhagia

Commonly, oestrogen and progesterone together (combined oral contraceptive pill) or, less commonly, progesterone alone (Depo-Provera) are the first-line treatments of this condition. Both medications decrease endometrial growth, thereby reducing menstrual loss. Indeed, after several injections with Depo-Provera, the majority of women become totally amenorrhoeic. Other long-acting progestin contraceptives (Norplant, Implanon, Mirena) are similarly effective in treating menorrhagia.

Prolonged bleeding

In the short-term management of this condition, continuous oestrogen or, more commonly, progesterone will usually stop the bleeding. Following hormone withdrawal, menstruation will ensue. When pathology has been excluded, cyclical therapy for 3–6 months is often necessary to regulate the cycle.

SUMMARY

The menstrual cycle is the result of complex hormonal and target organ interactions. The length of the cycle is regulated by ovarian events, but normal menstruation requires intact functioning of the whole: hypothalamus, pituitary, ovary and endometrium. The cyclical production of the steroids from the ovary (follicular/luteal phases) leads to the cyclical changes in the endometrium (proliferative/secretory phases). The main purpose of the endometrial changes is the preparation of a suitable environment for the implanting embryo.

6   Menstrual disorders

Janice Rymer

Expectations of the examiners

The candidate will be expected to have a basic knowledge of the physiology of the menstrual cycle. Menstrual disorders are common, and the initial assessment and management of these disorders are within the scope of general practice. However, the candidate is also expected to understand what specialist referral will involve and the subsequent management that would occur in hospital.

MENORRHAGIA

Definition

Menorrhagia is excessive menstrual bleeding that occurs with regular or irregular cycles. Median menstrual blood loss is 30–40 ml in total per period; > 80 ml is pathological.

Interesting facts

There has been a tenfold increase in the number of periods that women experience during their reproductive life (reducing family size, less lactation, early menarche, late menopause).

If menstrual loss is > 60 ml/month, a negative iron balance will potentially develop on a normal Western diet.

In routine clinical practice, objective measurement of menstrual blood loss is not used, so clinicians rely on the woman's assessment which has been shown to be inaccurate in approximately half of cases.

Pathophysiology

Menstrual bleeding can be ovulatory or anovulatory. In general, regular, painful periods are associated with ovulation, and irregular, painless periods with anovulation. The latter is more common in the extremes of menstrual life. There is now evidence that in women with proven menorrhagia, there are elevated levels of prostaglandins in the endometrium, and these women have an altered responsiveness to the vasodilator PGE_2. Progesterone inhibits prostaglandin production and oestradiol increases prostaglandin production. Ovulatory bleeding is associated with normal levels of these peripherally circulating hormones, so it is thought that altered prostaglandin synthesis is responsible for the increased menstrual loss. In particular the ratio of PGE_2 and prostacyclin to PGF_{2a} is significant, the former causing vasodilatation and inhibition of platelet aggregation and the latter promoting vasoconstriction and platelet aggregation.

In anovulatory cycles, oestrogen and progesterone levels are variable, causing irregular shedding of the endometrium.

Aetiology

1. Physiological, i.e. normal loss but interpreted as excessive. This commonly occurs in women who stop the oral contraceptive pill. Having been used to painless, light periods while taking the pill, they then revert to normal periods which are more painful and heavier.
2. Dysfunctional uterine bleeding (hormonal). This is a diagnosis which is made after pelvic pathology has been excluded.
3. Congenital, e.g. increased endometrial surface area, of which an example is a bicornuate uterus.
4. Traumatic, e.g. IUD.
5. Infective, e.g. chronic pelvic inflammatory disease.
6. Neoplastic, e.g. fibroids, endometrial polyps.
7. Metabolic, e.g. thyroid dysfunction.
8. Psychological factors.
9. Adenomyosis.
10. Blood dyscrasias.
11. Iatrogenic, e.g. drug ingestion, as seen in women on long-term anti-coagulation.

'Physiological' and 'dysfunctional uterine bleeding' account for 50% of all cases of menorrhagia.

Assessment

History is notoriously inaccurate but it is essential to distinguish menstrual bleeding from non-menstrual bleeding. The number of pads/tampons used does not equal amount lost, and a history of flooding or clots is unreliable. Objective measurement is impractical. Despite these limitations the diagnosis is based on the patient's own assessment of her menstrual loss.

Examination should include measurement of weight, a search for signs of endocrine disturbance and a pelvic examination, including a cervical smear if indicated.

Investigations

1. Full blood count. If anaemia is present, iron supplementation should be considered with medical treatment.
2. Thyroid function tests if any other stigmata of dysfunction exist.
3. Further tests are determined by history and examination: e.g. clotting disorders—clotting profiles, pelvic infection—endocervical swabs.

4. Vaginal ultrasonography. Transvaginal scanning can measure the thickness of the endometrium and detect abnormalites of the cavity, e.g. endometrial polyps. As the vaginal probe is so much closer to the pelvic organs, the uterus and ovaries can be more easily scanned. Fluid can be instilled into the uterine cavity to delineate polyps.
5. Endometrial biopsy. This should be performed if the menorrhagia is a recent phenomenon, if the woman is over 40 years of age, or if there is any intermenstrual bleeding. There are various techniques available. Outpatient endometrial sampling is becoming more popular and this involves a small diameter (2 mm) plastic cannula which is inserted through the cervical canal into the endometrial cavity. The inner plastic tube is withdrawn, creating a vacuum, and endometrial tissue is drawn into the plastic cannula. Dilatation and curettage has been replaced by hysteroscopy where the endometrial cavity can be visualized and biopsies appropriately directed. It must be remembered that, whatever form of endometrial biopsy is performed, the procedure is diagnostic not therapeutic, although some women may experience a few months of lighter periods after a formal dilatation and curettage.

Treatment

Any pathology that is found should be appropriately treated. One is then left with the treatment of dysfunctional uterine bleeding.

Anovulatory

In adolescents and premenopausal women the oral contraceptive pill can be prescribed, making the periods lighter, regular and less painful. Cyclical progestogens (e.g. medroxyprogesterone acetate 10 mg daily for 10 days) can be used to induce regular withdrawal bleeds. Likewise, in perimenopausal women, once the endometrium has been sampled, cyclical progestogens can also be used to induce regular withdrawal bleeding. If no withdrawal bleeding occurs, then there has been no oestrogenic stimulation of the endometrium; this indicates no ovarian function and the 'menopause' has occurred. If the woman is experiencing climacteric symptoms with menorrhagia, then it is appropriate to put her on hormone replacement therapy, remembering that she needs progestogens for at least 12 days of each calendar month.

Acute arrest for heavy bleeding. Start with a high dose of a progestogen and decrease, e.g. norethisterone 30 mg b.d. for 3 days, 20 mg b.d. for 3 days, 10 mg b.d. for 3 days, 5 mg b.d. for 10 days. Cessation of treatment will be followed by a withdrawal bleed.

Ovulatory

1. *Non-steroidal anti-inflammatory drugs.* These inhibit biosynthesis of the prostaglandins and reduce menstrual flow by about 30% in most women with menstrual blood loss greater than 80 ml/day. The advantage of this treatment is that it is only taken for a few days of each cycle, i.e. during menstruation.
2. *Antifibrinolytic drugs.* These probably act by reducing enhanced fibrinolytic activity found in the uterus in women with excessive menstrual blood loss.

Reductions are in the order of 50%. Side-effects are common, e.g. nausea and dizziness.

3. *Oral contraceptive pill.* The absolute contraindications must be ruled out and the relative contraindications considered. Ovulation is suppressed and the oestrogen levels remain constant. This inhibits endometrial growth, reducing menstrual loss.

4. *Hormone-releasing IUDs.* The progestogen released from this device affects the endometrium, making it atrophic. After 1 year of use most women have only scanty spotting of blood.

5. *Endometrial ablation or resection.* The endometrium is visualized hysteroscopically and destroyed with the laser or resectoscope. Newer ablature techniques include uterine thermal balloon, cryoablation, photodynamic therapy and microwave ablation. Some women become amenorrhoeic and the majority have reduced menstrual loss. Some women require further surgery as the long-term results can be disappointing. Microwave and endothermal balloon ablation can be done in the outpatient setting.

6. *Danazol.* The mechanism is uncertain but it induces atrophy of the endometrium as a result of low levels of circulating sex steroids. The normal dose is 200 mg daily. The disadvantages are that it requires daily dosage and has side-effects, e.g. weight gain, virilizing effects.

7. *Hysterectomy.* This is the definitive treatment but involves the risks associated with major pelvic surgery, e.g. pelvic thrombosis. Controlled trials have shown that postoperative psychological morbidity is similar to that seen preoperatively.

Summary

Menorrhagia is a common symptom which is difficult to assess objectively. As a generalization, heavy irregular bleeding is anovulatory and occurs in the extremes of reproductive life, and heavy regular bleeding is usually ovulatory. In dysfunctional uterine bleeding, hysterectomy should only be considered after failure of conservative medical treatment and local ablation techniques.

DYSMENORRHOEA

PRIMARY

Definition

Primary dysmenorrhoea is defined as painful periods for which no organic or psychological cause can be found.

Pathophysiology

There is an abnormally high production of endometrial prostaglandins which cause excessive uterine contractions. Dysmenorrhoea is generally associated with ovulatory cycles.

Assessment

History is important, as pain occurs with onset of menstruation and then declines. Examination must exclude obvious pathology.

Investigations

If diagnosis is made on history then no further investigation is needed. If treatment fails to improve symptoms then a laparoscopy is needed to exclude pathology.

Treatment

1. Non-steroidal anti-inflammatory agents are prostaglandin synthetase inhibitors and will decrease pain and reduce menstrual loss.
2. The oral contraceptive pill will inhibit ovulation. Primary dysmenorrhoea is usually associated with ovulation; thus the pill will relieve primary dysmenorrhoea.

SECONDARY

Definition

Secondary dysmenorrhoea is defined as painful periods where an organic or psychosexual cause can be found.

Aetiology

1. Pelvic inflammatory disease
2. Endometriosis
3. Ovarian tumour
4. Previous pelvic or abdominal surgery
5. Misplaced IUD
6. Past history of sexual abuse
7. Other psychological problems.

Assessment

History is important and may take time if psychosexual problems are present. Pelvic examination must be performed and swabs taken if indicated. Restricted mobility or fixed retroversion of the uterus suggests the presence of adhesions secondary to endometriosis, pelvic inflammatory disease or previous surgery.

Investigations

These will be guided by history, but laparoscopy is indicated in most cases.

Treatment

This depends on the cause. Often reassurance that the pelvis is normal is treatment in itself.

POLYCYSTIC OVARIAN SYNDROME

Definition
Polycystic ovarian syndrome (PCOS) is a common disorder that is almost always associated with either menstrual disturbance or hyperandrogenism.

Interesting facts
It was previously thought that anovulation was an essential feature of this syndrome but more than 80% of women who have hirsutism and regular cycles have PCOS on ultrasound. A polycystic ovary contains twice the number of FSH-sensitive follicles.

Aetiology
Controversial but recent evidence points to a gonadotrophin-dependent, intraovarian androgen excess. This is thought to be either due to a primary inherited abnormality of P450c17-α (enzyme in steroid pathway) or secondary to inherited or acquired hyperinsulinaemia. The insulin resistance is due to a receptor problem.

Biochemical investigations
The LH/FSH ratio and the serum oestradiol are raised. Testosterone and androstenedione are also characteristically elevated. A higher body mass index (BMI) is associated with increased serum testosterone and an increased prevalence of hirsutism. Hyperinsulinaemia is a prominent feature in obese patients with PCOS, and this enhances ovarian androgen production and inhibits hepatic synthesis of sex hormone binding globulin (SHBG), thereby increasing the exposure of hair follicles to free testosterone.

Hyperinsulinaemia also has an adverse effect on cardiovascular risk factors, e.g. decreased high-density lipoprotein (HDL), increased triglycerides and glucose, and raised blood pressure.

The high oestrogen levels may lead to hyperplastic changes of the endometrium, which in turn can lead to malignant change.

Appearance
The ovaries are typically enlarged, thickened and pearly white with sclerotic capsules and subcapsular follicular cysts. Bisection shows numerous cysts in the cortex, and on ultrasound scan a peripheral ring of follicles is seen.

Treatment
Hyperandrogenism
The mainstay of therapy is a combination of ethinylestradiol with either the anti-androgen cyproterone acetate or drosperinone, which is a spironolactone analogue, or a combined oral contraceptive pill containing a non-androgenic progestogen. These will give cycle control, reduce hyperandrogenic symptoms and provide contraception. Other therapies include:

1. Spironolactone 25–100 mg b.d.
2. Flutamide 250 mg b.d. days 5–25 of the cycle. (a non-steroidal pure anti-androgen)
3. Finasteride 5 mg daily (a prototype inhibitor of 5α-reductase, the cutaneous enzyme responsible for the conversion of testosterone to the more bioactive dihydrotestosterone)
4. LHRH analogue and addback therapy. Endogenous gonadotrophins are suppressed and then oestrogen and progesterone are 'added back'.

Anovulation

The management will depend on whether the woman wishes to conceive or not. If she does not then either the oral contraceptive pill or cyclical progestogen administration is suitable. If she wishes to conceive then initial treatment should be achievement of normal BMI, then clomifene and then gonadotrophin stimulation.

Metformin 500 mg b.d. is effective in the treatment of the obese patient with oligo- or amenorrhoea. Ovarian electrodiathermy has produced promising results with regard to inducing ovulation and significant conception rates in up to a year. This procedure has replaced wedge resection of the ovary.

Summary

PCOS is a complex and common syndrome and is a spectrum of disease from mild symptoms e.g. hirsutism with regular cycles to severe symptoms such as hirsutism, obesity and amenorrhoea. Women with PCOS may also be insulin-resistant and hyperinsulinaemic.

AMENORRHOEA

PRIMARY

Definition

Primary amenorrhoea is no menstruation by 14 years with growth failure or absence of secondary sexual characteristics, i.e. breast development and pubic hair growth, or no menstruation by 16 years when growth and sexual development are normal.

SECONDARY

Definition

Secondary amenorrhoea is absence of menses for 6 months (or six cycles) in a previously menstruating woman.

Aetiology
The causes can be divided into compartments:

1. Target organ and outflow tract dysfunction
2. Gonadal failure
3. Pituitary dysfunction
4. Hypothalamic dysfunction
5. Thyroid or adrenal dysfunction.

Assessment
The history should involve specific questioning about galactorrhoea, weight change, hirsutism, hot flushes, life crisis, possibility of pregnancy, recent gynaecological surgery and cyclical pain.

Investigations
1. Serum prolactin level (× 2)
2. Thyroid function tests if indicated
3. Serum FSH, LH, testosterone and SHBG levels
4. Karyotype if phenotype abnormal
5. Ultrasound scan of pelvis.

Treatment
See Figure 6.1. If the prolactin level is high then refer to a specialist centre for magnetic resonance imaging (MRI) of the pituitary fossa and bromocriptine or cabergoline if a microadenoma is present.

Thyroid disease should be treated appropriately. If both thyroid and pro-lactin levels are normal, then specialist referral would be appropriate at this stage. Management will involve a progestogen challenge test, e.g. 5 mg medroxyprogesterone acetate b.d. for 5 days. If this is followed by a with-drawal bleed, then anovulation is the diagnosis, most likely secondary to poly-cystic ovarian syndrome. In the absence of a withdrawal bleed, a raised FSH level indicates gonadal failure (i.e. menopause). If FSH is normal, then an oestrogen challenge test is performed, e.g. 2.5 mg conjugated oestrogens daily for 21 days, with the above medroxyprogesterone acetate regimen for the last 5 days. If there is no withdrawal bleed, then there is an outflow tract disorder, i.e. Asherman's syndrome, or cervical stenosis (assuming that the rest of the genital tract has been adequately examined and found to be normal). If there is a withdrawal bleed, then the problem is hypothalamic, but a CT is per-formed to check the pituitary fossa.

INTERMENSTRUAL BLEEDING

Definition
Intermenstrual bleeding is vaginal bleeding occurring between normal men-struation times.

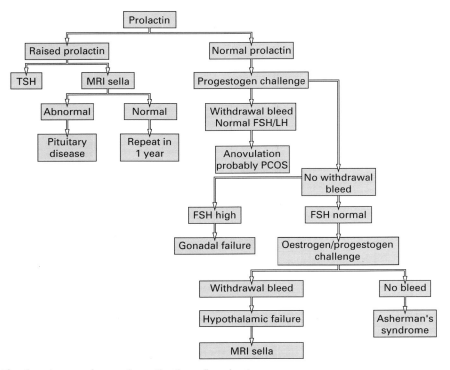

Fig. 6.1 Amenorrhoea—investigations flowchart.

Aetiology

Although classically associated with endometrial hyperplasia/carcinoma, intermenstrual bleeding may also occur with cervical carcinoma. Regular mid-cycle bleeding can occur in association with ovulation or the combined oral contraceptive pill.

Assessment

History is important, as a recent onset of intermenstrual bleeding is more suspicious of endometrial carcinoma (see Ch. 13).

Investigations

1. Cervical smear
2. Transvaginal scan
3. Endometrial biopsy/hysteroscopy is indicated in most cases, except those where changing the oral contraceptive pill rapidly corrects the disturbance.

Treatment

If the patient is on the oral contraceptive pill, she should take two pills on the days when the breakthrough bleeding is occurring, or change to a different pill preparation with a lower oestrogen content or a higher progestogen content.

POSTCOITAL BLEEDING

This is the classic symptom of cervical carcinoma so the cervix must be inspected and a cervical smear taken. Further management depends on the cytology result (see Ch. 13).

7

Endometriosis, dyspareunia and pelvic pain

Gregory Davis

ENDOMETRIOSIS

Expectations of the examiners

Endometriosis is a common condition that causes pain and infertility. The examiners will expect the candidate to have a sound knowledge of its presentation and methods of treatment.

Definition

Endometriosis is defined as the presence of functioning endometrial tissue outside the uterine cavity. Histological examination must confirm the presence of both glands and stroma.

Interesting facts

The reported incidence of endometriosis varies widely but is probably about 10% of menstruating white women and 25–50% of women presenting with infertility. It may be asymptomatic and an incidental finding at surgery for other reasons, or it may cause severe, chronic pelvic pain. The severity of the pain may be disproportionate to the extent of the disease.

Endometriosis may be present outside the uterus or within the myometrium (adenomyosis) or both. Adenomyosis is a histological diagnosis made after hysterectomy, usually for menorrhagia and dysmenorrhea.

Historically, endometriosis was described as presenting in infertile white women aged between 30 and 45 years of higher socioeconomic status. As the use of laparoscopy has become more widespread, this description has become less accurate. Users of the combined oral contraceptive pill are less likely to develop endometriosis.

Pathophysiology

Aetiology

Classically there are three theories concerning the pathogenesis of endometriosis:

1. *Retrograde menstruation.* Viable fragments of endometrium are known to reach the pelvic cavity during menstruation. In susceptible individuals these may implant, leading to intrapelvic distribution of endometrial deposits. Women with endometriosis have been shown to have a reduced 'immune response'. However, retrograde menstruation is common, not all women develop endometriosis, and this theory does not explain the development of endometriosis at distant sites.
2. *Lymphatic or vascular spread.* Small, viable endometrial 'emboli' can be recovered from the lungs and provide an explanation for the presence of endometriosis at peripheral sites.
3. *Metaplasia of coelomic epithelium.* In this theory it is proposed that the repeated inflammatory insult of menstrual fluid may lead to a differentiation of the primitive coelomic epithelium which constitutes the visceral peritoneum.

No single theory adequately explains the distribution of endometriosis and it is likely to be a combination of the above factors. It is not known what determines a woman's susceptibility to developing endometriosis but it is probably a result of immunological, genetic and physical components. If a woman has a first-degree female relative with endometriosis she has a six- to nine-fold increase in the risk of the disease. In addition, direct 'inoculation' may occur during surgery, leading to the development of endometriosis in hysterotomy, hysterectomy and caesarean section scars.

Site

Endometriosis commonly occurs in the dependent part of the pelvis: uterosacral ligaments, pouch of Douglas, pelvic side walls and ovaries. It is less commonly seen on other peritoneal surfaces of the abdominal cavity, in the bowel and bladder and in the umbilicus or scars from abdominal surgery. It has also been described in distant sites, e.g. lung, thigh and vulva.

Pathology

Commonly, endometriotic deposits consist of multiple small (< 1 cm), raised blue-black nodules which appear as if ink has been injected under the peritoneum. In more severe disease the nodules may be larger with variable amounts of surrounding fibrosis. If the ovary becomes involved then an endometrioma (or chocolate cyst) may form. In severe endometriosis there is extensive pelvic damage due to fibrosis and adhesion formation. In the latter situation the sigmoid colon may become adherent to the posterior cervix, leading to obliteration of the pouch of Douglas.

Microscopically, glands and stroma are present together with a variable amount of bleeding and fibrosis. These deposits may be out of phase with the woman's menstrual cycle but decidualize during pregnancy like normal endometrium.

Assessment

Women may present with symptoms due to the local effects of endometriosis or through the complications that have occurred as a result of the disease. Forty per cent of women with endometriosis present with the combination of dysmenorrhoea, dyspareunia and infertility.

History

Pain. Classically, endometriosis is associated with secondary dysmenorrhoea. The pelvic pain is directly related to the onset and duration of the menses and is usually progressive unless treated.

Dyspareunia. Intercourse may be painful on deep penetration throughout the menstrual cycle (see 'Dyspareunia' below).

Menstrual disturbance. Women with endometriosis will often give a history of increasingly heavy periods and, particularly, premenstrual spotting.

Complications

Infertility. Endometriosis may cause infertility in the absence of other symptoms. Even minimal disease is associated with infertility and is thought to be due to the release of prostaglandins and inflammatory cytokines that interfere with the oocyte at implantation. More severe disease causes adhesion formation and distortion of pelvic anatomy that further compromise fertility.

Lower genital tract. Uncommonly, deposits in the vagina or vulva may give rise to intermenstrual bleeding or dyspareunia.

Bowel. Endometriosis involving the bowel may cause cyclical rectal bleeding, stricture or rarely obstruction.

Bladder. The bladder is rarely affected but cyclical haematuria or frequency may occur if it is involved.

Abdominal wall. Deposits in the umbilicus or abdominal wounds may cause cyclical swelling and pain at the affected site.

Examination

Abdominal examination may reveal the presence of a mass (endometrioma) but this is uncommon. Abdominal wall deposits are usually tender and the diagnosis is made on the history and histology after excision. Pelvic examination may reveal nodules in the vagina or on the cervix that may bleed. On bimanual examination the uterus may be tender and/or fixed in retroversion by adhesions, and nodules on the uterosacral ligaments or in the pouch of Douglas may be palpable, particularly around the menses.

Investigations

Pelvic ultrasound scanning should be performed as 1 in 8 women with endometriosis will have an ovarian endometrioma at presentation and, if an endometrioma is present, more than 90% of these women will also have significant other endometriosis. The diagnosis is confirmed by laparoscopy. Involvement of other systems is investigated in the appropriate manner, e.g. cystoscopy and biopsy if bladder involvement is suspected. The extent of the disease is usually classified as mild (minimal), moderate or severe but a clear description with diagrams is more useful in case further laparoscopy at a later date is required. The American Fertility Society has produced a scoring system to assess the severity based on the size and extent of the lesions and the amount of adhesion formation.

Treatment

The treatment of endometriosis is controversial and both medical and surgical treatment have their advocates. It is the authors' opinion that all endometriosis should be excised surgically with the place of medical therapy being suppressive, either pre- or postsurgery.

Medical

Medical treatment is based on the prolonged inhibition of ovulation and was introduced because of the improvement in endometriosis that usually occurs during pregnancy. It is suppressive rather than curative. Meta-analysis of drug trials in the treatment of endometriosis has shown that all the agents described below are equally effective in temporarily relieving pain. In view of this, the safest, cheapest and easiest to take should be the agents of choice. Therefore, either progestin alone, medroxyprogesterone acetate, or the combined oral contraceptive pill are the agents of choice.

Danazol. 200–800 mg/day for 6–9 months. The actions of danazol are complex and it primarily prevents the mid-cycle surge of gonadotrophins. It is an androgen derivative and produces a high-androgen, low-oestrogen environment. Side-effects occur in 80% of women and are a result of: (1) low oestrogen—decreased breast size, hot flushes, vaginitis; or (2) high androgen—acne, oily skin, weight gain, hirsutism. Only 10% of women find the side-effects sufficiently troublesome to stop the drug but it should be stopped immediately if there is any deepening of the voice as this is irreversible.

Combined oral contraceptive. This is given continuously for 6–9 months. Weight gain is a more prominent side-effect than when the pill is given cyclically, but otherwise the side-effects are similar.

Medroxyprogesterone acetate. 20–30 mg/day is cheaper and has fewer side-effects. Breakthrough bleeding is a common problem which is treated with a 7-day course of oestrogen (e.g. ethinylestradiol 10 μg/day).

GnRH analogue. This long-acting agonist delivered intranasally, subcutaneously or via monthly implantation produces a state of hypogonadotrophic hypogonadism, achieving even lower levels of serum oestradiol levels than with danazol. The side-effects are those of oestradiol deprivation, and bone loss occurs. If long-term therapy is contemplated, then 'addback' therapy with continuous combined hormone replacement therapy or tibolone is recommended.

Surgical
Definitive surgery is required for the treatment of severe disease. The object of surgery is to restore normal anatomy and to remove all endometriosis. The only cure is the resection of all deposits which is usually performed laparoscopically. Many surgeons use medical treatment prior to surgery to improve the resectability of the lesions. Hormone replacement therapy can be used postoperatively with a minimal risk of growth in residual endometriosis.
Presacral neurectomy. This procedure can be performed for intractable dysmenorrhoea associated with endometriosis but its efficacy is questionable.

Follow-up
Medical therapy
This is usually effective in treating pain, particularly with minimal disease, but 5–20% of women will experience a recurrence of symptoms within a year and 50% within 5 years of stopping medication. Pregnancy rates of 50–75% are reported in both the treated and untreated groups and these rates probably reflect the fact that women with milder disease are often treated medically.

Surgery
The recurrence of pain after adequate surgery is less than 20% and this is improved with postoperative medical therapy for 6–12 months. Postoperative fertility is related to the severity of the disease, with 60% of women conceiving after surgery for moderate disease compared to 35% for severe disease. Fertility is greatest in the first 6–12 months after surgery and conception is unlikely after 2 years. After this time, assisted conception should be considered.

DYSPAREUNIA

Expectations of the examiners
This is a common symptom that may be managed by general practitioners without referral to a gynaecologist. The candidate must have an understanding of the physical causes, their diagnosis and the management of the physical and psychological aspects of this condition.

Definition
Dyspareunia is painful or difficult intercourse. It may be divided into: (1) superficial—pain at the onset of penetration; or (2) deep—pain during or after penetration has occurred.

Interesting facts

Dyspareunia is a common symptom but many women are reluctant to talk about it. Often there is a combination of physical and psychological factors contributing to the pain. Pain due to a physical problem often leads to fear of intercourse and lack of lubrication, which in turn makes intercourse more painful. This cycle may continue after the physical problem is cured. Both the physical and psychological aspects need to be addressed if the symptom is to resolve.

Pathophysiology

The causes of superficial dyspareunia are listed in Table 7.1. Pelvic pathology of any nature may lead to deep dyspareunia but the common causes are:

1. Endometriosis
2. Ectopic pregnancy
3. Pelvic inflammatory disease
4. Chronic pelvic pain syndrome (see below)
5. Ovarian cyst accident, e.g. haemorrhage, torsion.

Uterine prolapse and retroversion are commonly listed as causes but are unlikely to result in significant dyspareunia except where the uterus is involved in other pathology, e.g. endometriosis or adenomyosis.

Assessment

History

The onset and relationship of the pain to the woman's life events and menstrual cycle are important. The menstrual, contraceptive and obstetric history should be obtained in detail and a full sexual history taken. It is important to

Table 7.1 Causes of superficial dyspareunia.

Vulva	Anatomical
Vulvitis	Vaginal atresia
Atrophic	Imperforate hymen
Infective (candida, herpes, human	Contracture
papillomavirus)	Atrophy
Bartholinitis	Postsurgery
Dystrophy	Postradiotherapy
Neoplasm	
	Urethra
Vagina	Urethritis
Vaginismus	Urethral caruncle
Vaginitis	Urethral diverticulum
Atropic (postpartum, postmenopause)	
Infective (as for vulva)	

assess the woman's attitude to sexuality and the family history of attitudes to pain and sex. Acute dyspareunia suggests an organic cause, while chronic superficial dyspareunia is more suggestive of psychosexual dysfunction.

Examination
A very careful pelvic examination should be performed to exclude physical causes. The woman's attitude to the examination may reflect her underlying attitude to her sexuality (or a physical problem).

Investigations
Vaginal and endocervical swabs should be taken if indicated. Deep dyspareunia usually requires laparoscopy to make a diagnosis if a cause is not apparent on examination.

Treatment
Superficial dyspareunia
If the cause is organic, e.g. candidiasis, this is usually apparent on examination and should be appropriately treated. Vaginismus and other psychosexual dysfunction are usually treated with vaginal dilators combined with psychosexual counselling. This should be undertaken by a person with experience in this field.

Deep dyspareunia
Any organic cause should be treated appropriately. Unexplained or untreatable disease (e.g. due to previous surgery) may be improved by limiting penetration through the use of alternative positions during intercourse.

Follow-up
The treatment of physical disease causing superficial dyspareunia is usually successful provided that the woman has a supportive sexual partner. The outcome of psychosexual treatment is variable but pure vaginismus can usually be cured. The results of treatment of deep dyspareunia depend on the underlying cause. If no cause is found then it may become a chronic problem.

PELVIC PAIN

Expectations of the examiners
Pelvic pain is a common gynaecological problem and the candidate must understand how to approach it, exclude organic disease and deal effectively with the psychological aspects of this symptom.

Definition
Pain is localized to the pelvis but it may include lower abdominal and lower back pain.

Interesting facts

Twenty-five per cent of women referred to gynaecology outpatients complain of pelvic pain. The non-gynaecological causes include bowel (e.g. irritable bowel syndrome (IBS), appendicitis, diverticular disease) or urinary tract disease (e.g. urinary tract infection (UTI), ureteric calculus) and rarely spinal disease. In 30% of patients with pelvic pain no cause can be found at laparoscopy and these patients are characterized as having chronic pelvic pain (syndrome). Fifty per cent of women with chronic pelvic pain and a normal pelvic examination will have laparoscopic abnormalities. Only 15% of women with an abnormal pelvic examination will not have an abnormality on laparoscopy. Malignant gynaecological tumours may present with lower abdominal or pelvic discomfort. Significant pain is usually a late feature of advanced gynaecological malignancy.

Pathophysiology

All nerves from the pelvic organs ascend to the T10–L1 spinal segments but the pain is poorly localized and may be referred to the associated dermatome. The cause of the pain is unclear—acute distension of the fallopian tubes or ovaries causes pain (e.g. ectopic pregnancy) but chronic slow swelling may be asymptomatic (e.g. dermoid cyst). Venous congestion of the pelvis causing pain is a controversial issue and remains unresolved at present. Venous congestion is often striking in acute pelvic inflammatory disease, although whether this is the source of the pain is unknown. Dysmenorrhoea is caused by prostaglandin-induced myometrial contractions and anything that stimulates uterine contractions will cause pain (e.g. labour, incomplete abortion).

Assessment

History

A full history is fundamental in dealing with pelvic pain adequately and the pain should be defined as accurately as possible:

1. Site and radiation of pain
2. Character of pain (sharp, dull)
3. Duration and nature of onset
4. Periodicity of pain (constant, intermittent)
5. Severity of pain (e.g. effect on sleep, work, leisure)
6. Bowel patterns, abdominal bloating
7. Relationship to menstruation, food, movement, coitus, defaecation, micturition, posture
8. Any alleviating factors and effect of analgesics.

A full sexual history and a detailed social history focusing on stressful life events and current circumstances must be taken. While the history is being taken, an assessment of the woman's psychological status including mood and level of anxiety should be made.

Examination

A careful general and abdominal examination must be performed. If the pain is well localized, an organic cause is more likely. Similarly, abdominal guarding and rebound are unlikely to be elicited without underlying pathology. Pain of a gynaecological cause is usually most severe suprapubically. After speculum examination has been performed to exclude abnormality, a bimanual examination should be undertaken.

Investigations

Obvious gynaecological or non-gynaecological disease should be managed appropriately. Often the diagnosis is unclear and the only investigation of value in the absence of clinical findings is a laparoscopy.

Treatment

The treatment of any chronic pain disorder begins in the history-taking with the establishment of a rapport between the woman and doctor. In 30% of women with chronic pain, no abnormality can be detected and the pain may well be due to IBS or be 'psychosomatic'. Treatment should combine support, an attempt to increase the woman's awareness of how stress or emotions affect her pain, and analgesia. Initially, aspirin or paracetamol should be used or a prostaglandin synthetase inhibitor if dysmenorrhoea is a component. Once physical examination and laparoscopy have excluded a physical abnormality the therapeutic approach can shift to the perspective of how the woman is going to deal with the pain and still function in her normal life. Trained psychological support may also be beneficial when the woman has accepted that no physical cause can be found.

In women with chronic pelvic pain cognitive behavioural therapeutic approaches are often successful. Women who have admitted past or current sexual abuse require expert counselling and psychological support.

Follow-up

Women with pelvic pain need to be followed for 1–2 years, as a large proportion will have recurrent pain. This is a difficult management problem, particularly in those women who have had surgery for their pelvic pain (often including abdominal hysterectomy ± bilateral salpingo-oophorectomy). The corollary to this is that surgery should be avoided in the absence of obvious pathology.

8

Infertility

Michael Chapman

Expectations of the examiners

The candidate will be expected to have an organized approach to the investigation and management of the infertile couple. A basic understanding of reproductive endocrinology is necessary but the more complex aspects including detailed knowledge of sophisticated drug regimens are not essential.

Definition

Infertility can be defined as the failure to conceive after a period of 12 months of unprotected intercourse. The time period is arbitrary but relates to natural rates of conception, i.e. 80% of couples will be pregnant after 12 cycles.

During the second year of attempted conception 50% of those remaining will conceive spontaneously. Subsequently the chances of conception are in the order of 50% in the following 4 years. Any treatment for infertility must improve that background rate of conception.

The differentiation of infertility into primary (no previous pregnancies) and secondary (previous pregnancies) is useful in that the incidence of causes for each is different, e.g. secondary infertility is more likely to be due to tubal damage. Male factors are more likely in primary infertility.

Pathophysiology

The three major causes of infertility are:

1. Semen quality—40%
2. Ovulatory disorders—30%
3. Tubal problems—30%.

Other causes include:

1. In the male
   a. Impotence
   b. Retrograde ejaculation
   c. Antisperm antibodies
2. In the female
   a. Cervical factor (including antisperm antibodies)
   b. Endometriosis.

The diagnosis of unexplained infertility is reached after exclusion of the above causes accounting for 10–20% of cases.

Assessment

A detailed history from both partners can suggest the underlying problem(s). An assessment of the couple's general health and of their current life stresses, e.g. occupation, family problems etc., is useful to provide a background to the problem. Regularity of sexual intercourse, timing and any associated problems need to be explored with both partners. Infertility itself may contribute substantial psychological pressure and impair the ability to conceive.

Male

In the male, causes for poor semen quality should be sought:

1. Infections, e.g. mumps as an adult, gonococcal infection leading to blocked vasa deferentia
2. Operations, e.g. inguinal herniorrhaphy, orchidopexy
3. Drugs, e.g. antimitotic agents, β-blockers, alcohol (in excess), nicotine.

Information about previous pregnancies should be obtained from each partner separately. Examination should be performed to assess that the genitalia are normal. The size and consistency of the testicles should be noted as well as the presence of vasa deferentia and varicocele.

There is increasing evidence that microdeletions of the Y chromosome are involved in those men with severe oligospermia and azoospermia. Routine investigation has yet to become an accepted part of the assessment.

Female

In the female the history is aimed at providing evidence of ovulation. Signs and symptoms suggesting ovulation include:

1. Regular cycles
2. Mid-cycle pain (mittelschmerz)
3. Changes in vaginal discharge
4. Premenstrual symptoms, e.g. breast tenderness
5. Primary spasmodic dysmenorrhoea.

The reproductive history should be documented in detail. Factors suggesting tubal disease should be sought, i.e. pelvic inflammatory disease, previous pelvic or abdominal surgery, intrauterine device usage, chronic lower abdominal pain and secondary dysmenorrhoea. Full physical assessment including pelvic examination should be performed.

Investigations

Male

Semen analysis.   Instruction for collection should include 3 days' abstinence from ejaculation and rapid transport to the laboratory (< 1 hour) of a specimen obtained by masturbation.

Normal parameters (WHO criteria)
1. Volume: 2–5 ml
2. Concentration: > 20 million/ml
3. Motility: > 50%
4. Normal forms: > 30%

Specimens with subnormal parameters should be repeated in 4–6 weeks before final assessment of quality is made.

Diagnostic categories
1. Normal (as above)
2. Azoospermia (no spermatozoa seen)
3. Oligospermia (concentration < 20 million/ml)
   a. Severe
   b. Moderate
   c. Mild
4. Asthenospermia (decreased motility).

Further investigations should include: LH, FSH and testosterone.

Impaired semen quality is predominantly due to spermatogenic failure of unknown cause. The importance of varicoceles in male subfertility is controversial.

Postcoital test.   This test involves aspiration of a sample of cervical mucus around the time of ovulation within 6 hours of intercourse. A positive test, i.e. motile sperm in the cervical mucus, excludes a cervical problem and confirms vaginal intercourse has occurred. A negative test can be caused by many factors other than mucus hostility, e.g. poor timing and infection, and therefore its value is limited.

Female
Ovulation
Temperature charts.   The basal body temperature chart has a limited role but is worth recording for a maximum of two cycles to:

1. Define cycle length
2. Determine frequency of intercourse
3. Check biphasic pattern indicating ovulation (correlation with biochemical parameters of ovulation: 70–80%).

Serum progesterone.   This is taken 7 days prior to the menses, e.g. day 21 of a 28-day cycle or day 25 of a 32-day cycle. Serial measurements should be taken if the cycle is irregular. Values greater than 30 nmol/l indicate ovulation.

Other methods of assessment.   These include ultrasound monitoring, direct visualization of a corpus luteum at laparoscopy, and monitoring of serum LH levels to time ovulation.

Tubal patency

Hysterosalpingogram (HSG). HSG demonstrates intrauterine and tubal anatomy and patency but it provides little information about problems elsewhere in the pelvis, e.g. adhesions. It is an outpatient procedure but generally causes discomfort or pain. There is a small risk of introducing or reactivating infection.

Laparoscopy and dye instillation. This procedure demonstrates pelvic anatomy and pathology, e.g. adhesions, endometriosis, ovarian disease and tubal patency. It is an inpatient procedure requiring general anaesthesia, with an operative mortality of 1:16 000. The correlation of HSG and laparoscopy findings is 70–80% and therefore it may be necessary to perform both investigations. Most women have a laparoscopy and dye instillation initially, followed by an HSG if indicated. Hysteroscopy at the time of laparoscopy can show intrauterine pathology, such as adhesions, polyps or fibroids.

Rubella status. This should be checked prior to commencing treatment. Non-immune patients must be vaccinated and advised to avoid pregnancy for 3 months.

Treatment

Male

The outlook for azoospermia and oligospermia has been poor. Cold showers, loose underwear, varicocele ligation and hormonal strategies (except in hypopituitarism) have not been shown to be of any significant benefit. Micromanipulation techniques (intracytoplasmic sperm injection—ICSI) in conjunction with in vitro fertilization (IVF) have been successful in severe cases, offering hope in this group. Mild and moderate oligospermia may improve spontaneously and pregnancies do occur. Semen preparation can significantly improve the chances of conception with assisted reproduction techniques including intrauterine insemination in this group. Artificial insemination with donor semen is successful in 50–60% of cases (for 12 cycles) but is only acceptable to 60% of suitable couples.

Female

Ovulatory problems (see 'Amenorrhoea'). The use of ovulation induction techniques has substantially improved the chances of conception to almost normal rates. The first line of treatment is clomifene citrate, initially 50 mg from days 2 to 6 of the menstrual cycle. Clomifene increases FSH production by acting as an anti-oestrogen at the pituitary level. Serum progesterone levels should be checked to confirm ovulation. The use of other ovulation induction agents (gonadotrophins, LHRH analogues) is only appropriate in specialist units. The complications of ovulation induction agents include hyperstimulation and multiple pregnancy.

Tubal problems. The overall success rate of tubal surgery is 20–30%. In specialized centres, success rates in selected cases can be up to 50%.

In vitro fertilization. IVF produces a 'take home baby' rate of 15–30%. The procedure is used in cases of infertility due to tubal disease. It involves the induction of ovulation and collection of multiple ova (either by laparoscope or ultrasound guided needle aspiration) followed by extracorporeal fertilization. Embryos are replaced into the uterine cavity transcervically after 48 hours.

Unexplained infertility. This is an increasingly diagnosed situation. IVF, gamete intrafallopian transfer (GIFT) and intrauterine insemination (IUI) have been shown to enhance the pregnancy rate. GIFT involves ovulation induction and oocyte collection using the laparoscope. At the time of operation the oocyte and freshly washed semen are replaced into the fallopian tube where fertilization occurs. 'Take home baby' rates of 25–30% can be expected. IUI has rates of 10–15%/cycle.

Other problems. Cervical factors and antisperm antibodies are poorly understood and difficult to treat. Spontaneous pregnancies do occur and assisted conception can be useful.

The general practitioner's role in management

The initial investigation of an infertile couple (except for tests of tubal patency) can be performed in a general practice setting. In cases of straightforward failure of ovulation, treatment by the general practitioner with clomifene for 3–6 months is appropriate. Failure to conceive within this period necessitates specialist referral.

SUMMARY

Infertility is a common problem affecting 1:6 couples wishing to conceive. History is important and investigation should be structured to produce a diagnosis in a short time. Referral to specialist centres is mandatory if pregnancy is not achieved relatively quickly, as the psychological effects of infertility can aggravate the problem.

9

Congenital abnormalities of the female genital tract

Janice Rymer

Expectations of the examiners

A detailed knowledge of these abnormalities is not required but the candidate is expected to know the complications that may arise.

Definition

These are defined as anomalies of the female genital tract that are present at birth.

Interesting facts

Forty per cent of women with congenital abnormalities of the uterus also have renal tract anomalies. Congenital abnormalities of the genital tract are thought to be of polygenic aetiology rather than having a single genetic cause.

Pathophysiology

The paramesonephric (Müllerian) ducts are the precursors of the fallopian tubes, uterus and upper two-thirds of the vagina. The lower third of the vagina develops from the urogenital sinus. The paramesonephric ducts develop parallel to the mesonephric ducts from an invagination of coelomic epithelium. They progress caudally and cross in front of the mesonephric ducts, fusing to form a Y-shaped uterovaginal structure which projects into the urogenital sinus. Canalization of the paramesonephric ducts begins before fusion of the ducts and proceeds craniocaudally. The vaginal septum disappears before the uterine septum. The uterine fundus then bulges cranially to form a convex dome.

The classification of the congenital uterine anomalies may be based on the embryological developmental defect:

1. Failure of development, e.g. no paramesonephric duct development or unilateral development
2. Failure of paramesonephric duct canalization
3. Failure of fusion of paramesonephric ducts

4. Failure of median septum loss
5. Failure of fundal dome development
6. Failure of fusion of paramesonephric ducts with urogenital sinus
7. Failure of transverse septum loss between paramesonephric system and urogenital sinus.

See Figure 9.1.

Assessment

The following features are associated with congenital abnormalities of the uterus:

1. Primary amenorrhoea (cryptomenorrhoea)
2. Recurrent first trimester miscarriages
3. Recurrent second trimester miscarriages
4. Preterm labour
5. Abnormal fetal presentations in late pregnancy

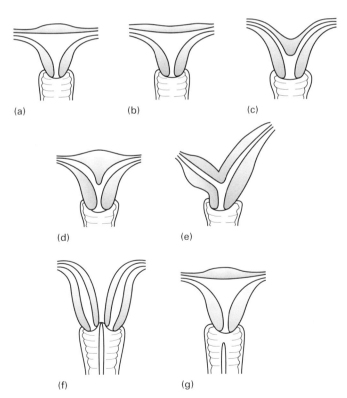

Fig. 9.1 Congenital abnormalities of the uterus and vagina. a, Normal uterus and vagina; b, arcuate uterus; c, bicornuate uterus; d, subseptate uterus; e, rudimentary horn; f, uterus didelphys; g, normal uterus with partial vaginal septum.

6. Intrauterine growth retardation (IUGR)
7. Incoordinate uterine action
8. Retained placenta.

As many of the above features can occur with other conditions, diagnosis is difficult. A high index of suspicion is needed and diagnostic procedures should be undertaken early. This is particularly important with vaginal atresia/imperforate hymen where severe endometriosis due to retrograde menstruation may occur before the diagnosis is made.

Investigations
1. Ultrasound.
2. Hysterography: dye is injected through the cervix and X-ray pictures are taken. The uterine cavity and tubal lumina can be seen.
3. Examination under anaesthesia
   a. Passing a dilator through the cervix: if a size 7 Hegar dilator can be passed through easily, then cervical incompetence may be present.
   b. Hysteroscopy: this is the best method of assessing the uterine cavity, and partial septums or double systems should be detected.
   c. During a manual removal of the placenta a uterine abnormality may be detected.
4. Laparoscopy ± dye insufflation.

Management
Each case must be dealt with individually and depends on:

1. Time of diagnosis
2. Previous obstetric history
3. Nature of the lesion
4. Mode of presentation.

In non-pregnant women
1. Cervical incompetence: this condition usually occurs after previous dilatation of the cervix; however, congenital cervical incompetence can occur. A cervical cerclage can be inserted prior to pregnancy, but most are performed at 14–16 weeks of pregnancy.
2. Hysteroscopic incision of the uterine septum: under direct visualization through a hysteroscope the uterine septum is divided, either surgically or by laser. The uterus remains arcuate.
3. Uteroplasty: the septum is surgically excised at laparotomy. Most operations reduce the size of the uterine cavity but the fundal dome is increased and these women must have caesarean sections in subsequent pregnancies.

During pregnancy
1. Cervical cerclage: this is ideally performed at 14–16 weeks. The suture is removed at 37 weeks. If the woman goes into spontaneous labour prior to this the suture must be removed.

2. Intrauterine growth restriction: placentation on the septum may result in IUGR and patients must be managed appropriately.

During labour

1. Incoordinate uterine action: if inefficient uterine action results because of congenital abnormality of the uterus this should be corrected with oxytocin.
2. Malpresentations or fetal distress: these are dealt with appropriately.
3. Vaginal septum: this can be excised if it prevents vaginal delivery.
4. Retained placenta: as the incidence of retained placenta is increased, active management of the third stage is required (see Ch. 26).

SUMMARY

As congenital abnormalities of the uterus are rare and difficult to diagnose, it is difficult to assess efficacy of the various forms of treatment. In cases of recurrent first trimester miscarriages, mid-trimester miscarriages, preterm labour and retained placentas, the index of suspicion should be high.

10

Hirsutism and virilism

Michael Chapman

Expectations of the examiners

Hirsutism is a common complaint which is not usually managed particularly well. The examiners will expect a limited understanding of the physiology of androgen metabolism. Candidates should have a knowledge of basic investigations, their interpretation and subsequent management. Specialist endocrinological referral will be part of the management in severe cases.

Definition

Hirsutism can be defined as excessive hair growth outside the normal female distribution. Difficulties have arisen in differentiating 'normal' from 'abnormal'.

Virilism is defined as masculinization of the female involving one or more of the following features: clitoral hypertrophy, muscle hypertrophy, breast atrophy, hirsutism, deepening of the voice.

Interesting facts

Hirsutism is common. Depending on the stringency of the definition, more than 10% of females could be deemed to be hirsute. Only a small proportion complain.

Management of the psychological effects of hirsutism is the most important aspect of this problem. In almost all cases the underlying hormonal imbalance is benign.

Virilism is extremely rare (< 1% of patients referred with hirsutism).

Pathophysiology

The physiology of the androgens is complex. There are many androgens with differing relative biological activities which are produced from a variety of sites. For example, dehydroepiandrosterone (DHEA) is produced predominantly by the adrenal gland and has a very weak biological activity when compared to testosterone. Dihydrotestosterone (DHT), which has greater biological activity, is produced by peripheral conversion of weaker androgens.

Binding of the androgens to sex hormone binding globulin (SHBG) and albumin reduces the availability of the free steroid which is required to activate the target cell.

In hirsutism, various disorders of androgen metabolism can occur. Production rates of the androgens can be increased from the ovary (e.g. in polycystic ovarian disease) or the adrenal gland (e.g. in the case of a tumour), or peripheral conversion can be enhanced (e.g. in obesity or increased precursor production). SHBG may be reduced in liver disease. Finally, there may be an increased sensitivity of target organs to normal levels of testosterone (e.g. hair follicles, clitoris).

Aetiology
1. Ovarian
    a. Polycystic ovarian disease
    b. Tumour, e.g. androblastoma, teratoma
2. Adrenal
    a. Androgen-secreting tumours
    b. Cushing's syndrome
    c. Congenital adrenal hyperplasia
3. Idiopathic
4. Rare causes
    a. Drugs
    b. Familial hypertrichosis
    c. Virilized intersexual disorders.

Assessment
Specific points in the history include:

Menstrual pattern
A regular menstrual cycle excludes a significant underlying hormonal disturbance. Oligo- or amenorrhoea should be investigated fully to look for polycystic ovarian disease and to exclude the rarer but potentially life-threatening hormone-secreting tumours.

Racial group and family history
Hair distribution varies substantially with racial group, e.g. Scandinavian women rarely have facial hair whereas in southern Mediterranean women it is common.

Drugs
Examples are danazol and testosterone implants.
    Examination should exclude endocrine disease and signs of virilism should be noted. The severity of the hirsutism should be assessed and specific enquiry should be made about previous local treatments.

Investigations
Plasma androgens
A normal or slightly elevated testosterone level suggests a benign cause for the hirsutism. High levels are strongly suggestive of an androgen-secreting

tumour. Raised serum DHEA and androstenedione levels indicate an adrenal origin of the excess androgens. Raised levels of 17-hydroxyprogesterone may indicate congenital adrenal hyperplasia.

SHBG
SHBG binds testosterone and reduces the free testosterone available to stimulate receptors in the hair follicles. A low level of SHBG is associated with a raised total testosterone level and a higher concentration of free testosterone.

Gonadotrophin levels
Raised LH levels and increased LH/FSH ratios are consistent with polycystic ovarian disease.

Transvaginal ultrasound will show polycystic ovaries in more than 80% of women with hirsutism.

Other
Further investigations of specific endocrine disorders should be performed as indicated.

Treatment
Serious conditions should be excluded.

Psychological
The benign nature of the condition should be explained and continuing support may be necessary.

Local treatment
This may be the most effective management and includes:

1. Bleaching agents
2. Plucking
3. Shaving
4. Depilatory creams
5. Waxes
6. Electrolysis: this is effective and permanent but it can be painful and occasionally leave scarring.

Drugs
1. Dexamethasone: adrenal (ovarian) suppression
2. Oral contraceptives: SHBG elevation
3. Cyproterone acetate: androgen receptor inhibition
4. Spironolactone: enzyme inhibition
5. GnRH analogues: pituitary downregulation leading to reduced ovarian production of steroids.

In general practice it is appropriate to use low-dose dexamethasone or oral contraceptives but further drug therapy should be prescribed after specialist referral.

It is important to emphasize that the pharmacological therapy of hirsutism is lengthy (12–24 months). Immediate improvement should not be expected.

SUMMARY

A detailed history and examination usually provide the diagnosis but basic investigations will confirm the presence of benign androgen excess. Reassurance can then be provided and advice about cosmetic treatment should be given. More severe cases should be managed by a gynaecologist or an endocrinologist.

11 Bleeding in early pregnancy

Gregory Davis

Expectations of the examiners

Bleeding in early pregnancy is common and candidates will be expected to distinguish between those women who can be managed at home and those requiring admission, depending on the clinical findings. In terms of clinical management, the important diagnostic decision is between threatened abortion and the remainder, but the terminology encourages examiners to ask about definitions.

Definitions

Abortion is defined as termination of pregnancy prior to 24 weeks' gestation, either spontaneous or induced.

Threatened miscarriage is defined as bleeding in early pregnancy without dilatation of the cervix or the passage of products of conception (POC).

Inevitable miscarriage is defined as bleeding in early pregnancy associated with cervical dilatation but without passage of POC. This is a term which was used prior to the introduction of ultrasound scanning in the routine management of bleeding in early pregnancy and is rarely used now.

Incomplete miscarriage is defined as bleeding in early pregnancy with cervical dilatation and the passage of POC.

Complete miscarriage is defined as bleeding in early pregnancy followed by the passage of all POC.

Missed miscarriage is defined as early pregnancy in which the fetus dies and the uterus fails to enlarge further. There may or may not be bleeding.

Septic abortion is defined as any abortion/miscarriage that becomes infected.

SPONTANEOUS ABORTION

Interesting facts

The commonly quoted incidence for miscarriage is 15% but incidence is probably much higher (40–60%) when very early pregnancies are included. These biochemical pregnancies present as slightly delayed periods which may be heavier than normal. Most spontaneous miscarriages occur prior to 12 weeks' gestation with a peak incidence at 7–8 weeks. The frequency of miscarriage increases with maternal age, smoking, polycystic ovarian syndrome and alcohol consumption.

Aetiology

1. *Fetal abnormalities*. These account for more than 50% of all spontaneous miscarriages and include chromosomal and developmental abnormalities. Chromosomal abnormalities (most commonly trisomy) are present in 80% of pregnancies in which a fetus is not present (otherwise known as a blighted ovum or an afetal sac).
2. *Uterine abnormalities*. Malformation of the uterus may interfere with normal development of the pregnancy. Abnormalities may be congenital or acquired, e.g. submucous fibroids or intrauterine adhesions from previous curettage (Asherman's syndrome).
3. *Systemic disease*. Most severe systemic diseases, e.g. connective tissue and renal disease, increase the rate of abortion. Any systemic infection or sustained pyrexia may cause abortion. Infections are not a common cause, but cytomegalovirus, toxoplasmosis and rubella are classically associated with an increased risk of abortion. Similarly, listeriosis and syphilis are uncommon causes of miscarriage in the second trimester.
4. *Drugs*. Cytotoxic drugs, particularly antimetabolites such as methotrexate, will cause abortion.
5. *Immunological*. There has been considerable debate on this subject and it is briefly reviewed in the section on recurrent miscarriage.
6. *Vascular*. An abnormal uterine arterial blood supply is associated with an increased risk of spontaneous miscarriage, possibly as a result of inadequate blood flow to the developing placenta.
7. *Psychological*. There is no convincing evidence that stress alone can cause miscarriage.

Assessment

History

1. Period of amenorrhoea.
2. Amount of bleeding.
3. Degree of pain.
4. Time of onset of pain in relation to bleeding (i.e. if pain precedes bleeding, ectopic pregnancy is more likely).
5. Passage of POC. Unless seen by an experienced clinician, this is very unreliable, as organized clot is difficult to distinguish from POC.

Examination

There are five clinical findings of relevance:

1. The cardiovascular status of the patient.
2. Abdominal findings. Although the uterus or lower abdomen may be tender, there should be no rebound tenderness and the pain is not usually unilateral. The exception is septic abortion where the whole of the lower

abdomen may be tender with guarding and rebound. The diagnosis is usually obvious as the woman is febrile and toxic.

3. State of the cervix—whether it is closed or starting to dilate.
4. Whether any POC are visible in the cervical os or vagina (remove at the time with sponge forceps and send for histology).
5. Uterine size should be equivalent to the expected size for the period of amenorrhoea.

Investigations

1. Ultrasound scan (USS). In the absence of confirmed POC or cervical dilatation, an USS is the definitive investigation in the management of abortion. If an intrauterine pregnancy is present, 45% will abort spontaneously. If a fetal heart is detected by ultrasound, 95–98% of these women will continue the pregnancy. A transabdominal ultrasound can reliably detect a live intrauterine pregnancy after 6 weeks' gestation and a transvaginal scan between 5 and 6 weeks.
2. Full blood count (FBC). This will assess blood loss and serve as a baseline.
3. Blood group and save. If bleeding is significant, blood may need to be cross-matched and transfused. Rhesus status must be known prior to discharge from hospital and anti-D given to Rhesus-negative women.
4. Septic abortions will require blood cultures and endocervical swabs. Further investigations will be required if the woman is septicaemic.

Treatment

Threatened miscarriage

There is no evidence that bed rest or progesterone supplementation affects the outcome of the pregnancy. Hospital admission is not necessary but may be appropriate in selected cases.

Incomplete, inevitable, missed miscarriage

May require admission to hospital and evacuation of the uterus (some early pregnancy assessment units are using more conservative management). Any products visible in the os at the initial examination should be removed with a pair of sponge-holding forceps. Failure to do so can allow the patient to go into 'cervical shock', i.e. cardiogenic shock thought to be related to vagal stimulation as a result of cervical dilatation. Ergometrine 0.5 mg i.m. may be useful in reducing blood loss and raising the blood pressure.

Septic abortion

The principles for the treatment of septic abortion are resuscitation, adequate antibiotic coverage and evacuation of the uterus when the patient's condition permits. Usually this means 12–24 hours of preoperative intravenous antibiotics, a broad-spectrum agent (such as a cephalosporin) and metronidazole, and gentamicin if the patient is septicaemic.

Evacuation of the uterus

This is usually performed with suction and completed with gentle curettage (preferably using a blunt curette) to ensure the uterus is empty. Particular care is necessary in septic abortion because of the increased risk of uterine perforation.

Complications

1. Immediate
   a. Haemorrhage
   b. Infection
   c. Uterine perforation
2. Delayed
   a. Infertility
   b. Asherman's syndrome—intrauterine adhesions occurring after curettage with complete or partial loss of the endometrium
   c. Cervical incompetence—whether this occurs after spontaneous abortion is debatable.

Follow-up

Anti-D immunoglobulin should be given to Rhesus-negative women. Suppression of lactation is not usually necessary before 20 weeks. Prior to discharge the causes and prognosis should be discussed with the woman (and partner if possible). After miscarriage in the first pregnancy the chance of miscarriage in the next pregnancy is about 15–20% and slightly higher, 25–30%, after the first two pregnancies miscarry. The emotional reaction to miscarriage is variable and some women require full bereavement counselling. The Miscarriage Association is a support group which many women find helpful (contact: Clayton Hospital, North Gate, Wakefield, West Yorkshire). Avoidance of pregnancy for at least 6 months may be recommended for psychological reasons, but each couple must be dealt with on an individual basis.

RECURRENT MISCARRIAGE/RECURRENT PREGNANCY LOSS

Definition

These are defined as loss of three or more pregnancies at less than 24 weeks' gestation with no more than one living child from the current partnership.

Interesting facts

The incidence of recurrent miscarriage (RM) is quoted as 2–5% of those couples who have conceived. The mean gestational age of miscarriages in women with RM tends to be greater than in sporadic miscarriage. If the couple have had a live child the incidence of RM is halved. The likelihood of a successful pregnancy following three consecutive miscarriages is about 75%.

Aetiology

The aetiology of RM can be different according to the gestation at which the pregnancy losses occurred. The majority occur in the first trimester.

First trimester loss

Polycystic ovarian syndrome. Fifty to sixty per cent of women with RM have been found to have polycystic ovaries on ultrasound scanning. An association with a raised LH concentration has been found, although the mechanism whereby this abnormality may cause RM is not understood. Suppression of LH prior to pregnancy does not improve pregnancy outcome.

Antiphospholipid syndrome (APS). Antiphospholipid antibodies (lupus anticoagulant and anticardiolipin IgG and IgM antibodies) are present in 15% of women with RM. These are detected by measuring anticardiolipin antibodies (ACA) and lupus anticoagulant (LA). Anticardiolipin antibodies are associated with the development of systemic lupus erythematosus (SLE), although the majority of women with RM who are anticardiolipin antibody-positive are asymptomatic. It is thought that these antibodies are a marker for poor implantation and may be associated with a poor obstetric history, e.g. placental abruption, intrauterine growth restriction as well as miscarriages in both the first and second trimesters. Other autoimmune diseases such as rheumatoid arthritis do not seem to be associated with an increased risk of RM.

Chromosomal. The majority of the embryos of women with RM are chromosomally normal. Approximately 5% of partners with RM are found to have a structural chromosomal abnormality, most commonly a balanced translocation.

Endocrine. Uncontrolled diabetes mellitus and hypothyroidism are associated with an increased risk of miscarriage. There is no evidence that controlled diabetes increases the risk of miscarriage but thyroid disease has been found to be an association in 1–2% of women with RM.

Immunological. It had previously been thought that some women with RM were unable to mount an adequate immune response to prevent their fetus being rejected by the maternal immune system. They were then 'immunized' with their partners' leukocytes in order to develop an immune response. While the initial study showed a significant improvement in outcome, subsequent studies did not confirm these findings. The treatment has been abandoned in the majority of centres particularly as there is a risk of transfusion reaction and transmission of infection.

Thrombophilic disorders. Increased rates of RM have been reported in women with inherited thrombophilias—antithrombin III and proteins S and C deficiencies, and hyperhomocysteinaemia. These abnormalities are also associated with poor outcomes in later pregnancy (similar to APS above), with increased rates of placental abruption, growth restriction and intrauterine death.

Second trimester loss

Cervical incompetence. True cervical incompetence is uncommon. The classic history is of painless loss of one or more pregnancies after 16 weeks. It is not usually preceded by spontaneous rupture of the membranes or infection. It is usually associated with a past history of trauma to the cervix, particularly termination of pregnancy or cone biopsy. Incompetence is rare after a loop excision or laser ablation of the cervix. The diagnosis should be made on the basis of the history of previous pregnancy loss.

Uterine abnormalities. These affect 2–3% of women with RM. It is unclear whether these abnormalities truly cause fetal loss as they are found as commonly in women with a normal reproductive history.

Assessment

History of pregnancy loss
1. How many losses?
2. What gestation?
3. Was a beating fetal heart seen prior to the loss or was the sac empty?
4. Were the losses preceded by bleeding and/or pain?
5. Were they all with the same partner?
6. How many living children/other obstetric history?
7. Ease of conception
8. Menstrual cycle length.

Medical/surgical history
1. History of systemic disease
2. Previous surgery to cervix
3. Family history of miscarriage.

Examination
1. General for endocrine/SLE in particular
2. Pelvic examination (rarely positive).

Investigations
1. Days 5–8 of cycle: LH, FSH, testosterone, SHBG to exclude PCOS
2. Screen for diabetes or thyroid disease only if clinically indicated
3. Rubella (important to vaccinate prior to conception if non-immune)
4. Anticardiolipin antibodies, lupus anticoagulant, thrombophilia screen (APS, SLE)
5. Chromosomes of both partners
6. Ultrasound scan (PCOS, uterine abnormality)
7. Haemoglobinopathy screen of both partners if from West Africa or of Mediterranean/Asian origin (α-thalassaemia, sickle cell disease).

Treatment
All groups require psychological support and regular ultrasound scans in early pregnancy to confirm that all is going well or to detect fetal demise at the ear-

liest possible opportunity. This has been shown to be as effective as any other treatment offered. Recent meta-analysis shows that progesterone supplementation does not improve the outcome of this condition.

PCOS
Weight loss in overweight women with PCOS has been shown to reduce fetal wastage significantly. However, ovulation induction has not been shown to improve the outcome.

APS
The use of aspirin 75 mg/day and heparin 5000 IU b.d. during pregnancy is associated with significantly better pregnancy outcomes than aspirin alone, which is significantly better than placebo. Appropriate specialist units should administer this treatment. Many women with inherited thrombophilias are being treated similarly although there is little evidence to support this as yet.

Chromosomal
These couples should be referred to a geneticist for counselling.

Immunological
As there is no evidence that immunization with paternal cells improves pregnancy outcome and there are risks associated with the practice, it should be actively discouraged.

Cervical incompetence
Cervical cerclage is indicated where cervical incompetence is suspected. The Shirodkar suture that involved reflection of the bladder off the cervix and placement of a suture around the cervical–isthmic junction has been replaced by the McDonald suture. This is a simpler technique where a four-bite suture encircling the cervix as high as possible is inserted. The suture is removed at 37 weeks. In women who miscarry despite this technique, a transabdominal approach has been used to place a suture around the cervix at the level of the internal os with good results. In this case the baby is delivered by caesarean section leaving the stitch in place.

THERAPEUTIC ABORTION

Definition
Therapeutic abortion is medical termination of pregnancy prior to 24 weeks' gestation.

Features
Since the 1967 Abortion Act, termination of pregnancy is possible in England and Wales providing it is carried out (in a licensed place) by a registered medical

practitioner and two registered medical practitioners have signed the appropriate consent form (Certificate A). The grounds for abortion under the Act are:

A. The continuance of the pregnancy would involve risk to the life of the pregnant woman greater than if the pregnancy were terminated.
B. The termination is necessary to prevent grave permanent injury to the physical or mental health of the pregnant woman.
C. The pregnancy has NOT exceeded its 24th week and the continuance of the pregnancy would involve risk, greater than if the pregnancy were terminated, of injury to the physical or mental health of the pregnant woman.
D. The pregnancy has NOT exceeded its 24th week and the continuance of the pregnancy would involve risk, greater than if the pregnancy were terminated, of injury to the physical or mental health of any existing child(ren) of the family of the pregnant woman.
E. There is substantial risk that if the child were born it would suffer from such physical or mental abnormalities as to be seriously handicapped.

The vast majority of therapeutic abortions are carried out on the basis of the second reason—risk to the physical or mental health of the pregnant woman. In 1997–1999, abortions constituted 20% of total births and abortions, i.e. about 1 in 5 pregnancies was terminated.

The rate of legal terminations in 1997–1999 was approximately 15.4/1000 women aged 15–44. Most NHS hospitals provide a termination service and there are a number of private clinics and private gynaecologists who also provide this service.

Assessment

Assuming that the practitioner follows the woman's (and partner's, if present) wishes, three pieces of information are required:

1. Is she pregnant and, if so, what is the gestation?
2. Does the woman definitely want an abortion?
3. Is she fit for an anaesthetic?

Abortion services should provide counselling so that each woman can be adequately assessed and have the opportunity to discuss the decision in a supportive environment. As most women are referred by their general practitioner, they should have discussed it with him/her and the referring doctor should sign the medical consent form which the woman can bring with her.

History
1. Pregnancy
   a. Period of amenorrhoea
   b. Menstrual cycle
   c. Previous contraception
   d. Symptoms of pregnancy
2. Past medical and obstetric history.

Examination
1. Physical examination
2. Uterine size.

Investigations
1. Ultrasound scan if < 8 or > 14 weeks' gestation to confirm gestation
2. FBC
3. Blood group and antibody screen.

Methods
Most terminations of pregnancy in England and Wales are carried out under general anaesthesia but in other countries local anaesthesia is used up to 12 weeks' gestation. The latter has the advantage of avoiding the risks of general anaesthesia and reducing blood loss, but requires greater support by staff.

Prior to 12 weeks
Suction aspiration. This is used routinely up to 12 weeks' gestation. The cervix is dilated and a semirigid plastic suction catheter is inserted into the uterus. Most operators check that evacuation is complete with sponge forceps and *gentle* curettage.
RU486. The progesterone antagonist, RU486, in association with a prostaglandin pessary, is 99% effective in termination of pregnancy prior to 8 weeks' gestation without recourse to operation. Provided that anti-abortion opinion allows its general introduction, it represents the biggest single advance in the field since the 1967 Act.

After 12 weeks
Dilatation and evacuation. After 12 weeks' gestation, instrumental destruction of the pregnancy and removal of the pieces is employed, often in conjunction with suction aspiration to reduce the uterine volume. A bolus of 5–10 IU of oxytocin is often given intravenously during or after the procedure. This method is commonly used up to 16 weeks' gestation and by a few operators up to 20–22 weeks.
Prostaglandins (PGs). These are used for second trimester terminations, usually after 16 weeks. They may be administered as repeated, frequent vaginal pessaries, infused extra-amniotically into the uterine cavity, or given as an intra-amniotic bolus injection. PG by any route, but particularly if inadvertently given intravenously, may cause systemic side-effects of nausea, vomiting, sweating, bronchospasm or diarrhoea. Usually these symptoms are not prominent but resuscitation equipment and adrenaline (epinephrine) must be readily available.

PGs are used for most late terminations but the terminations may be prolonged (12–48 hours) and require considerable analgesia. Often an oxytocin infusion is added to accelerate the onset of labour (despite the relative insensitivity of the uterus to oxytocin until the third trimester).

Mifepristone and gemeprost are becoming popular (mifepristone 600 mg orally and then 1 mg gemeprost 36–48 hours later).

Hysterotomy.   This is very rarely used in modern practice. The major reason for avoiding its use is the risk of rupture of the uterine scar in subsequent pregnancy.

Complications

The risk of complications is directly related to the experience of the operator and the gestation of the pregnancy. Complications include:

1. Immediate
   a. General anaesthesia.
   b. Uterine perforation—usually this is minor and the woman can simply be observed overnight in hospital, but evidence of continuing bleeding necessitates laparoscopy or laparotomy and closure of the uterine defect.
   c. Incomplete evacuation leading to haemorrhage or infection.
2. Delayed
   a. Infertility due to postoperative infection.
   b. Asherman's syndrome (see above).
   c. Cervical incompetence (see above).
   d. Psychological—the response is very variable but can be prolonged and significant. Future subfertility is often attributed (both correctly and incorrectly) to previous termination of pregnancy.

Follow-up

In practice, very few centres follow up their patients despite the frequency of emotional difficulties that most women experience after termination of pregnancy. In those that attempt to, attendance by the women postoperatively is sporadic.

EXTRAUTERINE PREGNANCY

Definition

Extrauterine pregnancy is defined as implantation of a pregnancy outside the uterine cavity, the majority in the fallopian tube (95%).

Interesting facts

In the 1997–1999 Maternal Mortality report for the United Kingdom, ectopic pregnancy was the third commonest cause of maternal mortality (12 cases). The initial diagnosis is incorrect in 25–50% of cases. Its incidence (1 in 100 pregnancies) has doubled in the past 20 years and varies in different groups, e.g. 1 in 30 pregnancies in the West Indies and in 5% of pregnancies resulting from assisted conception.

The diagnosis is usually made late and delay between admission and operation is common. The classic symptoms of ectopic pregnancy are abdominal pain, amenorrhoea and irregular vaginal bleeding. The diagnostic problem is that these symptoms are also associated with spontaneous miscarriage and pelvic inflammatory disease, the two commonest alternative diagnoses. Shock is present in 15–25% of cases. It is unclear how many would or do resolve spontaneously.

Predisposing factors

Pelvic inflammatory disease (PID). Histological evidence for previous pelvic infection can be found in 30–50% of ectopic gestations. Evidence suggests that previous infection increases the risk of ectopic pregnancy about 10 times. It is widely believed that the recent increase in ectopic pregnancy is related to the increasing prevalence of PID and assisted conception techniques.

Tubal surgery. Any form of surgery to the tubes including sterilization increases the ratio of ectopic to intrauterine pregnancy.

Previous tubal pregnancy. The risk of a subsequent pregnancy implanting ectopically is increased 20-fold even if salpingectomy has been performed. This is presumably because the predisposing pathology (i.e. tubal damage) is bilateral.

Infertility. Pregnancy in subfertile women, whether spontaneous or after assisted conception techniques (e.g. IVF), is more likely to implant ectopically. In many cases this is due to pre-existing tubal disease.

Intrauterine devices. The overall incidence of ectopic pregnancy in IUD users is lower than normal. However, if pregnancy occurs, the ratio of ectopic to intrauterine pregnancies is 1:20.

Progestins. The low-dose progestogen-only pills have a similar effect to IUDs in that they increase the ectopic to intrauterine pregnancy ratio while not affecting, or slightly reducing, the overall incidence of ectopic pregnancy.

Assessment

The most important aid to diagnosis is a high level of suspicion—all women in the reproductive age group who present with one or any combination of the symptoms, i.e. abdominal pain, vaginal bleeding and amenorrhoea, should be assumed to have an ectopic pregnancy until proven otherwise.

History

1. Pain
   a. *Usually* unilateral but may be bilateral
   b. Usually starts prior to the bleeding
   c. May radiate to the shoulder tip
2. Bleeding
   a. Classically dark red and described as 'prune juice'
   b. Usually not as heavy as in spontaneous miscarriage
   c. May pass a decidual cast, mimicking POC
3. Amenorrhoea: *absent* in 25% of cases.

Examination
1. Cardiovascular status—may be shocked
2. Abdomen—unilateral tenderness usually with rebound but may present with a rigid abdomen if significant blood loss
3. Uterus enlarged, cervical excitation is usually present and a mass may be palpable, although in half of these cases the ectopic pregnancy will be on the opposite side.

Investigations
In the collapsed, shocked patient, no investigations are required prior to surgery. In less obvious cases the following investigations are necessary.

Pregnancy test
Sensitive tests for HCG will be positive in almost all ectopic pregnancies.

Ultrasound scan
If an intrauterine pregnancy is detected, the diagnosis of ectopic pregnancy can virtually be excluded. The coexistence of intrauterine and ectopic pregnancies is rare (1 in 30 000) except in assisted conception (1 in 5000). The problem arises in pregnancies at 4–6 weeks' gestation where the sac is not visible. Transvaginal ultrasound scanning allows earlier detection of an intrauterine pregnancy and should be preferred to transabdominal pelvic ultrasound.

Laparoscopy
All women who present with pain and bleeding, a raised HCG and no intrauterine pregnancy on ultrasound should have an urgent laparoscopy. Where the diagnosis is uncertain (HCG < 1500, no intrauterine pregnancy), the woman should be kept in hospital and the serum HCG repeated after 48 hours. In a viable intrauterine pregnancy the HCG doubles in 48 hours and therefore a slowly rising or static HCG is indicative of an ectopic or non-viable pregnancy. In these circumstances laparoscopy and uterine curettage are usually indicated. Undiagnosed unilateral pain (without a positive pregnancy test or raised serum HCG) which does not resolve within 24–48 hours should also be investigated by laparoscopy to exclude ectopic pregnancy and other causes of pelvic pain.

Other investigations
1. FBC
2. Crossmatch.

Treatment
Resuscitation
An i.v. line and resuscitation should be initiated, en route to theatre in severe cases.

Surgery

The operation of choice is controversial. Progressively more of the surgery for ectopic pregnancies is performed laparoscopically, although the serum HCG should be followed postoperatively to ensure that it falls appropriately, as the persistence of trophoblast is more common than after laparotomy. When the woman is shocked laparotomy is usually preferred. There is debate over whether the tube should be conserved or removed. The intrauterine pregnancy (IUP) rate is similar after salpingectomy (excising the tube) or salpingotomy (opening the tube). However, persistent trophoblast is more common after salpingotomy, and the current RCOG recommendations are to perform a salpingectomy if the other tube is normal. If the other tube is abnormal then the RCOG recommend salpingotomy. Persistent trophoblast is usually treated with methotrexate. There is no evidence that removal of the ovary on the same side affects the prognosis for future fertility in any way.

Surgery for extratubal pregnancies (e.g. ovarian or intra-abdominal pregnancies) should achieve a balance between removing the pregnancy and damaging the site of implantation. Haemostasis is often a major problem.

Medical

In women wishing to avoid surgery who are asymptomatic with a presumptive diagnosis of ectopic pregnancy (rising HCG, empty uterus on ultrasound ± pelvic mass) methotrexate has been used successfully. Favourable prognostic signs are absence of symptoms, HCG < 10 000 IU, tubal mass < 2 cm, no fetal heart seen, and no or little free fluid in the abdomen. In these circumstances medical therapy can be expected to be effective in about 80% of cases. Apart from failure to treat the ectopic pregnancy adequately, the other disadvantages of medical therapy are the necessity for prolonged follow-up and, often, prolonged bleeding.

Expectant

Not all ectopic pregnancies require treatment. Studies that have looked at expectant management of ectopic pregnancy have shown that about 70% will resolve spontaneously. However, the women in these studies were selected for low-risk status: low levels of HCG which then declined, tubal mass < 2 cm, absence of symptoms. Expectant management can therefore be offered in this clinical situation provided that the woman understands the risks involved and is prepared to return promptly should symptoms develop.

Anti-D

It is recommended that all Rhesus-negative women be given anti-D after treatment of ectopic pregnancy.

Prognosis

1. Immediate postoperative complications are uncommon. Persistent trophoblast occurs more commonly after laparoscopic salpingotomy (5–10%) than salpingectomy (< 1%). Therefore after the former procedure, medical

therapy or expectant management, the HCG should be followed weekly until it is undetectable. Tubal rupture may occur despite falling levels of HCG and women should be warned to return if pain increases. Routine postoperative management and follow-up should be undertaken.

2. Future pregnancy: the IUP rate after surgery is about 50% and the repeat ectopic rate is 10–15%. The figures are similar after methotrexate although on much smaller numbers as yet.

3. Undiagnosed ectopic pregnancy may result in tubal abortion into the peritoneal cavity with subsequent reabsorption of the products or, rarely, abdominal implantation. Chronic bleeding from an ectopic pregnancy can lead to a pelvic haematocoele—a pelvic haematoma surrounded by inflammatory change and adhesions.

HYDATIDIFORM MOLE

Definition
Hydatidiform mole is a benign tumour of trophoblast.

Features
The incidence in the UK is lower (1 in 2000 pregnancies) than in South East Asia (1 in 200 pregnancies). The aetiology is unknown and there are two types which are genetically and clinically dissimilar: complete (classic), in which no fetus is present; and partial, where a fetus (or fetal material) is present. Complete moles are rare. The cells contain 46 chromosomes of *paternal* origin and they may lead to choriocarcinoma. Partial moles are more common; they have 69 chromosomes (triploid), of which the additional haploid set are again paternal in origin and probably do not give rise to choriocarcinoma. A mole may become 'invasive' and penetrate the uterus and/or metastasize, particularly to the lungs. Hydatidiform mole is distinct from choriocarcinoma, which is a malignant tumour of trophoblast.

Pathology
Complete mole
There is a triad of microscopic features:

1. Hyperplasia of both syncytiotrophoblast and cytotrophoblast
2. Villous oedema forming multiple small collections of fluid 'cisterns'
3. Absence of fetus.

Partial mole
The placenta shows *focal* hyperplasia which is usually confined to the syncytiotrophoblast, and focal villous swelling with cistern formation. The fetus usually dies early and the only remnants may be the presence of erythrocytes in placental vessels. The diagnosis may be difficult as villi are often swollen in aborted tissue so the diagnosis rests with the pathologist. Where a fetus is

present, multiple congenital abnormalities are evident, consistent with the triploid state.

Assessment

Moles usually present with irregular vaginal bleeding in pregnancy. The massive production of HCG may lead to exaggerated symptoms of pregnancy.

History
1. Amenorrhoea
2. Bleeding
3. Hyperemesis (25–30%)
4. Passage of grape-like vesicles
5. Rarely, metastatic spread: haemoptysis, pleuritic pain.

Examination
1. Pre-eclampsia may develop early (15–20%).
2. Uterus is usually larger than dates (55%), but may be smaller (15–20%).
3. Fetal heart is usually absent.
4. Theca lutein cysts in the ovaries may be palpable (10–20%).

Investigations
1. Ultrasound: scanning reveals a typical 'snow storm' appearance in the uterus. A fetus is not usually identified.
2. HCG is usually significantly elevated.
3. Chest X-ray to exclude pulmonary metastasis.

Treatment

Suction evacuation
Complete molar pregnancies are usually evacuated easily because of the lack of fetal parts unless the uterus is very large. The risk of perforation is increased. Curettage may need to be repeated if bleeding persists or HCG levels are still elevated 6 weeks after initial evacuation and ultrasound scanning suggests abnormal intrauterine contents.

Medical termination
Medical termination should be avoided in complete molar pregnancies because of the theoretical risk of embolization. In partial moles medical termination may be used as the risk of persistent trophoblastic disease requiring chemotherapy after partial molar pregnancy is small (0.5%).

Follow-up

All patients with molar pregnancy should be registered at a screening centre for trophoblastic disease. Meticulous follow-up of all women with molar pregnancies is essential. Estimations of HCG should be performed as indicated by the screening centre but usually continue for 6–24 months depending on the risk profile of the individual woman. Any rise or plateau in the HCG levels requires chemotherapy as outlined below under choriocarcinoma. These cases (10% of the total) usually become evident between 3 and 6 weeks after evacuation.

Prognosis

The mortality from trophoblastic disease is 6–8 women per year in the UK. The incidence of a subsequent molar pregnancy is 1 in 74. Pregnancy should be avoided until HCG levels have been normal for 6 months and oral contraception is not recommended until HCG levels return to normal. In subsequent pregnancies, women are asked to attend early for exclusion of molar pregnancy by ultrasound and an HCG should be performed 3 weeks after delivery.

CHORIOCARCINOMA

Definition

Choriocarcinoma is defined as a malignant tumour of trophoblast.

Interesting facts

Choriocarcinoma may follow normal or molar pregnancy but is a thousand-fold more common after molar pregnancy, i.e. a woman presenting with choriocarcinoma has an equal chance of the preceding pregnancy being normal or molar. One in 30 moles becomes choriocarcinoma and it is vastly more common in South East Asia.

Local extension is frequent and metastatic spread is usually vascular to the lungs (70%) or brain.

Treatment

1. Methotrexate and folinic acid plus evacuation of the uterus or hysterectomy.
2. Resistant or high-risk cases require combination chemotherapy.
3. Invasive mole and choriocarcinoma are treated similarly, the treatment depending more on risk factors such as age and degree of spread than histology.
4. Follow-up of HCG levels is required similar to that in molar pregnancy.

Prognosis

Remission can be expected in all women except the few with metastases other than pulmonary. Pregnancy after choriocarcinoma is possible after 2 years free of disease and is managed in a similar way to pregnancy following other trophoblastic disease.

12   Benign conditions of the female genital tract

Adam Rodin

Expectations of the examiner

The candidate is expected to be familiar with benign lesions of the female genital tract as they are very common. An understanding of management and when to refer is essential.

Interesting facts

Benign lesions of the female genital tract are common and may be congenital or acquired. Occasionally, they are manifestations of systemic disease.

THE VULVA

Abnormal appearance of the external genitalia at birth may represent an intersex state; further discussion of intersex is beyond the scope of this book. Clitoromegaly may occur in certain virilizing conditions.

PRURITUS VULVAE

Vulval irritation can occur at any age and may be an extremely distressing symptom. It is most commonly caused by *Candida albicans* infection (see Table 12.1).

Management of this complaint is aimed at identifying the cause and then treating appropriately. A history is taken and a physical examination is performed to look for generalized causes of pruritus. The vulva is inspected, a gentle speculum examination is performed and microbiological swabs are taken prior to digital examination. Glycosuria should be excluded and blood tests should be performed as clinically indicated. Skin biopsies should be taken if epithelial changes are suspected.

Table 12.1 Causes of pruritus vulvae.

Local causes	General causes
Infection	Skin diseases, e.g. eczema, psoriasis
Candida albicans	Medical conditions, e.g. diabetes mellitus,
Herpes genitalis	hypothyroidism, liver disease, chronic
Genital warts	renal failure, Crohn's disease,
Other sexually transmitted diseases	polycythaemia
Threadworms, pubic lice, scabies	Drug reactions
Atrophic vulvitis	Psychogenic
Vulval dermatoses	
Tumours	

VULVAL DERMATOSES AND INTRAEPITHELIAL NEOPLASIA

Benign lesions can coexist with squamous intraepithelial neoplasia in the vulval skin. These include lesions which were previously termed vulval dystrophies. A new classification of these conditions is now in use and the term 'dystrophy' should not be used.

Classification of vulval dermatoses and intraepithelial neoplasia
1. Squamous hyperplasia (previously hyperplastic dystrophy without atypia)
2. Vulval intraepithelial neoplasia (previously hyperplastic dystrophy with atypia)
3. Lichen sclerosus
4. Lichen sclerosus with squamous cell hyperplasia (previously mixed dystrophy)
5. Other dermatoses.

Assessment
Pruritus vulvae is the commonest symptom and on examination the vulva appears atrophic and white plaques (leukoplakia) may be present. Fusion of the labia may occur with stenosis of the introitus. The changes do not extend into the vagina. The diagnosis is confirmed by histological examination of skin biopsies. Colposcopic examination of the vulva may be required.

In lichen sclerosus there is thinning of the epidermis and hyperkeratosis and chronic inflammation in the dermis. Squamous hyperplasia is characterized by thickening and hyperplasia of the epidermis.

Treatment
This depends on the histological diagnosis. For treatment of vulval intraepithelial neoplasia, see Chapter 13. In lichen sclerosus treatment is with corticosteroid cream. Topical oestrogen and testosterone preparations have also

been used. There is a low risk of malignancy in lichen sclerosus but because of this, follow-up is advised. In cases of intractable pruritus vulvae, simple vulvectomy may be required.

VULVAL LUMPS AND SWELLINGS

Lumps and swellings of the vulva are common and in the majority of cases are benign. Any skin condition may affect the vulva (see Table 12.2).

Bartholin's gland swellings

The Bartholin's glands are paired structures which lie deep to the posterior ends of the labia minora posteriorly. The duct on each side opens between the labium minus and the hymen and is about 0.5 cm long. Normally the gland cannot be palpated. Obstruction of the duct results in accumulation of secretions and cyst formation. Women present with a painless vulval swelling. A Bartholin's abscess is painful and women present with a tender, red and sometimes fluctuant lump.

Treatment of both cysts and abscesses is by marsupialization. This involves making an elliptical incision into the roof of the cyst, draining the cavity and suturing the cyst wall to the skin to allow continuing drainage. Excision of the Bartholin's gland is rarely performed.

Urethral caruncle

This term is applied to any reddened area involving the posterior margin of the urethral orifice and is thought to be due to prolapse of the posterior urethral wall. Caruncles are often symptomless and are usually found in postmenopausal women. They occasionally cause bleeding and dyspareunia.

Treatment with topical oestrogen cream is usually effective but sometimes surgical excision is necessary.

Causes of vulval ulceration

See Chapter 39.

Table 12.2 Causes of swellings of the vulva.

General causes	Specific causes
Sebaceous cyst	Bartholin's gland: cyst/abscess
Haematoma	Urethral caruncle
Varicose veins	Endometriosis
Benign tumours, e.g. lipoma, papilloma,	Carcinoma of the vulva
fibroma, hidradenoma	Inguinal hernia
Malignant tumour: primary/secondary	Hydrocele of canal of Nuck

THE VAGINA

VAGINAL SEPTUM

See Chapter 9.

VAGINITIS

See Chapter 39.

VAGINAL CYSTS

These are usually remnants of the lower portion of the mesonephric (Wolffian) duct and occur anterolaterally in the vagina. They are usually asymptomatic and require no treatment.

THE CERVIX

The vaginal portion of the cervix is covered by stratified squamous epithelium and the endocervical canal is lined by columnar epithelium. Before puberty, the squamocolumnar junction is in the endocervical canal. During adolescence, the ovarian hormones cause eversion of the lower part of the cervical canal so that columnar epithelium appears on the ectocervix. The columnar epithelium is exposed to the acid environment of the vagina and is replaced by stratified squamous epithelium (squamous metaplasia). If the process of squamous metaplasia results in the obstruction of cervical glands, retention cysts may form which are known as nabothian follicles.

CERVICAL ECTROPION

Eversion of the lower cervical canal occurs during adolescence, during pregnancy and while taking the combined oral contraceptive pill, and the characteristic appearance of the cervix in these circumstances is known as cervical ectropion. The florid appearance of the cervix in these situations gives rise to the term 'erosion'; however, this term is a misnomer and should be avoided.

Ectropion may also result from cervical tears sustained during childbirth. Cervical ectropion is usually asymptomatic, but occasionally causes excessive vaginal discharge or postcoital bleeding. A cervical smear should be taken. Treatment is rarely necessary but women with persistent symptoms can be treated with cryocautery as an outpatient procedure.

CERVICITIS

Chronic cervicitis is a non-specific condition which is difficult to define. It is a common clinical diagnosis which is rarely confirmed by bacteriology.

CERVICAL POLYPS

These develop from the endocervix and protrude from the external os into the vagina. They are covered by columnar epithelium which often undergoes squamous metaplasia. They are usually asymptomatic, but the dependent part of the polyp may ulcerate causing intermenstrual and postcoital bleeding. They may also cause an increase in vaginal discharge. Cervical polyps are rarely malignant.

Cervical polyps should be avulsed and sent for histological examination. Their base should be cauterized to prevent regrowth and an endometrial biopsy should be taken at the same time to exclude other causes of irregular vaginal bleeding.

THE BODY OF THE UTERUS

POLYPS

Various types of polyp form in the cavity of the uterus, including:

1. Endometrial polyps (adenomatous)
2. Fibroid polyps
3. Placental polyps.

Endometrial polyps are the most common; they may be multiple in premenopausal women but are usually single in postmenopausal women. Occasionally they extrude through the cervix causing dysmenorrhoea. They may be symptomless but usually present with abnormal vaginal bleeding. Menorrhagia and intermenstrual bleeding may occur and in the older woman there may be postmenopausal bleeding. If the polyp has passed through the cervix there may be postcoital bleeding. Ideally, endometrial polyps should be removed under direct vision using a hysteroscopic resectoscope. The polypoid tissue must be sent for histological examination to exclude malignancy.

UTERINE FIBROIDS

Fibroids or leiomyomata are the commonest tumours of the female genital tract and are present in at least 20% of women over the age of 30 years. Their aetiology is unknown but their growth is oestrogen-dependent and they regress after the menopause. Fibroids are associated with nulliparity in white women and are more prevalent in Afro-Caribbean women.

Fibroids are mainly derived from smooth muscle but also contain some fibrous tissue elements. They form well-defined tumours with a false capsule and may be found in various sites; intramural fibroids lie within the uterine wall, subserous fibroids project from the peritoneal surface of the uterus, and submucous fibroids encroach on the uterine cavity, sometimes distorting it and increasing its surface area. Subserous fibroids may become pedunculated and a submucous fibroid may become extruded to form a fibroid polyp. Only 2% of fibroids arise in the cervix.

Fibroids are usually multiple and vary in size from seedlings to large tumours. They may undergo various types of degenerative change:

Hyaline degeneration. This is the commonest change and it occurs as the fibroid outgrows its blood supply. Areas liquefy and cysts form.

Calcification. This occurs in postmenopausal women.

Infection. Subserous or pedunculated fibroids may become infected by spread from adjacent structures. Ascending infection may complicate submucous fibroids.

Red degeneration. This occurs during pregnancy when the blood supply is insufficient to support growth of the fibroid; the cut section of the fibroid appears red.

Malignant change (leiomyosarcoma) is rare (< 0.5% of fibroids) but may be suspected when there is rapid or painful enlargement of fibroids.

Assessment

The majority of fibroids are asymptomatic and are detected at routine pelvic examination. The commonest symptom is menorrhagia which is particularly associated with submucous fibroids. Some women present with abdominal distension and others complain of pressure symptoms such as increased frequency of micturition and stress incontinence. Pain is an unusual feature but occasionally fibroids present as an acute abdomen following torsion of a pedunculated fibroid or haemorrhage into a large fibroid. Fibroids do not cause infertility unless they are obstructing the cornua of the uterus.

Pelvic examination reveals an enlarged and often irregular uterus which may be palpable per abdomen. The main differential diagnosis is from ovarian tumours where the uterus should be detected separately from the pelvic mass. The presence of ascites is highly suggestive of ovarian pathology. In practice, it may be difficult to distinguish between the two clinically.

Investigations

Ultrasonography may be useful to distinguish between uterine and ovarian pathology. Abnormal vaginal bleeding should be investigated by hysteroscopy and endometrial biopsy. A cervical smear should be performed.

Blood tests may reveal an iron deficiency anaemia. Large fibroids are rarely associated with polycythaemia due to erythropoietin production.

Treatment

Conservative management

Conservative management is appropriate in the following situations:

1. Uterus smaller than 16 weeks' gestation
2. Asymptomatic
3. During pregnancy
4. Menopause approaching
5. Fertility required.

Medical treatment of fibroids using GnRH analogues has produced disappointing results. Fibroids regress during treatment but rapidly regrow when therapy is discontinued. Duration of treatment is limited by bone loss due to oestrogen deficiency.

Surgery

Surgery is indicated in the following situations:

1. Fibroids causing symptoms
2. Uterus > 16 weeks' size
3. Rapid growth in fibroids
4. Recurrent miscarriage/fibroid-related complications in previous pregnancy (see below)
5. Diagnosis uncertain.

Hysterectomy is the definitive procedure. Myomectomy can be technically difficult and regrowth of fibroids after this procedure is common. Myomectomy should be reserved for women who wish to retain fertility and for those who decline hysterectomy. Submucous fibroids can be resected hysteroscopically. Pedunculated and subserous fibroids may be removed laparoscopically.

Fibroid embolization

This is a non-surgical procedure performed by an interventional radiologist and involves embolization of the uterine arteries. The technique leads to significant shrinkage of the fibroid in most cases with good symptomatic improvement. The complication rate is low but severe sepsis may follow the procedure.

Fibroids in pregnancy

Fibroids may be detected for the first time in pregnancy. They may cause the uterus to feel large for dates. They do not usually influence the outcome of the pregnancy but they may be associated with some complications:

1. Recurrent miscarriage: submucous fibroids distort the uterine cavity and may be associated with repeated early pregnancy loss.
2. Pain: red degeneration may occur in large fibroids causing pain and localized uterine tenderness; torsion of a pedunculated fibroid may occur.

3. Malpresentations/abnormal lie.
4. Obstructed labour (rare).
5. Postpartum haemorrhage.

Surgical treatment of fibroids is not undertaken during pregnancy, except in the rare situation when a pedunculated fibroid undergoes torsion. Red degeneration is treated with rest and analgesia.

THE OVARIES

Functional cysts of the ovaries are common and they usually cause no symptoms. Follicular cysts are rarely >5 cm in diameter and are usually diagnosed by ultrasound in women with anovulatory cycles and those receiving fertility treatment. Corpus luteal cysts are associated with short periods of secondary amenorrhoea followed by heavier than usual bleeding. Multiple theca lutein cysts are characteristically associated with trophoblastic disease and hyperstimulation associated with fertility treatment. Functional cysts usually resolve spontaneously and should be followed up by ultrasonography. Persistent cysts should be removed laparoscopically and examined histologically.

ENDOMETRIOSIS

See Chapter 7.

OVARIAN NEOPLASMS

See Chapter 13.

13 Gynaecological oncology

Antony Hollingworth

Expectations of the examiners

Candidates are expected to understand the natural history of the common gynaecological malignancies, and to know their mode of presentation and the principles of their management. An appreciation of the role of screening will be important for the general practitioner.

Gynaecological malignancies are not common. All gynaecological malignancies occur at less than half the rate of breast cancer in England and Wales. The ratio of malignancies is 6:1 for breast and ovary; it is 9:1 for breast to endometrium. This means that an average GP will see 1 case of ovarian cancer every 5+ years and 1 case of endometrial cancer every 7–9 years.

Screening

The criteria for introducing a screening test were formulated by Wilson and Jungner and, of the 10 listed, at least seven need to be fulfilled before a test should be introduced. The criteria are as follows:

1. The condition sought should be an important health problem.
2. There should be an accepted treatment for patients with recognized disease.
3. Facilities for diagnosis and treatment should be available.
4. There should be a recognizable latent or early symptomatic stage.
5. There should be a suitable test or examination.
6. The test should be acceptable to the population.
7. The natural history of the condition, including development from latent to declared disease, should be adequately understood.
8. There should be an agreed policy on whom to treat as patients.
9. The cost of case-finding (including diagnosis and treatment of patients diagnosed) should be economically balanced in relation to possible expenditure on medical care as a whole.
10. Case-finding should be a continuing process and not a 'once and for all' project.

Screening for the different types of gynaecological malignancy will be discussed where appropriate.

THE VULVA

VULVAL INTRAEPITHELIAL NEOPLASIA

The incidence of vulval intraepithelial neoplasia (VIN), though difficult to assess, appears to be on the increase. It is a premalignant lesion although its malignant potential for transformation to vulval cancer is not as great as that of cervical intraepithelial neoplasia (CIN) to cervical cancer.

The average age of presentation is 38 years. In premenopausal women < 50 years, the disease may be multicentric and multifocal and coexist with CIN. The disease is usually a single focus in postmenopausal women (> 50 years). The most common site is the labia minora.

Predisposing features include:

1. Coincidental CIN
2. Previous genital tract infections, e.g. warts, herpes simplex, gonorrhoea, *Trichomonas vaginalis*
3. History of immunosuppression.

Women may present with the following symptoms:

1. Local discomfort
2. Superficial dyspareunia
3. Pruritus
4. Local red spot
5. White lesion
6. Asymptomatic (noted at time of colposcopy).

If there is a suspicious lesion then a biopsy must be taken.

Histological appearance

VIN1   Thickened epidermis and nuclear atypia confined to the lower third of the epithelium

VIN2   Marked nuclear atypia in the lower half of the epithelium

VIN3   Carcinoma in situ, marked nuclear atypia extending through the full thickness of the epithelium.

Treatment

Treatment depends on the site and size of the lesion(s), as well as the age and general condition of the patient. Follow-up is essential as recurrences do occur. Treatment methods include:

1. Local destruction
    a. Laser vaporization
    b. Cryotherapy
    c. 5-fluorouracil (5-FU) cream

2. Excision methods
   a. Wide local excision
   b. Simple vulvectomy
   c. Skinning vulvectomy with skin grafting.

CARCINOMA OF THE VULVA

Vulval carcinoma accounts for about 4% of all genital tract tumours.

Incidence
In 1998, 851 new cases of vulval carcinoma were reported in England and Wales (Office of Population Censuses and Surveys—OPCS). Deaths from this disease numbered 321 in 2000.

Age
Most tumours occur in the 65–70-year age group, though there is an increasing number of cases in younger women with multifocal premalignant changes in the lower genital tract.

Geography
There is no obvious geographical distribution.

Predisposing factors
A history of vulval irritation may be a predisposing factor. In younger women, there may be some relationship to human papillomavirus. VIN may progress to invasive disease. Any woman with a history of lichen sclerosus should be reviewed regularly as she is also at risk.

Staging
I Lesion confined to the vulva, maximum diameter 2 cm; no suspicious groin nodes
II Lesion confined to the vulva, diameter > 2 cm; no suspicious groin nodes
III Lesion extends beyond the vulva with no suspicious nodes or lesion confined to the vulva with suspicious nodes
IV Lesion of any size with obviously positive nodes *or* lesion involving rectum, bladder, urethra or bone or all cases with pelvic or distant spread.

Microscopic appearance
The majority of tumours are squamous in origin (85%). The rare types include melanomas, basal cell carcinomas, sarcomas, and adenocarcinomas of the Bartholin's gland. The spread is slow with local tissue infiltration, before metastasizing to the inguinal and femoral nodes. There may be spread to the

contralateral lymph nodes. Pelvic node spread is late and carries a poor prognosis.

Symptoms

The majority of women present with irritation or pruritus, a mass or an ulcer. Other symptoms may include vulval pain, bleeding or discharge. Most tumours are ulcerative, though some may be exophytic. Death is usually due to infection, general debility or haemorrhage. The majority of lesions occur on the labia (70%).

Prognosis

The 5-year survival rate is as follows:

Stage I	70%
Stage II	50%
Stage III	30%
Stage IV	10–15%.

Treatment

The preoperative investigations of patients with vulval carcinoma will reflect the age and general medical condition of the patient. All patients need an examination under anaesthesia (EUA), with a full thickness biopsy and fine needle aspiration of any suspicious nodes.

Surgical

In the case of small lesions (stage I), a wide local excision or simple vulvectomy may be the most appropriate treatment with regular follow-up. Otherwise, the treatment of choice is radical vulvectomy with bilateral groin node dissection.

Radiotherapy

This treatment is reserved for local recurrence or nodal disease as it is usually poorly tolerated by the patient.

Chemotherapy

In some centres, mitomycin C and 5-FU have been used in conjunction with radiotherapy to good effect in large tumours.

THE CERVIX

CERVICAL INTRAEPITHELIAL NEOPLASIA (CIN)

Cervical premalignant disease (CIN 1–3) and invasive disease are thought to be part of a continuum:

CIN1 → CIN2 → CIN3 → Microinvasion → Frank invasion

The further the disease progresses to the right along this continuum, the less likely it is to regress. The evidence for these statements is that the epidemiological features of CIN and invasive disease are similar and also that progression studies have demonstrated the progression of CIN1 to CIN3, and CIN3 to invasive carcinoma.

The transformation zone

The cervix is lined by two types of epithelium: stratified squamous and columnar epithelium. The latter is one cell thick and is translucent, which accounts for its red appearance (ectropion) on visualization with the naked eye. In the prepubertal stage, the squamocolumnar junction (SCJ) is within the endocervical canal. As a result of growth of the cervix at the time of puberty, there is eversion of the columnar epithelium. The columnar epithelium may be stimulated to undergo metaplastic change to squamous epithelium. This area is known as the transformation zone (TZ) which, described simply, is the area where one type of epithelium (columnar) has transformed to another type (squamous). This metaplastic epithelium is susceptible to external agents (see 'Predisposing factors' in 'Cancer of the cervix' below) and may become *dys*plastic (abnormal epithelium).

Pathology

CIN is divided into three grades. In each case the basement membrane is intact. Figure 13.1 shows the abnormal changes seen in CIN1–3. The three grades are:

CIN1   Nuclear atypia confined to the basal third of the epithelium
CIN2   Nuclear atypia present in the lower two-thirds of the epithelium
CIN3   Nuclear abnormalities occuring throughout the full thickness of the epithelium.

Screening

Screening for premalignant disease of the cervix is by cytology. Cells are collected from the squamocolumnar junction by means of an Ayre's spatula, and are spread onto a glass slide and fixed with alcohol. The slide undergoes an automated staining process. The slides are screened for *dys*karyotic (abnormal nuclei) cells. The nucleocytoplasmic ratio is altered in abnormal cells, ranging from mild to moderate to severe changes. In the latter, there is hardly any cytoplasm surrounding an enlarged nucleus.

The current screening guidelines are for women between the ages of 20 and 64 years. The frequency of screening is dependent on local protocols but women should be screened at least every 5 years and optimally every 3 years. Screening annually does not significantly increase the detection of disease. The NHS cervical screening programme (NHSCSP) prevents between 1100 and 3900 cases per year.

The current criteria for referral of a woman to a colposcopy clinic include moderate dyskaryosis, severe dyskaryosis, possible invasive disease, glandular

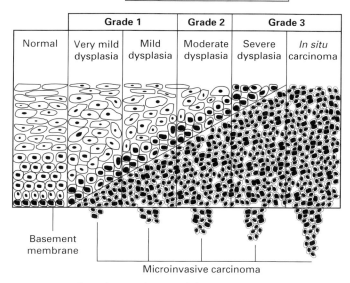

Cervical intraepithelial neoplasia

Fig. 13.1 Precursors to invasive carcinoma of the cervix. The diagram illustrates abnormal changes in the cervical epithelium in CIN1–3. Microinvasion is shown as crossing the basement membrane.

neoplasia, three consecutive inadequate smears or a suspicious-looking cervix. If the woman has had two borderline or mildly dyskaryotic smears 6 months apart then referral is also indicated.

ThinPrep

Forty-seven per cent of fully invasive cervical cancers in women below 70 years of age occurred despite an adequate screening history, which suggests that there may be problems with the sensitivity of the test. This may be due to sampling or reading errors or the fact that screening is poor at detecting glandular lesions.

A significant contributing factor to a false negative smear is that much of the cellular material on the collection device (spatula) does not make it onto the slide. ThinPrep is a way of reducing the number of inadequate smears and improves the detection of high-grade lesions. The cells are collected in the same way but are then rinsed in a vial of fixative. By a series of manoeuvres the cells are collected across a disposable filter membrane before being screened in the usual way.

Colposcopy

Colposcopy is an aid to diagnosis. The cervix is visualized through a colposcope and 5% acetic acid is used to bathe the cervix. In abnormal epithelium there is a relative excess of nuclear material (protein) and a relative lack of cytoplasm (glycogen). As a result, the epithelium appears white and may show a mosaic pattern or punctation. Aqueous iodine solution may also be used; this is taken up by normal glycogenated epithelium. In an abnormal epithelium, the area is iodine-negative. The affected area is biopsied and the histology of that sample gives the diagnosis.

Treatment

1. Local ablative techniques, which will treat the whole of the TZ
   a. Laser vaporization
   b. 'Cold' coagulation
   c. Diathermy
   d. Cryocautery, which should only be used in HPV or CIN1
2. Excision techniques
   a. Laser cone biopsy
   b. Large loop excision of the TZ
   c. Cold knife, i.e. surgical under general anaesthetic
   d. Hysterectomy depending on other possible indications.

The lesion must fulfil the following criteria before local ablative techniques can be undertaken:

1. The whole lesion must be visible.
2. There must be no suspicion of invasion.

Adequate follow-up is important with regular cytology, usually following NHSCSP guidelines. Ideally a cytobrush smear should be taken to ensure that cells from either side of the SCJ have been sampled.

HUMAN PAPILLOMAVIRUS (HPV)

This is a DNA virus and more than 80 different types have been identified. Types 6 and 11 cause genital warts and are of low malignant potential. HPV 16 and 18 are considered oncogenic. There are ongoing studies looking at the role of HPV testing within the cervical screening programme. The clearest role at present is in the management of women with borderline or mildly dyskaryotic smears which, if positive for high-risk types (HPV 16 and 18), would suggest referral for colposcopy instead of repeat cytology.

The potential exists for HPV testing as the sole method in older women; it may be useful for post-treatment surveillance. There is a potential for the woman to collect the sample herself. The other major advantage of this type of screening is that it may be automated. However, it is not known how long a negative result will afford protection against development of an abnormality.

CARCINOMA OF THE CERVIX

The majority of these tumours are squamous in type (90–95%); adenocarcinoma accounts for 4–8%, while the remainder are rarer tumours including sarcomas, lymphomas and melanomas.

Incidence
In 1998, 2594 new cases of cervical cancer were reported (OPCS), making cervix the third commonest genital tract tumour (after ovarian cancer) in England and Wales. In 2000 there were 1106 deaths from the disease.

Age
The median age for cervical cancer is 52 years. There has been an increase in the number of younger women (20–35 years) developing the disease and the prognosis is worse in this age group.

Geography
On a worldwide basis, cervical cancer is the second commonest malignancy in women after breast cancer. It is much more common in the developing than the developed world.

Predisposing factors
1. Sexual activity is a key event in the development of cervical cancer, especially an early age of first intercourse. Other factors are the number of sexual partners and a 'high-risk' male partner with many previous sexual contacts.
2. There is no definite association with the oral contraceptive pill, though sexual mores may be affected by its availability and use.
3. Smoking affects the local immunity of the cervix, making it more sensitive to oncogenic change.
4. HPV is the current contender for aetiological agent in cervical cancer. There are over 60 types of HPV, and HPV 16, 18 and 33 have been associated with CIN and cancer.

In the past, herpes simplex type II virus was thought to be linked with cervical cancer but this is no longer the case.

Staging
0   CIN
I   Carcinoma confined to the cervix:
    Ia1 Microinvasive disease with a depth of invasion < 3 mm and
       < 7 mm diameter of horizontal spread
    Ia2 Microinvasion with a depth of invasion of < 5 mm from the
       epithelial base and < 7 mm horizontal spread and no marked
       lymph space invasion
    Ib All other cases

II Carcinoma extends beyond the cervix but not to the pelvic side wall; it may involve the upper two-thirds of the vagina:
  IIa No obvious parametrial involvement
  IIb Obvious parametrial involvement
III Carcinoma extends to the pelvic side wall
IV Carcinoma extends beyond the true pelvis, or involves the bladder or rectum.

Microscopic appearance

The majority (90–95%) of tumours are squamous carcinomas with the cells being described as keratinizing, large cell non-keratinizing, or small cell non-keratinizing. Most of the remaining tumours are adenocarcinomas. The method of spread of cervical tumours is direct invasion and lymphatic permeation, which dictates the methods of treatment.

Symptoms

Invasive disease may be initially asymptomatic and, if not detected at the time of routine cytology, will present with intermenstrual, postcoital or postmenopausal bleeding, plus or minus offensive discharge. Pain is usually a sign of advanced disease.

Prognosis

The 5-year survival rate is as follows:

Stage I   Up to 90% when microinvasive disease is included
Stage II   55%
Stage III 30–35%
Stage IV   < 10%.

Treatment

All patients with cervical carcinoma need a preoperative full blood count and an intravenous urogram (IVU) or other assessment of the renal tract. An examination under anaesthetic is important for accurate staging to determine treatment modality, and a biopsy is necessary.

A CT scan may be performed for assessment of lymphatic spread; however, an MRI scan will give a much better anatomical view of the extent of the disease and allow appropriate planning for treatment.

Surgery

1. The treatment of microinvasive disease is controversial but most authorities would suggest that cone biopsy can be used if the depth of invasion is < 3 mm and there is no lymphatic involvement.
2. Radical hysterectomy with a cuff of vagina, the parametrium and pelvic node dissection plus or minus conservation of the ovaries is the treatment of choice for stages Ib and IIa.

3. Radical trachelectomy, which involves removal of the cervix up to the internal os plus parametrial tissue, is being used for younger women wanting to preserve their fertility.

Radiotherapy
This is used for stages Ib and IIa if the patient is not suitable for surgery. Stages IIb onwards, radiotherapy is the mainstay of treatment.

Chemotherapy
This may be used for palliation. HRT may be used in women who have had radiotherapy. Regular follow-up is essential, as most recurrences will occur within the first 2 years of treatment.

The future for treatment of this disease may be in the use of a combination of chemotherapy and radiotherapy.

CARCINOMA OF THE BODY OF THE UTERUS

The majority of tumours of the uterus are adenocarcinomas of the endometrium. Sarcomas account for up to 4% of all uterine tumours. Screening for endometrial carcinoma is not a practical proposition. However, any woman presenting with postmenopausal bleeding or discharge, or abnormal bleeding after the age of 40 years, needs investigation. This may include endometrial sampling, hysteroscopy, and dilatation and curettage.

Incidence
In 1998, 4086 new cases were reported in England and Wales (OPCS). In 1999 there were 671 deaths due to endometrial cancer. These figures placed uterine cancer second in frequency of genital tract tumours after ovarian cancer.

Age
Eighty per cent of cases occur in postmenopausal women, with a median age of 60 years. Less than 5% of cases occur before the age of 40 years.

Geography
In the USA and parts of Australia, endometrial cancer is the most common genital tract malignancy.

Predisposing factors
Endometrial carcinoma is oestrogen-dependent, so a history of unopposed oestrogen administration or, less commonly, oestrogen-secreting tumours of the ovary may be significant.

Obesity is a risk factor as androgens are converted to oestrogens in the peripheral fat, leading to an increase in the serum oestrogen concentration.

Other associations include nulliparity, late menopause, a history of diabetes or previous pelvic radiotherapy for cervical cancer.

Endometrial hyperplasia will develop in 20% of women who have been using unopposed oestrogens for 12 months. Hyperplasia can be divided into simple, complex and complex with atypia. The risks of developing endometrial cancer are 1% in simple hyperplasia and 3% in complex hyperplasia, but 22% in complex hyperplasia with atypia.

Staging

I   Carcinoma confined to the body of the uterus:
    Ia   Confined to the endometrium
    Ib   Confined to the uterine body with invasion of less than half the myometrium
    Ic   Confined to the uterine body with invasion of more than half the myometrium
II   Carcinoma involving the body of the uterus and the cervix but not extending beyond the uterus
III Carcinoma extending beyond the uterus but not beyond the true pelvis
IV   Carcinoma extending outside the true pelvis or involving the mucosa of the bladder or rectum.

Microscopic appearance

Most of the endometrial tumours are adenocarcinomas and are graded according to differentiation. Grade 1 is well differentiated, grade 2 moderately differentiated and grade 3 poorly differentiated.

These tumours spread locally to the cervix or via the fallopian tubes to the ovaries, or invade the myometrium. There is also lymphatic spread to the pelvic and para-aortic nodes.

Sarcomas can occur in the uterus but are very uncommon with an incidence of 2/100 000 women. They account for < 4% of all uterine tumours and are highly malignant with a poor response to radiotherapy and chemotherapy. The risk of a fibroid becoming malignant is < 0.1% but this should be considered if the fibroids are growing rapidly.

Symptoms

In postmenopausal women, carcinoma of the uterus usually presents early with vaginal bleeding or discharge. The disease in pre- or perimenopausal women usually presents with irregular vaginal bleeding.

Prognosis

The 5-year survival rate is as follows:

I   72%
II   56%
III 32%
IV   10%.

Treatment

The majority of tumours (90%) will present at stage I or II. Depth of invasion of the tumour is the most important predictive index of the disease, with the most likely place of recurrence being the vault.

Surgery

Total abdominal hysterectomy with bilateral salpingo-oophorectomy is undertaken once the diagnosis has been made. This is also the treatment for sarcomas.

Radiotherapy

1. Radiotherapy is used as an adjunct following surgery to prevent vault recurrence.
2. Radical radiotherapy is employed in women who are unsuitable for surgery.
3. Radiotherapy serves as palliation in advanced cases.

Chemotherapy

Progestogens have been used for recurrent disease or to reduce bleeding prior to surgery. Cytotoxic agents are used for disseminated or recurrent disease. Regular follow-up is essential.

CARCINOMA OF THE OVARY

Ovarian carcinoma is the commonest gynaecological tumour in England and Wales, and usually presents in more advanced stages because of its lack of specific symptoms. As a result the outlook in terms of survival remains poor.

Incidence

In 1998, 5529 new cases of ovarian cancer were reported. In 2000 there were 3909 deaths (OPCS).

Age

The incidence increases with the woman's advancing age.

Geography

It is more common in the developed than in the developing world.

Predisposing factors

1. Continuous ovulation may be important, i.e. nulliparity, early menarche and late menopause. The combined oral contraceptive pill (OCP) is thought to be protective. There is evidence that ovulation induction agents may also increase the risk of ovarian cancer.

2. Other possible risk factors include talc and the mumps virus.
3. In a small number of cases (10%), there is a family predisposition.

Staging

This is done at the time of laparotomy.

I Tumour confined to the ovaries:
  Ia Confined to one ovary, capsule intact and no ascites
  Ib Confined to both ovaries, capsule intact and no ascites
  Ic Confined to one or both ovaries with ascites or positive peritoneal washings
II Tumour involving one or both ovaries with pelvic extension:
  IIa Spread to the uterus and/or tubes
  IIb Spread to other pelvic tissues
  IIc IIa or IIb with ascites or positive peritoneal washings
III Tumour involving one or both ovaries with intraperitoneal spread outside the pelvis or tumour limited to the pelvis with extension to the small bowel or omentum
IV Tumour involving one or both ovaries with distant spread, i.e. extra-abdominal.

Microscopic appearance

Ovarian cancer spreads directly to involve the pelvic peritoneum, and is carried upwards to cover the peritoneal surfaces of the diaphragm, liver, bowel and omentum. Lymphatic and blood-borne spread occurs in the later stages of the disease. Differentiation of the tumours ranges from well differentiated through moderate to poorly differentiated. Some tumours are reported as borderline in that they have histological features of malignancy but no stromal invasion.

It is important to remember that ovarian tumours may be primary or secondary:

1. Primary types
   a. Epithelial tumours (85%), adenocarcinomas which include serous, mucinous, endometrioid and clear cell
   b. Germ cell tumours (2%)
   c. Sex cord tumours (6%)
   d. Miscellaneous including sarcomas and lymphomas
2. Secondary types account for about 6% of cases and the most common primary sites include breast, stomach, colon and lung.

Symptoms

The majority of patients (70%) present in the late stages of the disease. Most of the symptoms are vague and include abdominal discomfort, increasing girth, pressure symptoms, urinary frequency, weight loss and very occasionally menstrual problems. When a patient presents, in addition to carrying out an abdominal examination, it is important to palpate the supraclavicular region for lymph nodes, to examine the chest and breasts, and to perform both rectal and vaginal examinations.

Prognosis
The approximate 5-year survival rate is as follows:

I   70–75%
II   45%
III 20%
IV   5%.

Management
Routine preoperative bloods tests should be done. The serum CA125 level is a useful tumour marker in about 80% of cases and may be used to assess the response to treatment. Ultrasound or CT scan of the abdomen and pelvis may be useful but the final tissue diagnosis and staging will be by laparotomy.

Surgery
Staging laparotomy is used, involving peritoneal washings, total abdominal hysterectomy, bilateral salpingo-oophorectomy plus omentectomy, and as much debulking as possible. This may not be appropriate in stage Ia if fertility is a consideration.

Radiotherapy
This may be used for remaining disease, though it is ineffective if the bulk is large and its role in treatment is controversial. It may be useful for palliation to reduce symptoms from tumour bulk or metastasis.

Chemotherapy
Adjuvant combination chemotherapy has largely taken the place of radiotherapy. It is used in patients when the extent of the disease is greater than stage 1. The NICE guidelines recommend the combination of paclitaxel (Taxol) and a platinum agent. Cisplatin, etoposide and bleomycin are used for germ cell tumours.

Regular follow-up is important, as most recurrences will occur within the first 2 years of presentation. If the woman's disease has recurred more than 12 months after original treatment, then she is likely to respond to further chemotherapy.

Screening
The difficulty in screening for ovarian cancer arises from not knowing its natural history. Tests that have been used include pelvic examinations, serum CA125 levels and diagnostic ultrasound. The sensitivity of these tests is poor and they do not convey any prognostic value. These tests are useful if the patients are involved in trials or in the small percentage of women with a family history of ovarian cancer.

A. GYNAECOLOGY

14

The menopause and hormone replacement therapy

Adam Rodin and Janice Rymer

Expectations of the examiners

The candidate is expected to understand the basic physiology of the menopause. A knowledge of the long-term effects of ovarian failure and a detailed understanding of the management of women on hormone replacement therapy are needed.

THE MENOPAUSE

Definition

The menopause is defined as the cessation of menstruation and marks the end of a woman's reproductive potential. It is a retrospective diagnosis usually made after 12 months of amenorrhoea.

Interesting facts

The average age of the menopause in the UK is 51 years. The main determinant of age at menopause appears to be genetic but environmental factors may have an effect. For example, there is evidence that smokers have an earlier menopause. Interest in menopause-related problems has grown due to the increase in mean female life expectancy, which is now 82 years (in the UK).

The average woman spends 38% of her life after the menopause, and in the UK postmenopausal women number more than 9 000 000 and comprise 18% of the total population. The short- and long-term problems associated with the menopause cause significant morbidity and mortality and have important economic implications. Women who do not suffer the 'acute' symptoms of the menopause remain at risk of long-term complications.

Physiology

The menopause is the result of ovarian failure and is preceded by a transition phase known as the climacteric which is of variable duration. The climacteric is characterized by increasing resistance of the ovarian follicles to stimulation by the gonadotrophins. Total oestrogen output by the ovaries declines and therefore gonadotrophin levels increase. Anovulation becomes more frequent and as a result progesterone deficiency occurs; this may lead to prolonged or irregular vaginal bleeding. These changes commence 10–15 years before the menopause and some women complain of symptoms of oestrogen deficiency during the climacteric. The menopause may occur prematurely (< 40 years) and it may follow surgery (bilateral oophorectomy) or radiotherapy.

Prior to the menopause, the main oestrogen is 17β-oestradiol which is secreted by the ovaries. This is converted to oestrone which has one-tenth the potency of 17β-oestradiol, and then to oestriol. In the postmenopausal woman, ovarian 17β-oestradiol production ceases and oestrone becomes the primary oestrogen. The major source of oestrone after the menopause is the peripheral conversion in adipose tissue of androstenedione which is produced by the adrenal cortex (70%) and the ovary (30%). After the menopause, the ovary continues to secrete androgens, mainly testosterone and androstenedione. FSH and LH levels plateau 2–3 years after the menopause and begin to decline after 5–10 years.

The effects of oestrogen deficiency

Oestrogen deficiency is responsible for the characteristic features of the menopause syndrome. Most systems are affected but the manifestations vary between individuals. Vasomotor instability affects 75% of women and 25% are severely affected. Hot flushes and night sweats may continue for more than 5 years in 25% of women. Flushes can be socially disabling and may interfere with daily activities while night sweats result in interrupted sleep and progressive fatigue. The mechanism of menopausal vasomotor instability is uncertain but a hypothalamic mechanism has been suggested.

Atrophy occurs in all oestrogen-sensitive tissues, notably the urogenital tract, breasts and skin. In the vagina, there is flattening and thinning of the epithelium which may result in atrophic vaginitis. Women may complain of vaginal dryness, pruritus and dyspareunia. Atrophic vaginitis is a common cause of postmenopausal bleeding. Loss of glycogen from the epithelial cells leads to the disappearance of the lactic acid-forming Döderlein's bacilli and, as a consequence, the pH of the vagina changes and it becomes alkaline. Postmenopausal women are, as a result, more prone to vaginal infection. The bladder and urethra, which are lined by transitional epithelium, undergo similar changes to the vagina. The supporting structures of the genital tract lose tone and prolapse may become apparent. Breasts become atrophic with a reduction in adipose tissue and lobules.

The psychological effects of the menopause may be the direct result of oestrogen deficiency on the central nervous system. They may also be triggered by distressing physical symptoms or clustering of life events. Common symptoms including depression, anxiety and panic attacks. Poor concentration and loss of short-term memory are often troublesome.

The long-term consequences of the menopause are:

Osteoporosis.   Postmenopausal osteoporosis is a major health care problem. The important fracture sites are the vertebrae and the femoral neck. Twenty-five per cent of women over 60 will suffer vertebral crush fractures. The incidence of fractured neck of femur is increasing, although the reasons for this trend are unclear. Twenty per cent of women who suffer this type of fracture die from complications and many of those that survive never return to full mobility.

Following the menopause, bone mineral is lost from the skeleton at an accelerated rate for about 5 years and then becomes more gradual. Women who have an early menopause or who have had amenorrhoea (either weight- or exercise-related) during their potential reproductive years are at greater risk of osteoporosis in later life.

Other risk factors include being Caucasian, having a positive family history or having a history of prolonged steroid treatment.

Cardiovascular disease.   Premenopausal women have a lower risk of cardiovascular disease compared to men of the same age group. This effect is partly due to the influence of oestrogen on the lipid profile (raises high-density lipoprotein or HDL-cholesterol and lowers low-density lipoprotein or LDL-cholesterol). Oestrogen also acts as an arterial vasodilator increasing blood flow to the myocardium and central nervous system. Following the menopause the protective effect of oestrogen is lost and the prevalence of cardiovascular disease in men and women is similar.

Assessment

The diagnosis is usually straightforward and is based on the history. Common presenting symptoms are listed in Table 14.1.

It is important to elicit how the symptoms are interfering with everyday activities and relationships. Diagnosis may be less obvious in women who have premature ovarian failure and in women who have undergone hysterectomy with conservation of the ovaries. A medical history should exclude contraindications to hormone replacement therapy. Smoking should be discouraged. General physical examination should include breast examination,

Table 14.1   Common presenting symptoms of the menopause.

Physical	Psychological
Hot flushes	Depression
Night sweats	Anxiety/panic attacks
Exhaustion	Irritability
Joint pains	Lethargy
Dysuria	Poor memory
Vaginal dryness	Poor concentration
Dyspareunia	Decreased libido

and height, weight and blood pressure should be recorded. Pelvic examination should include a cervical smear if indicated.

Investigations
Blood tests are rarely helpful but in cases where the diagnosis is in doubt, measure serum gonadotrophins and/or oestradiol. Oestradiol < 70 pmol/l and FSH/LH > 15 IU/l are found in menopausal women. Endometrial biopsy is not performed as a routine but it is mandatory in women with postmenopausal bleeding or irregular bleeding. Mammography should be offered to women over 50 years.

Non-invasive methods are used to measure bone density in the lumbar spine and femoral neck. Dual energy X-ray absorptiometry is the most popular technique. CT scanning may also be used, and ultrasound techniques are available.

Treatment
Hormone replacement therapy (HRT) is the most appropriate treatment for women with menopause-related problems. Randomized controlled trials (RCTs) have shown that high-dose progestogens and clonidine relieve vasomotor symptoms. The decision to commence HRT should be made after full discussion with the patient.

Indications for HRT include:

1. Menopause-related symptoms
2. Early menopause
3. Prevention of osteoporosis.

Contraindications to oestrogen replacement therapy are:

1. Carcinoma of the breast
2. Carcinoma of the endometrium
3. Liver disease (porphyria, active hepatitis)
4. Inherited thrombophilia.

Hypertension is not a contraindication to therapy but blood pressure should be stabilized before HRT is commenced. For HRT in women with a history of thromboembolic disease, see 'HRT and venous thromboembolism' below.

In the case of HRT in women who have had carcinoma of the breast or endometrium, careful discussion should centre on quality of life issues. Each case should be individualized and if a woman is prepared to accept the theoretical risk of disease recurrence by taking HRT, then it is her right to choose what she deems right for her quality of life.

Oestrogen therapy
'Natural' oestrogens (17β-estradiol, estradiol valerate, conjugated equine oestrogens) are commonly used. Tibolone is a synthetic steroid which has oestrogenic, progestogenic and some androgenic activity. Ethinylestradiol and other synthetic oestrogens have now been superseded by natural preparations.

Oestrogen should be given continuously and may be administered orally or parenterally. The pharmacodynamics and biochemical effects of exogenous oestrogens can vary markedly with the route of administration. Oral therapy is the most widely used. Oestrogen delivered by this route first passes through the liver. This has several effects:

1. Hepatic metabolism removes a large proportion of a given dose.
2. Oestrogen may influence the synthesis of various hepatic products and this may have beneficial or adverse effects; oral oestrogen favourably alters the HDL/LDL ratio by elevating plasma HDL-cholesterol; oral therapy may increase renin substrate production and a parenteral route of administration may be more appropriate in hypertensives; similarly antithrombin III production may be depressed, and parenteral administration may be advisable in women with clotting disorders.
3. Concurrent drug therapy (e.g. with anticonvulsants) may result in induction of hepatic enzymes leading to rapid inactivation of oestrogen.

The parenteral route avoids the first pass effect and is particularly suitable for hypertensives and women with a history of thromboembolic disease (see 'HRT and venous thromboembolism'). It is a convenient method following hysterectomy. Subcutaneous implants of estradiol (25 mg, 50 mg or 100 mg) are inserted under local anaesthesia into the anterior abdominal wall or buttock. Testosterone (25 mg, 50 mg or 100 mg) may be added to improve libido and energy levels. The procedure is repeated every 6–10 months. Vaginal administration of oestrogen may result in blood levels comparable to those seen after oral therapy and endometrial hyperplasia may occur with unopposed long-term use. Oestrogen can be administered transdermally via skin patches or creams which are convenient and effective. An intranasal preparation is also available.

Whichever type of oestrogen and route of administration are chosen, the dose prescribed must be adequate to prevent bone loss. 'Bone sparing doses' are as follows:

Conjugated equine oestrogens	0.625 mg a day
Estradiol valerate	2.0 mg a day
Transdermal estradiol patch	50 μg/24 hours
Subcutaneous estradiol implant	50 mg/6 months.

Progestogen therapy
Prolonged administration of oestrogens to postmenopausal women is associated with an increased risk of development of endometrial hyperplasia and cancer. This risk can be avoided by adding a progestogen for 10–12 days each calendar month in sequential regimes. Daily administration of a lower dose of progestogen provides the same protection in continuous combined regimens. Progestogenic side-effects can be reduced by using the minimum dose of progestogen. Progestogens are usually administered orally but can be given parenterally via transdermal patches, vaginal gel or the progestogen-containing intrauterine system (IUS).

Unwanted effects of progestogen are:

1. Withdrawal bleeding, which occurs in 90% of women on sequential regimes
2. 'Premenstrual' symptoms
3. Alterations in the lipid profile, which may counteract the favourable effect of oestrogen.

Tibolone therapy

Tibolone is a synthetic steroid with oestrogenic, progestogenic and androgenic activity. It does not cause endometrial proliferation and it obviates the need for withdrawal bleeds. It is effective in preventing bone loss and improving libido.

Selective oestrogen receptor modulators

Raloxifene is the first of a new class of non-hormonal compounds which act by selectively stimulating oestrogen receptors in different tissues. Tamoxifen and clomifene (clomiphene) are chemically similar. Raloxifene acts as an oestrogen agonist in the skeleton and cardiovascular system and an antagonist in the breast and uterus. It is effective in preventing osteoporosis and has a beneficial influence on the lipid profile. It does not relieve symptoms of oestrogen deficiency. It appears to have a protective effect with regard to developing oestrogen receptor-positive breast carcinomas.

Approaches to treatment

For the purposes of treatment, women can be classified into two groups: those who have a uterus and those who have previously undergone hysterectomy. Women should be fully counselled before starting treatment and they should be warned about common side-effects.

Women with a uterus. The regimen used must not cause endometrial proliferation. There are four main options:

1. Continuous oestrogen + cyclical progestogen 12/28 days. The majority of women will have withdrawal bleeds on this regimen.
2. Continuous oestrogen + continuous progestogen. The majority of users will be amenorrhoeic but some bleed irregularly, particularly in the first 6 months.
3. Tibolone. As with continuous combined therapy, irregular bleeding may occur within the first few months, but usually less than with continuous combined.
4. Insertion of IUS. A progestogen-containing IUD is inserted and oestrogen can be administered orally or parenterally. The local progestogen release induces an atrophic endometrium. The IUS is effective for 5 years.

Women without a uterus. These women can be given continuous oestrogen either orally or parenterally.

Delivery systems available. Women can be offered their HRT either orally, transdermally (patch, gel, cream) subcutaneously, nasally or vaginally (rings, creams, gels, pessaries).

Follow-up of women on HRT

Women should be reviewed 3 months after treatment is commenced. Symptoms should be discussed and enquiries should be made about the pattern of vaginal bleeding (in those with a uterus). Weight and blood pressure should be recorded at each visit. Subsequently, women should be reviewed every 6 months. Smears should be taken as necessary and annual breast examination should be performed. Mammography can be repeated every 2–3 years. Unscheduled vaginal bleeding must be investigated promptly with an endometrial biopsy and transvaginal ultrasound scan, endometrial biopsy ± hysteroscopy.

There is no consensus about the optimum duration of HRT and treatment must be tailored to suit the needs of the individual. To obtain significant protection from osteoporotic fractures, a minimum course of 5 years' treatment is recommended.

Advantages of HRT

1. Relief from menopausal symptoms.
2. Prevention of bone demineralization; oestrogen therapy halts bone loss and protects against osteoporotic fractures. It is most effective if it is commenced shortly after the menopause to avoid the period of accelerated bone loss associated with ovarian failure. Epidemiological evidence suggests that treatment for 5 years is associated with a 50% reduction in hip fractures.
3. Recent evidence suggests that HRT may decrease the risk of developing Alzheimer's disease.
4. It was previously thought that HRT may protect against cardiovascular disease, however two recent trials, namely the HERS and WHI, have refuted this. The HERS showed no benefit of HRT for women who had pre-existing HRT and the WHI study showed that in the HRT group there was an increased incidence of cardiovascular disease. HRT is not now recommended for the primary and secondary prevention of cardiovascular disease.

HRT and cancer

The continuous combined oestrogen and progestogen therapies may be more protective than sequential therapies in reducing the risk of endometrial cancer to below that in an untreated population. There is no association between HRT and carcinoma of the cervix. Colorectal cancers are no more common in HRT users and there is some evidence for a protective effect from HRT.

HRT and breast cancer

There has been much concern and speculation about the relationship between HRT and breast cancer. There is evidence for a small increase in risk of breast cancer related to duration of HRT use. Women who commence HRT at 50 and continue for 5 years have a cumulative excess risk of breast cancer of 2 cases/1000 women. The excess risk is 6 cases after 10 years and 12 cases after 15 years of HRT use. This elevated risk is lost 5 years after stopping HRT.

HRT and venous thromboembolism

Prior to 1996 the literature on HRT and venous thromboembolism was largely reassuring. More recent studies have suggested an increased risk of venous thromboembolism in HRT users. The risk of venous thromboembolism in women aged 45–64 years is 1 per 10 000 per year. HRT users have a threefold increased risk at 3 per 10 000 per year. Prior to commencing HRT women should be asked about their personal and family history of venous thromboembolism and, if indicated, a thrombophilia screen should be performed.

SUMMARY

The average woman spends more than one-third of her life after the menopause. The long-term sequelae of the menopause have important medical implications. The benefits of HRT in improving menopausal symptoms and preventing osteoporosis are well recognized but this must be balanced out against the increased risk of breast cancer and venous thromboembolism. Women must be fully counselled before commencing HRT.

15 The premenstrual syndrome

Adam Rodin

Expectations of the examiners

The candidate should have a basic understanding of the premenstrual syndrome (PMS) and the management of women with this condition.

Definition

PMS is defined as distressing physical and psychological symptoms which occur during the premenstrual phase of the menstrual/ovarian cycle and regress at the onset of menstruation.

Interesting facts

PMS was first described by Frank in 1931. He reported a small group of women with tension, depression and irritability occurring 7–10 days before menstruation and relieved by the onset of 'the menstrual flow'. This condition remains poorly understood. Estimates of the prevalence of PMS in the general population vary from 5% to 95%.

Pathophysiology

The aetiology of PMS is unknown. It is likely that PMS is not a homogeneous condition but is due to a combination of physical, psychological, genetic and environmental factors. A variety of mechanisms have been proposed in PMS but they remain unproven. Popular hypotheses include progesterone deficiency, fluid retention, vitamin deficiency, hypoglycaemia or defective prostaglandin metabolism. The link between PMS and cyclical ovarian activity is certain and the condition characteristically commences after pregnancy or discontinuation of the combined contraceptive pill with the resumption of ovarian activity.

Assessment

Diagnosis is based on the history. Symptoms are many and varied and any body system may be involved. Patterns of symptoms vary between women and the severity of symptoms may vary from cycle to cycle. Common symptoms are listed in Table 15.1.

Table 15.1 Symptoms of premenstrual syndrome.

Physical	Psychological
Breast discomfort	Irritability
Bloating	Anxiety
Weight gain	Tension
Acne	Depression
Headache	Insomnia
Pelvic pain	Change in libido
Change in bowel habit	Poor concentration

In addition, there may be behavioural changes, and pre-existing medical conditions such as epilepsy, asthma or herpes may be exacerbated. If the history is suggestive of PMS, confirmatory evidence can be obtained by prospectively assessing symptoms over three cycles. Various methods have been used ranging from self-grading of severity of symptoms to the use of visual analogue scales. Blood tests are of no value in the diagnosis of PMS.

Treatment

A variety of approaches have been used and these are summarized in Table 15.2.

The placebo response in PMS may exceed 90% and consequently it is difficult to prove the effectiveness of any active treatment. The choice of first-line treatment will be influenced by the severity of symptoms. In mild cases, vitamin B6 or γ-linolenic acid may be helpful. The combined contraceptive

Table 15.2 Treatments used in premenstrual syndrome.

Drug treatment	Psychological
Hormonal	Psychotherapy
Progesterone	Hypnosis
Combined pill	
LHRH analogues	**Other**
Estradiol implants	Diet
Danazol	Acupuncture
Non-hormonal	Bilateral oophorectomy
Diuretics	Radiation menopause
Vitamins B6, A, E	
Cabergoline	
Prostaglandin synthetase inhibitors	
Psychoactive drugs	
γ-Linolenic acid	

pill or dydrogesterone 10 mg b.d. on days 12–26 of the cycle can be prescribed for moderately affected women.

In severe cases, inhibition of the ovarian cycle is the approach of choice. This can be achieved by using subcutaneous oestradiol implants combined with cyclical oral progestogen to prevent the development of endometrial hyperplasia. LHRH analogues are extremely effective but because of the suppression of ovarian oestrogen production they are not appropriate for long-term use unless 'addback' therapy is instituted.

If single symptoms predominate, it may be preferable to try a therapy aimed at alleviating that specific complaint: for example, bromocriptine for breast pain and diuretics for bloating. Counselling or psychotherapy may be beneficial in women with PMS.

SUMMARY

PMS is associated with cyclical ovarian activity and does not occur before puberty, during pregnancy or after the menopause. Most women experience adverse symptoms prior to menstruation. The aetiology of PMS is unknown and treatments are non-specific. In severe cases, ovarian suppression is the treatment of choice.

16   Urinary incontinence

Janice Rymer

Expectations of the examiners

The candidate will be expected to have a basic knowledge of the physiology of micturition and of the various types of incontinence. In particular, the candidate should be able to distinguish between stress and urge incontinence, and manage appropriately.

Definition

Incontinence is defined as the involuntary loss of urine which is a social and hygienic problem and is objectively demonstrable.

Causes

Whenever the intravesical pressure is greater than the intraurethral pressure loss of urine will occur.

The three commonest causes of incontinence are genuine stress incontinence, detrusor instability and overflow incontinence. Although urinary fistulas are a rare cause in the UK, they are a common cause in developing countries.

STRESS INCONTINENCE

Definition

Stress incontinence is defined as involuntary loss of urine coinciding with a rise in intra-abdominal pressure (e.g. during laughing, coughing or, jumping).

Pathophysiology

Control of micturition depends on two main factors:

1. A competent sphincter mechanism able to resist the changes in intra-abdominal pressure
2. The capacity to inhibit a bladder contraction until it is convenient to micturate.

Urine leakage occurs when the intravesical pressure exceeds the maximum urethral pressure. Most commonly the urethral 'occlusive forces' have been diminished by childbirth trauma, surgical damage and/or menopausal

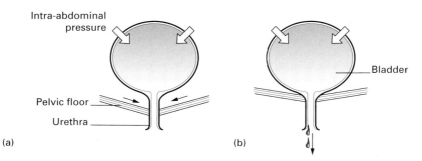

Fig. 16.1 Stress incontinence. a, Normally an increase in intra-abdominal pressure will be transmitted to the bladder and to the urethra, thus maintaining continence. b, If there is an alteration in the position of the bladder neck and most of the urethra is below the pelvic floor, then an increase in intra-abdominal pressure will increase the intravesical pressure but not the urethral pressure, so that urine will be lost.

atrophy, and this deficiency is aggravated by descent of the proximal third of the urethra below the level of the pelvic floor (see Fig. 16.1). In addition, a chronically raised intra-abdominal pressure such as in chronic bronchitis or obesity will aggravate the condition.

Assessment

History

History is important to determine whether this is pure stress incontinence or whether an element of urgency is present. A full obstetric and gynaecological history must be obtained especially concerning previous incontinence and repair procedures. Chronic constipation, chronic bronchitis, smoking and diuretics are associated with stress incontinence and should be specifically asked about. Classically the incontinence occurs synchronously with the rise in intra-abdominal pressure. Most patients find incontinence a social and hygienic problem.

Examination

General and abdominal examination should be performed. To assess the stress incontinence, the patient should be examined in the Sims position with a full bladder. The labia are parted, noting any excoriation, the patient is asked to cough, and loss of urine and vaginal wall descent are noted. A Sims speculum is inserted along the posterior vaginal wall and the anterior wall is observed, again with coughing. Descent of the cervix is observed and traction may be applied using a sponge forceps on the anterior lip of the cervix. The speculum is gradually withdrawn and any laxity of the posterior vaginal wall is noted. A bimanual examination should be performed. The value of Bonney's test (elevation of the bladder neck) at the time of examination is debatable.

Investigations

MSU.   This should be performed to exclude a urinary tract infection.

Urodynamic investigation.   This should be performed in all cases to exclude voiding difficulties and detrusor instability. (Operations to correct genuine stress incontinence may aggravate detrusor instability.)

Treatment

Local causes.   These should be treated appropriately, e.g. infection.

Conservative therapy.   This is predominantly used for women with mild genuine stress incontinence or in women who have not completed their family.

Pelvic floor exercises (± interferential therapy ± faradism).   These may be helpful, ideally under the guidance of a physiotherapist, and vaginal cones may be a useful adjunct.

Surgery.   This the mainstay of treatment and there are various options. Suprapubic operations are more effective for curing stress incontinence. The choice of operation depends on the degree of uterovaginal descent and the general health of the patient:

1. *Colposuspension.* This is an abdominal procedure in which sutures are placed periurethrally and lateral to the bladder neck, from above, and then sutured to the iliopectineal ligament (Burch), or the periosteum overlying the symphysis pubis (Marshall–Marchetti–Krantz).
2. *Tension-free vaginal tape (TVT) procedure.* This procedure uses a knitted prolene mesh tape placed at the mid-urethra, the aim being to have the tape lying free at rest and only exerting sufficient pressure on the urethra during a cough to prevent leakage of urine.
3. *Anterior colporrhaphy.* This is a vaginal procedure where the anterior wall of the vagina is elevated and any excess tissue is removed. It is a good operation to repair a cystocele but has a high failure rate for genuine stress incontinence.
4. *Sling procedures.* These can be performed abdominally or vaginally, using synthetic material or fascia lata to elevate the urethra. The sling is then attached to the rectus sheath. They have a high success rate but also a high complication rate, e.g. long-term voiding difficulties.
5. *Stamey procedures.* A long needle is inserted abdominally and a suture is placed either side of the bladder neck to elevate it. The suture is secured to the rectus sheath. These procedures are reserved for elderly patients or repeat procedures.
6. *Injectables.* GAX collagen or macroplastique is injected paraurethrally to build up bulk around the sphincter.
7. *Artificial sphincter.* This is a complex operation which is considered an end-stage operation.

Ring pessaries.   If there is associated uterovaginal prolapse, these can be used in cases not fit for anaesthetic.

Summary

Genuine stress incontinence is a common problem which may be socially embarrassing and unhygienic. A careful history and examination are essential to make the correct diagnosis. Urodynamic investigations must be performed to enable an accurate diagnosis. Conservative treatment can be helpful but the definitive treatment is surgery, with the Burch colposuspension being the operation of choice.

URGE INCONTINENCE

Definition
Urge incontinence is defined as involuntary loss of urine caused by uninhibited detrusor contractions.

Interesting facts
Detrusor instability more commonly produces the classic triad of symptoms: namely, urgency, frequency and nocturia (passing urine at night). Whether or not the patient leaks will depend on the integrity of the urethral sphincter mechanism. Urge incontinence may be precipitated by a urinary tract infection or gynaecological surgery.

Pathophysiology
In this condition the urethra functions normally but the bladder contracts in an uninhibited fashion, and if the intravesical pressure exceeds the urethral pressure, incontinence results.

Aetiology
1. Idiopathic
2. Secondary to an upper motor neurone lesion
3. Secondary to previous incontinence operations.

Assessment
History
History involves determining the severity of the following symptoms: frequency, urgency and nocturia.

Examination
Examination is usually uninformative, but should include a full neurological examination.

Investigations
1. Urine microscopy and culture.
2. Urodynamics: a normal bladder can be filled to at least 500 ml with an intravesical pressure rise of less than 10 cm of water. Normally, detrusor

activity is suppressed with posture changes, sudden rises in intra-abdominal pressure and rapid filling. Cystometry measures intravesical pressure during bladder filling.

3. Detrusor instability is confirmed by a sensation of discomfort or a detrusor contraction (pressure rise > 15 cm water) during filling, coughing or standing.

Treatment

Bladder drill

This requires patient motivation for success. The aim is to increase the interval between episodes of micturition progressively. The usual interval should be determined, and the patient should then be instructed to pass urine at this frequency even if she has no desire to void. Once she has accomplished this, with no accidents, she should increase the time in 15-minute increments. This may take a few days, but once this is achieved, increase again and again until an interval of 3 hours is achieved. Essentially the bladder is 'retrained'. Ideally this should be done with the woman as an inpatient and with biofeedback, but few units have these facilities. Fluid restriction and frequency volume charts may be useful.

Drug therapy

Anticholinergic agents are the mainstay of treatment. They have the side-effect of causing a dry mouth and blurred vision. They include:

1. Oxybutynin: anticholinergic and direct smooth muscle relaxant effect; good for all symptoms of detrusor instability
2. Tolterodine: antimuscarinic; may be as effective as oxybutinin but with fewer adverse effects
3. Propantheline: anticholinergic; effective for diurnal frequency
4. Imipramine: anticholinergic and central nervous system effect; good for nocturia and nocturnal enuresis
5. Desmopressin: antidiuretic hormone analogue; prevents the patient producing urine at night, which is when it is taken; good for nocturia and nocturnal enuresis
6. HRT: good for patients with irritative bladder symptoms, especially in conjunction with other medication.

Surgery

The Clam cystoplasty results in long-term voiding problems and is reserved for intractable detrusor instability.

Summary

Detrusor instability produces the symptoms of urinary urgency, frequency and nocturia. Cystometry is essential to confirm the diagnosis, and bladder drill is the treatment of choice. One must be cautious with drug therapy as urinary retention can be precipitated.

OVERFLOW INCONTINENCE

Definition
Overflow incontinence is defined as frequent involuntary loss of small volumes of urine, usually precipitated by changes in posture. The urinary stream is slow with hesitancy, and after micturition there may be a sensation of incomplete emptying.

Pathophysiology
Overflow incontinence may be caused by obstruction to bladder outflow or bladder atony. Urine leakage occurs when the intravesical pressure exceeds the maximum urethral pressure in the absence of detrusor activity. Frequency may occur due to decreased functional capacity.

Aetiology
Detrusor hypotonia
1. Lower motor neurone lesions (e.g. diabetes)
2. Drugs with anticholinergic side-effects
3. Secondary to pain (e.g. herpes), which pushes the patient into retention and then overdistends the bladder and results in detrusor damage.

Outflow obstruction
1. Pelvic mass
2. Uterovaginal prolapse
3. Inflammation
4. Constipation
5. Incontinence surgery.

Assessment
History
This will provide the symptoms as above. Overflow incontinence may have been precipitated by a recent event.

Examination
This may reveal a palpable mass. The passage of a urethral catheter will reveal a large residual urine.

Investigations
1. MSU.
2. Cystometry will reveal a large residual urine with a delayed first sensation, and enlarged bladder capacity. In detrusor hypotonia the voiding pressure will be reduced whereas in obstruction it will be raised. With time the detrusor compensates so that all patients may present with a reduced voiding pressure and a reduced peak flow rate regardless of cause.

Treatment

1. If drug ingestion is causing the problem, the drug regimen must be altered.
2. Urine infection should be treated.
3. Treat constipation.
4. Instruct the patient to double void.
5. If detrusor hypotonia is the problem, then try cholinergic agents such as bethanechol.
6. If outflow obstruction is the cause, then treat the cause (e.g. pelvic mass). If it is due to urethral stenosis, then perform a urethrotomy.
7. In failed cases teach clean intermittent self-catheterization.
8. Some patients who are not dextrous may require a long-term in-dwelling catheter.

Summary

Overflow incontinence can be due to either detrusor hypotonia or outflow obstruction. The two may present in a similar manner but require different treatments.

TRUE INCONTINENCE

Definition

True incontinence is defined as continuous urine leakage most commonly due to a fistulous track between the vagina and either the ureter, the bladder or the urethra.

Interesting facts

Congenital abnormalities are rare, e.g. ureteric ectopy which presents in infancy.

A very low urethrovaginal fistula can cause intermittent incontinence.

Aetiology

1. Prolonged labour
2. Carcinoma
3. Surgery
4. Radiotherapy.

Assessment

There is a history of urine continuously draining from the vagina. Examination is best performed in the Sims position, with a Sims speculum. Colouring the urine and placing tampons in the vagina may aid location of the fistulous track.

Investigations

A micturating cystourethrogram and/or an intravenous pyelogram (IVP) may help location.

Treatment

1. Wait—some fistulae will heal spontaneously if given enough time with continuous bladder drainage.
2. Surgery.

FUNCTIONAL INCONTINENCE

Definition

The patient complains of intermittent or continuous incontinence but all investigations reveal no evidence of abnormality. Reassurance is helpful, and referral to a psychiatrist may be indicated.

17

Uterovaginal prolapse

Adam Rodin

Expectations of the examiners

The candidate is expected to have a basic understanding of the support structures of the female genital tract. The candidate should be aware of the clinical features of different types of prolapse and should be competent in the appropriate examination. Management options should be clearly understood but details of surgical repair techniques are not required.

Definition

Uterovaginal prolapse is defined as descent of a pelvic organ or structure into and sometimes outside the vagina.

Interesting facts

Uterovaginal prolapse is a common gynaecological problem which accounts for a large proportion of major gynaecological surgery. It is caused by a failure of the support structures of the genital tract.

Causes of uterovaginal prolapse

1. Congenital (rare), e.g. connective tissue disorder
2. Acquired (common).

Parity

Childbirth is the principal risk factor for uterovaginal prolapse. Many factors contribute but surprisingly little is known about which components of pregnancy and labour are implicated in the causation of prolapse. The considerable weight of the pregnant uterus may play a part and, in addition, the effects of prolonged labour, pushing before full dilatation and genital tract trauma may be of importance. Multiparity increases the risk of subsequent prolapse.

Raised intra-abdominal pressure

Conditions which result in chronic elevation of intra-abdominal pressure may cause or aggravate prolapse. They include:

1. Chronic cough
2. Chronic constipation

3. Intra-abdominal masses
4. Heavy lifting.

Prolapse commonly becomes clinically apparent after the menopause. Oestrogen deficiency results in atrophy of the vaginal skin and laxity of the uterine supports leading to prolapse which was initiated by childbirth many years before.

The support structures of the female genital tract

The main supports of the uterus and the upper vagina are the cardinal ligaments (transverse cervical ligaments) and the uterosacral ligaments. These are formed from condensations of the endopelvic fascia. The cardinal ligament fans out from the lateral cervix and upper vagina to reach the lateral walls of the pelvis. The uterosacral ligaments pass posteriorly, lateral to the rectum and upwards to insert onto the sacrum. Anteriorly, the fascia runs from the cervix and under the bladder to reach the pubic symphysis (the pubocervical ligament). The round ligament does not have a support function.

The pelvic floor is the other important support for the female genital tract. It comprises the levator ani muscles which each have three components: ischiococcygeus, iliococcygeus and pubococcygeus. It is thought that damage to the levator ani in childbirth may be one of the major events predisposing to later prolapse.

Types of prolapse (see Fig. 17.1)

Prolapse of the anterior vaginal wall and bladder is known as a cystocele. This may be accompanied by prolapse of the urethra or urethrocele.

Prolapse of the rectum and posterior vaginal wall is known as a rectocele.

An enterocele is a hernia of the pouch of Douglas through the posterior vaginal fornix. There is a peritoneal sac which may contain small intestine. Enterocele is usually associated with uterine prolapse but may occur in isolation or after hysterectomy. It is a recognized complication of colposuspension procedures.

Uterine prolapse

Uterine prolapse is usually associated with anterior and posterior vaginal wall prolapse. There is descent of the cervix and uterine body into the vagina. Three stages of uterine prolapse are recognized:

1. First degree, in which there is descent of the cervix but it does not reach the vaginal introitus
2. Second degree, in which the cervix reaches the introitus
3. Third degree prolapse or procidentia, in which the cervix and body of the uterus lie outside the introitus.

Vault prolapse

Vault prolapse is an inversion of the vaginal vault that can occur after hysterectomy.

Fig. 17.1 Types of prolapse in the female reproductive system. 1, Urethrocele; 2, cystocele; 3, uterine prolapse; 4, enterocele; 5, rectocele.

Clinical features

Prolapse is often asymptomatic and may be detected at routine screening. It commonly presents as a vaginal swelling which may cause discomfort. The swelling is often worse at the end of the day and may disappear when the patient is recumbent. The patient may be aware of a dragging sensation in the pelvis.

Cystocele is sometimes associated with urinary symptoms. Stress incontinence may occur but is not necessarily associated with a cystocele (see Ch. 16). Incomplete voiding may leave an increased volume of residual urine in the bladder, increasing the chances of urinary tract infections.

Rectocele may be associated with difficulty in defaecation. Patients may sometimes need to reduce the posterior wall prolapse digitally before the rectum can be emptied. Enterocele may present with small bowel obstruction secondary to incarceration. This is a very rare complication.

Procidentia may be associated with decubitus ulceration of the cervix. Rarely, bilateral ureteric obstruction occurs and chronic renal failure has been reported.

Assessment

History

From the history it is important to ascertain the degree to which the prolapse is causing interference with daily activities and impairing quality of life. Specific questions must be asked about urinary and bowel symptoms. Postmenopausal women must be asked about vaginal bleeding and premenopausal women must be questioned about menstrual disorders. If surgical repair is being considered it is essential to record whether the woman is sexually active.

Further questions must be asked about chronic conditions which may aggravate prolapse, e.g. chest disease and smoking. The success of surgical repair in these women may be prejudiced. Record the patient's occupation and social circumstances, as work involving heavy lifting is unsuitable after surgical repair.

Examination

General physical examination. This should be carried out to assess whether the patient is fit for anaesthesia and to exclude conditions which may aggravate prolapse, e.g. chest disease, abdominal masses. (A thorough abdominal examination must always be performed prior to a pelvic examination.)

Pelvic examination. Ask the patient to turn to the left lateral position for examination with a Sims speculum. Separate the patient's buttocks with assistance if necessary. Ask the patient to cough. Insert the blade of the Sims speculum along the posterior vaginal wall and retract to display the anterior vaginal wall. Ask the patient to cough again to assess the degree of prolapse of the anterior vaginal wall and note any stress incontinence. (Remember the patient's bladder may be empty and she may have stress incontinence but it may not be demonstrable.) Support the anterior vaginal wall with a sponge forceps and ask the patient to cough again while continuing to support the anterior vaginal wall with the sponge forceps. One can then observe for cervical descent. The patient is asked to bear down again and the speculum is then removed slowly. While anterior vaginal wall support is maintained, the top of the vaginal vault and the posterior vaginal wall can be visualized sequentially to detect the presence of an enterocele or a rectocele respectively. A bimanual examination should then follow.

When discussing the examination findings anterior and posterior wall prolapse is usually described as 'mild, 'moderate' or 'severe'. These descriptions are highly subjective.

Treatment

Treatment is not indicated when prolapse is found at routine examination and is asymptomatic.

General measures which should be considered include weight reduction, stopping smoking and HRT. Aggravating conditions, e.g. chest infections, should be treated when possible before definitive treatment.

Surgery is the mainstay of treatment for uterovaginal prolapse. In some women conservative measures may be more appropriate.

Conservative management

1. Indications
   a. Patient's choice
   b. Unfit for surgery
   c. Temporary problem, e.g. in pregnancy

2. Methods
   a. Pelvic floor exercises (only suitable for minor degrees of prolapse)
   b. Pessaries.

Many devices have been used. The ring pessary is now in common use. It is inserted to occupy the posterior fornix and the lower part of the anterior vaginal wall, and works by putting redundant vaginal skin on stretch. Use of this pessary is effective for anterior vaginal and uterovaginal prolapse but less effective for posterior wall prolapse. It should be changed every 6 months and may cause erosion of the skin of the vaginal walls.

Surgical repair
The choice of repair procedure will be influenced by the preference of the gynaecologist. These are guidelines:

Cystocele/urethrocele.   Anterior colporrhaphy ± bladder neck support.
Rectocele.   Posterior colporrhaphy.
Enterocele.   Hernia sac identified and opened. Contents reduced and neck tied. Sac excised. Combined with posterior repair.
Vault prolapse.   Sacrocolpopexy. Sacrospinous fixation.
Uterovaginal prolapse.   Vaginal hysterectomy ± repair.

The Manchester (Fothergill) repair is occasionally used. This involves amputation of the cervix, approximating the cardinal ligaments in front of the cervical stump, and anterior and posterior colporrhaphies. The uterus is conserved and reproductive potential is retained in younger women.

SUMMARY

Uterovaginal prolapse is common in postmenopausal women and is usually caused by childbirth. Symptoms may be influenced by the type of prolapse present. Surgical repair is usually the treatment of choice.

18 Minimal access surgery

Barry Auld

Expectations of the examiners

Whilst a detailed knowledge of this kind of surgery is not required, some general understanding of these new procedures is expected. One should be able to give a basic explanation of the techniques involved and some indication of the pattern of recovery and the expected outcome. An appreciation of the potential risks and benefits of this form of surgery, particularly in comparison to conventional surgical techniques, is also appropriate.

Definitions

In gynaecology minimal access surgery encompasses two therapeutic approaches. Hysteroscopic surgery comprises a range of procedures carried out within the uterine cavity. When performed under direct vision these require hysteroscopy, although several newer procedures to achieve endometrial ablation avoid this. Laparoscopy allows surgery within the abdomen and pelvis, avoiding the need for a laparotomy incision. This therefore minimises much of the postoperative recovery and morbidity of a larger wound.

Interesting facts

It is now considered that up to 80% of all classic gynaecological operations can be carried out endoscopically. Continuing technological advances maintain the evolution and refinement of these procedures.

HYSTEROSCOPIC MINIMAL ACCESS SURGERY

Technique of hysteroscopy

Hysteroscopy allows inspection of the uterine cavity via the cervix using CO_2 gas or fluid to distend the uterine cavity. Diagnostic hysteroscopy is performed with a narrow diameter scope (2–5 mm) which often permits insertion without dilatation of the cervix, thus avoiding general anaesthesia and enabling the procedure to be performed in an outpatient setting. Operative hysteroscopy is usually performed under general anaesthesia when the insertion of a wider diameter instrument is required, as in transcervical endometrial resection.

Contraindications and complications

Contraindications to hysteroscopy are pregnancy and the presence of acute pelvic infection. Uterine perforation is a complication which may follow any form of instrumentation but in operative hysteroscopy it carries a greater risk of damage to intra-abdominal viscera or blood vessels. Less serious complications are pelvic infection, excessive absorption of fluid distension media and anaesthetic complications.

Operative hysteroscopy

Hysteroscopic surgery is indicated for a number of conditions:

1. Uterine septum
2. Uterine synechiae (Asherman syndrome)
3. Endocervical/endometrial polyp
4. Fibroid polyps
5. Submucous fibroids
6. Dysfunctional uterine bleeding
7. Retrieval of IUD.

Most of the above conditions are treated hysteroscopically either using electrocautery techniques or by laser.

The main interest and practice of hysteroscopic surgery have been in the treatment of dysfunctional uterine bleeding.

Endometrial ablation

Historically many techniques have been used to remove the endometrial lining of the uterus. The operation of dilatation and curettage (D&C) removes only the superficial endometrium, which then regenerates. Endometrial ablation aims to remove the endometrium to a depth where the basal layer is destroyed and the underlying myometrium is exposed. Total endometrial ablation should result in amenorrhoea. It was the expectation of this outcome, performed as a day case procedure and without the need to remove the uterus, that has led to the current enthusiasm for this procedure.

Hysteroscopically two techniques were favoured: transcervical resection of the endometrium (TCRE) performed with electrocautery, and laser endometrial ablation (LEA) in which the endometrium is destroyed by energy from

Table 18.1 Comparison of the outcomes from TCRE and LEA (%).

Operation	TCRE	LEA
Totally amenorrhoeic	35	60
Improved menstruation	50	32
No improvement in menstruation	15	8
Requiring hysterectomy	16	—

the Nd:YAG laser. Ablation of the endometrium using rollerball electrocautery is an alternative hysteroscopic technique. The treatment of dysfunctional uterine bleeding has now progressed to second and third generation devices which use differing modalities of energy to achieve ablation but with which the procedure is carried out without hysteroscopic guidance. Two technologies are gaining acceptance. In balloon ablation a catheter with an inflatable balloon is inserted into the uterus. The balloon is filled with a fluid which is then heated to a temperature sufficient to destroy the endometrial layer. Microwave endometrial ablation uses a probe which can be manipulated within the uterus to deliver microwave energy. Both these techniques have the opportunity to be used in an outpatient setting.

Patient selection
The success of these procedures depends on patient selection. Women under the age of 40 years are more likely to have a poor outcome, often with recurrence of their symptoms. The ideal patients are women approaching the menopause who wish to avoid hysterectomy. The uterus should be of a normal size. Fibroids which significantly enlarge the uterus or distort the contour of the cavity are also a contraindication. Symptoms of pelvic pain and dysmenorrhoea may suggest the presence of adenomyosis. In adenomyosis the pockets of intramyometrial endometrium allow regeneration of the endometrium and thus recurrence of symptoms. These patients may therefore not be suitable. It is mandatory to have sampled the endometrium before ablation to exclude a histological abnormality. Finally, these patients should have completed their family.

Pretreatment for endometrial ablation
Suppression of the endometrium improves the outcome but if surgery is to be carried out on unprepared patients it is more effective in the postmenstrual phase when the endometrium is thinnest. Regimens for endometrial suppression are:

1. Medroxyprogesterone acetate 30–50 mg daily for 6 weeks
2. Danazol 600 mg daily for 6 weeks
3. GnRH analogue (goserelin implant 3.5 mg) 1 month before surgery.

Pregnancy and sterilization
Most women will be sterile following the procedure, but sterility cannot be guaranteed and occasional pregnancies have been reported. Of greater concern is the risk that pregnancy may establish ectopically in the fallopian tube, particularly in its intramural segment. For this reason laparoscopic sterilization should be considered at the time of the endometrial ablation/resection.

Complications of endometrial ablation
A perforation rate in the order of 1.3% is quoted but only a very few of these cases are associated with major trauma involving damage to great vessels, bowel and ureter. Emergency hysterectomy is only rarely required. Other

serious complications occur at a rate of about 0.2% and include water intoxication, pulmonary oedema, and haemorrhage requiring blood transfusion. A minor complication is prolonged vaginal bleeding and discharge associated with postoperative infection. A long-term complication is the sequestration of endometrial tissue in a walled-off pocket, thus forming a haematometra.

Results

The outcome of endometrial ablation can be assessed in terms of whether there is total amenorrhoea, a reduction in menstrual flow and return of cycle regularity, no change or even a deterioration in menstrual symptoms. Results for endometrial ablation are approximately similar irrespective of the technique of ablation used. Total amenorrhoea is the outcome in about 50% of treatments while 40% will have an improvement in their menstruation. One long-term outcome measure is the number of women who will subsequently require a hysterectomy for recurrent symptoms. Early data suggested that about 15% of these women would eventually require hysterectomy but it may be that this figure is somewhat higher.

Conclusions

The results of endometrial ablation have shown that it is a viable alternative to hysterectomy in a proportion of women. Currently an unanswered worry hangs over this technique regarding the presentation of malignancy in women who have had this operation, although the risk is very small. If the use of ablative techniques delays or masks the presentation of endometrial carcinoma, allowing it to progress, then in the long term its use may be limited.

LAPAROSCOPIC MINIMAL ACCESS SURGERY

Gynaecologists have been using the laparoscope as a diagnostic tool for many years. The use of the laparoscope to perform more complex operative procedures has been relatively recent. General surgeons have far more rapidly assimilated the benefits of laparoscopic surgery into their practice. The range of surgical procedures open to a laparoscopic approach now covers almost all aspects of gynaecological surgery. Operations which can be performed laparoscopically are listed below:

1. Tubal sterilization
2. Assisted reproductive procedures
3. Ovarian drilling (for polycystic ovarian syndrome)
4. Adhesiolysis
5. Surgery for endometriosis
6. Uterosacral ligament transection
7. Tuboplasty, fimbrioplasty, neosalpingostomy
8. Treatment of ectopic pregnancy
9. Ovarian cystectomy

10. Salpingo-oophorectomy
11. Myomectomy
12. Hysterectomy (supracervical and total) with combined vaginal approach
13. Colposuspension and sacrocolpopexy
14. Presacral neurectomy
15. Pelvic lymphadenectomy
16. Radical hysterectomy
17. Pelvic floor repair.

Laparoscopic treatment of endometriosis

Data are accumulating to suggest that laparoscopic treatment of endometriotic deposits is more effective than medical treatment, and that a combination of both treatments may be best of all. The surgical approach avoids the side-effects of medical therapy, particularly when pregnancy is actively sought. In patients with ovarian endometriomas (chocolate cysts), it is possible to remove these laparoscopically. Surgical treatment has resulted in pregnancy rates as high as 80%. It is also claimed to be an effective treatment for those patients who also complain of pelvic pain and dysmenorrhoea resulting from endometriosis. It is becoming established that severe endometriosis is best dealt with laparoscopically if a conservative approach to fertility is required. This form of laparoscopic surgery, which often involves infiltrating deposits of endometriosis sometimes affecting the bowel, requires a high degree of skill.

Laparoscopy for tubal infertility

Laparoscopic surgery to restore normal tubal anatomy and patency to a hydrosalpinx (neosalpingostomy) has been shown to achieve pregnancy rates of the order of 60% when the endosalpinx of the tube is healthy.

Laparoscopic treatment of ectopic pregnancy

Advances in the use of transvaginal ultrasound and quantitative HCG testing mean that increasingly ectopic pregnancy is being diagnosed early, usually before tubal rupture has occurred. This allows a more conservative approach with preservation of the tube. The patient may be discharged from hospital the next day but requires continued follow-up of serum HCG levels. Static or rising levels indicate the presence of residual trophoblastic tissue which can be treated by systemic therapy with methotrexate and folinic acid. Subsequent intrauterine pregnancy rates are reported of between 20% and 83%, with recurrent tubal pregnancies of between 10% and 22%.

Laparoscopic treatment of polycystic ovarian syndrome

As an alternative to classic open wedge resection, the ovaries are now drilled ('pepperpotting') laparoscopically using a diathermy needle. These multiple holes in the ovaries destroy the androgen-producing stroma which leads to a restoration, albeit temporary, of normal ovarian activity. Ovulation rates of 75% have been reported with pregnancy rates of 50–75% in women previously unresponsive to clomifene. The effect may only last for 3–6 cycles, however.

Laparoscopic oophorectomy and ovarian cystectomy

Ultrasound assessment of all adnexal masses is essential regardless of the age of the patient. Masses should be less than 10 cm in diameter with distinct borders and no evidence of irregular solid parts, thick septae, ascites or matted bowel loops. The serum CA125 concentration should be less than 35 IU/ml. At laparoscopy the abdominal cavity is fully inspected for evidence of malignant disease. If concern exists about the risk of malignancy or if the contents of the cyst are toxic (dermoid cysts), ovarian tissue can be placed inside a retrieval bag and the bag closed by means of a drawstring to avoid spillage before removal. If the tissue bulk is too large to remove through a small trocar point a posterior colpotomy in the vagina will allow removal via this route. Oophorectomy is sometimes practised as an adjunct to treatment for breast cancer or to relieve pain in women with residual or entrapped ovarian syndrome.

Laparoscopic hysterectomy and laparoscopically assisted vaginal hysterectomy

Interesting facts

In the UK some 73 000 hysterectomies are performed annually, of which 75% are abdominal and 25% vaginal. Abdominal hysterectomy prolongs the hospital stay and the morbidity from abdominal surgery is significantly greater than from vaginal surgery. The laparoscopic approach to hysterectomy offers the opportunity to convert the outcome for hysterectomy from that associated with abdominal surgery to an outcome similar to that of vaginal hysterectomy or even better.

Reich first described laparoscopic hysterectomy in 1989. He differentiated between two levels of laparoscopic hysterectomy. In true laparoscopic hysterectomy (LH) the laparoscopic approach is used to secure all the pedicles down to the level of the uterine arteries and below. In laparoscopically assisted vaginal hysterectomy (LAVH) the laparoscopic approach is used to secure only the upper pedicles and the uterine arteries are secured from the vaginal end.

It is now clear that most surgeons in practice rarely remove the ovaries via the vaginal route. One of the benefits of LAVH therefore is that when the ovaries need to be removed at the time of hysterectomy then LAVH will avoid an abdominal operation. Similarly, laparoscopy may facilitate a vaginal hysterectomy when there are adhesions in the pelvis which can be dealt with laparoscopically and without which a vaginal operation would not have been possible.

Technique of laparoscopic hysterectomy

The laparoscope is inserted in the usual subumbilical position once a pneumoperitoneum has been achieved with carbon dioxide. Further trocar points are inserted, either two or three, usually low down in the suprapubic area. Major vascular pedicles can be secured by electrocautery, endosuturing techniques or disposable endostapling devices which simultaneously insert rows of parallel haemostatic staples and divide the pedicle between these rows.

Such instruments add to the costs of the operation but reduce the length of operating time.

Following the laparoscopic procedure the vaginal approach is used to secure the remaining vascular pedicles. The uterus and adnexal structures are removed through the vagina which is then repaired in the normal fashion. A final laparoscopic inspection is made to ensure haemostasis.

Results and complications of laparoscopic hysterectomy

The early experience of this operation suggests a long-term outcome similar to that of abdominal hysterectomy but with a reduced perioperative morbidity. The major advantage is in terms of shortened hospital stay (1–3 days) and shortened recovery to normal activities (21 days). Most patients are pleased with the cosmetic outcome and particularly appreciate the minimal postoperative pain they experience.

Any laparoscopic operation carries a risk of damage to internal structures. These risks reflect the skill and learning curve of the surgeon and the degree of difficulty in relation to any existing pathology encountered. Despite this the risks of laparoscopic hysterectomy remain low, probably less than 1% and usually in the form of uncontrollable haemorrhage or damage to the bowel or urinary tract. The major complication most commonly recognized is ureteric injury which usually occurs in laparoscopic hysterectomy when the uterine arteries are divided.

Conclusions

The main drawbacks of laparoscopic surgery are the capital costs needed to set up the necessary facilities and the considerable learning curve needed to acquire the skills to carry out these operations. The risk of complications which may be serious should encourage lengthy preoperative counselling of patients regarding the possibility of undergoing a laparotomy.

In all these procedures the avoidance of a laparotomy incision benefits the patient by a less painful, more speedy recovery, which in turn shortens the length of hospital stay and hastens the return to normal activities. The surgical outcomes of most of these procedures are the same as their laparotomy counterparts. In theory, however, a potential benefit of laparoscopic surgery is the avoidance of the inevitable handling of tissues necessary at open laparotomy. Also tissue damage is much reduced, resulting in less postoperative adhesion formation and fewer complications overall. The consequences of this are that laparotomy is a less justifiable approach in many instances and we must expect that laparoscopic surgery will become increasingly normal for most gynaecological procedures.

DEBATE

The next generation of gynaecological surgeons will need to retain all the skills of traditional gynaecological surgery, whilst developing the very specialist skills necessary to perform minimal access procedures. As with cancer surgery it may well be that more advanced techniques of laparoscopic surgery become located in specialist tertiary centres where resources and skills can be brought together.

19

Prepregnancy counselling and prenatal diagnosis

Gregory Davis

PREPREGNANCY COUNSELLING

Expectations of the examiners

Candidates will be expected to know the range of disorders in which prepregnancy care is of benefit and the principles of management of the common conditions.

Definition

Prepregnancy counselling is the discussion and investigation of medical conditions either past or present which may influence fetal or maternal health in future pregnancies.

Interesting facts

Because of the emotional and financial cost of special care for infants or mothers with medical conditions, preventive medicine should be as widely practised as possible. Counselling is indicated in women with medical illnesses that may become complicated because of pregnancy or in those who may be at risk of giving birth to an infant with a genetic or environmentally induced birth defect.

Assessment

An increasing number of women are seeking advice prior to pregnancy with questions concerning diet, smoking, alcohol, drugs and exercise. In low-risk women, 500 μg of folic acid daily until 14 weeks of pregnancy is recommended to reduce the incidence of neural tube defects (NTD). All women wishing to conceive should receive supplementation at least 6 weeks prior to conception and there is some evidence that the addition of other vitamins and minerals can reduce the incidence of NTD even further. In women at increased risk of having a baby with NTD (previous affected baby, parent with NTD) a daily dose of 5 mg of folate is recommended. Smoking, alcohol and drugs

Table 19.1 Indications for prepregnancy counselling.

Maternal conditions

Diabetes and other metabolic endocrine disorders

Essential or secondary hypertension

Specific maternal infections, e.g. herpes, human immunodeficiency virus (HIV)

Risk of genetic disease, e.g. maternal age, family history of genetic abnormalities

Drug exposure, either prescription or illicit

Abnormal maternal nutrition, either obesity or subnormal weight

Chronic medical problems, e.g. renal disease, SLE, heart disease, epilepsy, neurological disorders

Previous obstetric history

Previous pregnancy loss, e.g. stillbirth, recurrent miscarriage

Previous preterm delivery, growth retardation

Previous infant with congenital anomaly or mental retardation

Previous adverse delivery experience

(both prescription and illicit) should be avoided. Prescription drugs should be reduced to minimal essential levels and changed to those known to be safe in early pregnancy if possible. There is no evidence that exercise adversely affects either conception or development (unless excessive exercise induces anovulation and amenorrhoea).

All these questions can be answered by the general practitioner but women with more specific problems, as outlined in Table 19.1, should be referred to an obstetrician. Some of these problems can then be dealt with by the obstetrician directly, e.g. previous adverse delivery experience, but others will require referral for further medical evaluation or genetic counselling. The obstetrician then remains the contact point for the woman, and can discuss with her the options given by the physician or geneticist. Ideally, the woman should make an informed choice either to conceive or, rarely, to avoid conception.

Follow-up

It is essential that prepregnancy counselling is followed by consultation early in the pregnancy to confirm the presence of a viable intrauterine pregnancy, to allow accurate dating of the pregnancy and to arrange for prenatal diagnostic investigations if appropriate (see following section).

PRENATAL DIAGNOSIS OF FETAL ABNORMALITIES

Expectations of the examiners

Candidates will be expected to have a knowledge of the basic methods of prenatal diagnosis and the risks of common congenital disorders. They should also be familiar with the use and interpretation of routine prenatal screening tests for congenital anomalies.

Definition
Prenatal diagnosis is the detection of fetal disease or abnormality prior to delivery.

Interesting facts
Serious congenital abnormalities now account for 20% of perinatal deaths, are present in 2% of all births, and account for 30% of all paediatric admissions to hospital. Prenatal diagnosis is required in up to 10% of all pregnancies and, although it has been described as 'preventive medicine', in reality many affected fetuses are terminated, thereby removing them from the perinatal mortality statistics. However, some parents prefer to know if their child is abnormal prior to delivery in order to prepare themselves adequately for the birth.

Pathophysiology
Congenital abnormalities can be divided into four groups:

1. Chromosomal abnormalities arise during gamete formation or early in embryonic cleavage. They account for 60% of spontaneous abortions. Common examples are the trisomies 21 and 18, and Turner syndrome 45XO. The incidence of many chromosomal disorders increases with maternal age.
2. A single gene defect accounts for many autosomal recessive diseases such as inborn errors of metabolism.
3. Structural abnormalities may result from multifactorial influences but some may occur in association with chromosomal abnormalities (e.g. duodenal atresia and cardiac defects in Down syndrome) or drugs (e.g. phocomelia with thalidomide).
4. Environmental factors causing abnormality are mostly drugs or infections. Congenital infections are uncommon but may cause developmental abnormalities, intrauterine death or neonatal illness. Infections in this category include rubella, syphilis, listeria, cytomegalovirus and toxoplasma.

Incidence of common congenital abnormalities
Down syndrome (trisomy 21)
Overall incidence is 1 in 650 live births (LB). (see Table 19.2).

Neural tube defects
The overall incidence of NTD in the UK is difficult to determine as many affected fetuses abort or are terminated. The birth prevalence varies from 3 to 5 in 1000 total births in the north and west of the country to 2 in 1000 total births in the south and east. The recurrence rate is 1 in 30 after one affected child, rising to 1 in 5 after three affected children. The risk of an NTD in the

Table 19.2 Incidence of Down syndrome.		
Maternal age	Approximate risk of affected child	Risk of recurrence
20	1 in 2000	1 in 100
30	1 in 900	(irrespective of age)
35	1 in 365	
40	1 in 110	
42	1 in 70	
46	1 in 25	

offspring of one affected parent is 5%; this rises to 30% if both parents are affected. Fifty per cent of affected fetuses have anencephaly (which is incompatible with life), 45% spina bifida and 5% encephalocoeles. There are varying degrees of handicap but of those born with open spina bifida, 70% will die within the first 5 years and only 10% will be free of major handicap.

Congenital heart disease
The incidence of serious congenital heart disease is 8 per 1000 live births of which 50% are major defects. The recurrence risk is 1 in 50 and there is a 5% risk of having an affected child if one parent is affected.

Cystic fibrosis
Cystic fibrosis is inherited as a classic autosomal recessive trait with a birth prevalence of 1 per 2500. Males are sterile due to obliteration of the vas deferens but females can reproduce. The risk of an affected woman having an affected child is 1–2%.

Antenatal screening
Ninety per cent of congenital anomalies will arise in women who do not have any risk factors and screening is therefore important. Routine screening tests are:

1. Nuchal translucency scanning at 11–13 weeks
2. Serum screening for Down syndrome at 14–20 weeks
3. Ultrasound at 18–20 weeks
4. Testing for rubella immunity
5. Testing for sickle cell disease in Afro-Caribbean women
6. Haemoglobin electrophoresis to detect thalassaemia in Mediterranean and Asian women.

Nuchal translucency scanning
Increased nuchal thickness measured at 11–13 weeks is strongly associated with aneuploidy. The measurement is entered into an algorithm with maternal age to give a risk of Down syndrome and other chromosome anomalies.

In the original report on this technique, 80% of Down syndrome fetuses and 70–80% of other chromosome abnormalities were detected. More recently, the addition of serum screening for pregnancy-associated placental protein A and HCG to the nuchal translucency measurement has been reported to increase the detection of Down syndrome to 90%. There is a 5% false positive result, meaning that 5% of women tested will be found to have an increased risk but the fetus will be normal.

Biochemical screening for Down syndrome

In this test the serum values of AFP, HCG and oestriol in combination with maternal age are used in an algorithm (similar to the nuchal translucency scan) to derive a risk estimate for Down syndrome. If the risk is higher than the risk of Down syndrome for a woman aged 35, then amniocentesis for karyotyping is offered. This test is based on the observation that in Down syndrome pregnancies, AFP and oestriol levels are low, while HCG levels are usually higher than average. This test should detect about 60% of babies with Down syndrome. It remains controversial because, on a population basis, the same number of normal babies will be lost due to complications of amniocentesis as cases of Down syndrome detected.

Routine morphology scan

This is performed at 18–20 weeks to confirm gestation and to exclude major fetal structural abnormalities. The fetus is carefully scanned with particular attention to the head, spine, four-chamber view of the heart, kidneys, bowel, presence of a bladder, and moving limbs of normal length. Ninety per cent of NTD (the commonest structural abnormality) will be detected in this manner and it is rare to miss a major NTD.

Maternal serum α-fetoprotein (AFP) levels

Serum AFP is raised in a large number of conditions, including NTD, twin pregnancy, abdominal wall defects in the fetus, fetal death and fetal hydrops. Low levels of maternal AFP have been shown to be associated with chromosomal abnormalities in the fetus. The use of AFP screening has largely been superseded by the routine use of a morphology scan at 18–20 weeks' gestation.

Testing for sickle cell disease and thalassaemia

In women who are known to carry the trait or have these or rarer haemoglobinopathies, haemoglobin electrophoresis is performed on the partner's blood. If the partner is a carrier and hence the fetus is at risk of having the disease, then fetal DNA can be obtained by chorionic villus sampling (CVS) or amniocentesis and the specific mutations sought.

Rubella immunity

Most women should be immune to rubella through the nationwide immunization of teenage girls and now of children. Non-immune women are identified and immunized either before pregnancy or immediately after birth. Pregnancy must be avoided for 3 months after immunization because of the small risk of rubella syndrome in the fetus.

Identification of risk groups

Women at risk of having a fetus with congenital abnormality are outlined in Table 19.3 and should be referred early in pregnancy for prenatal diagnosis.

Investigations

Methods

Ultrasound scan. This is used to detect structural abnormalities in the central nervous system, gastrointestinal tract, urinary system, skeleton and heart. In addition, cleft lip and palate can be detected if a specific search is made. Routine ultrasound screening for structural abnormalities is performed at 18–20 weeks, which is a compromise between performing the procedure early (so that safer termination of pregnancy may be carried out) and late (when the structural details become more obvious).

Amniocentesis. Removal of liquor under ultrasound guidance for the culture of desquamated fetal fibroblasts permits karyotyping and the detection of enzyme defects. It takes 2–3 weeks for the cells to proliferate sufficiently for investigation and culture is unsuccessful in < 1% of cases. It is ideally performed between 15 and 18 weeks when sufficient liquor is available. Amniocentesis at earlier gestations, particularly 10–13 weeks, appears to carry a higher risk of miscarriage. The risk of pregnancy loss after the procedure is

---

Table 19.3 Women at risk of having a fetus with congenital abnormality.

History
Previous abnormal child/fetus
Family history of abnormality
Maternal age > 35

Current pregnancy
Maternal diabetes (4 × risk)
Consanguineous relationship (2–3 × risk)
Exposure to teratogens—drugs, radiation
Suspicious findings on routine ultrasound scan
Breech presentation (4 × risk)
Oligohydramnios
Polyhydramnios
Severe growth restriction
Twin pregnancy (2 × risk)
Maternal infection with known teratogenic pathogen, e.g. rubella, CMV

1% higher than the background loss rate at any given gestation.

Chorionic villus sampling. CVS involves aspirating placental tissue under ultrasound guidance with a needle either transcervically or transabdominally. Karyotyping and other investigations can be performed immediately on placental tissue, reducing the delay between the procedure and the result. It is also carried out earlier in pregnancy (10–13 weeks), permitting earlier and safer termination of pregnancy if necessary. Fetal loss secondary to the procedure is 2% and probably improves as the operator gains experience.

Cordocentesis. Ultrasound-guided sampling from the umbilical cord permits the direct assessment of the fetal blood, e.g. rapid karyotyping, acid–base status, electrolytes and pathogens, and is possible after 18 weeks' gestation. Because of the invasive nature of this technique, its use is restricted to at-risk fetuses—e.g. severe growth restriction, suspected congenital infection—in specialist units. It is used routinely for intrauterine transfusions of fetuses with haemolytic disease. Rates of fetal loss are approximately 3% but figures for the risk of the procedure are difficult to interpret because of the high-risk group in which the procedure is used.

Fetoscopy. An alternative method for sampling fetal blood or tissue is to do so under direct vision using a fine laparoscope. Fetal losses from this procedure were reported to be about 5% but the technique has been largely superseded by cordocentesis for this purpose. The main use of fetoscopy now is laser ablation of superficial anastomoses in uncommon cases of twin-to-twin transfusions.

Laboratory investigations

Chromosome analysis. Either nuclei are stained immediately (CVS, cordocentesis), or the cells are cultured (CVS, amniocentesis) and the nuclei then stained. Duplication of chromosomes and gross rearrangements (e.g. translocations) are then detectable. The commonest chromosomal abnormalities which survive until term are the trisomies (21 Down syndrome, 18 Edwards syndrome, 13 Patau syndrome) and Turner syndrome (45XO).

Enzyme defects. It is only possible to test for these defects when the fetus is known to be at risk of an inborn error of metabolism for which the genetic mutation is known, i.e. where the parents have had an affected infant previously or screening has revealed the parents to be carriers.

Tests on fetal blood. Rapid karyotyping, FBC, platelet count and other haematological indices can be measured directly on fetal blood. This is only of value after fetal viability (24 weeks' gestation) and is used to assist in the management of severely compromised fetuses (structural abnormality, severe growth restriction).

DNA analysis. Using these methods, abnormal genes are detected in two ways, either directly or indirectly (linkage studies). Direct detection is only possible where the specific mutation has been identified, e.g. sickle cell disease or cystic fibrosis. Some of the more common conditions for which mutations are known are listed in Table 19.4.

Table 19.4 Inherited conditions for which genetic testing is available.	
X-linked recessive	Phenylketonuria
Duchenne muscular dystrophy	Sickle cell anaemia
Fragile X syndrome	Thalassaemia
Haemophilia A and B	
	Autosomal dominant
Autosomal recessive	Huntington's chorea
Cystic fibrosis	Neurofibromatosis

Management of at-risk couples

Irrespective of whether at-risk couples opt for termination of pregnancy or not, genetic counselling is of value. General practitioners and obstetricians should be familiar with the risks and preliminary management of the conditions for which women are routinely screened in antenatal clinics. For at-risk couples, most practitioners will need to involve a medical geneticist and/or genetic counsellor, although the management principles are the same.

These principles include:

1. Knowledge of which couples are at risk from their history or clinical features. It is important that the diagnosis of the affected member(s) of the family is accurate before proceeding further.
2. The natural history of the disease.
3. The range of its clinical manifestations.
4. Possibility and risks of treatment.
5. Accuracy of diagnosis and prognosis.
6. Possibility of detecting carriers.
7. Psychological implications.
8. Likelihood of recurrence and management in subsequent pregnancy.

It is important that information, which is often quite complex, is presented to the parents in a way that they can understand. Although it is difficult to present information in an unbiased manner, this should be the goal. Genetic counselling has been shown to fail to educate at-risk couples adequately in 40% of cases, so repeated visits may be necessary. Other clinicians involved in their care should avoid confusing the situation if they are not fully conversant with the disorder. Couples will often experience grief that must be dealt with before information can be passed on. Most couples then regard the problem in terms of how it will affect their relationship, their immediate family and their financial status.

Follow-up

The need for close follow-up of affected pregnancies is self-evident. If an affected child is delivered, then ongoing paediatric care is usually necessary and the couple then need to return for information on the prognosis for the affected child and recurrence risk in future children. Couples that have opted for termination of pregnancy attend for the results of the post-mortem (if possible) and to discuss again the possibility and management of subsequent pregnancy.

20   Antenatal care

Gregory Davis

Expectations of the examiners

The routine management of pregnancy and the assessment of obstetric risk are fundamental to the appropriate care of pregnant women and the examiners will therefore expect candidates to have a comprehensive grasp of all aspects.

Definition

Antenatal case has been defined as 'a planned program of observation, education, and medical management of pregnant women directed toward making pregnancy and delivery a safe and satisfying experience' (American College of Obstetricians and Gynecologists).

Interesting facts

At least 80% of pregnant women would deliver healthy babies without any antenatal care and very few of the measures used routinely in antenatal care have been properly evaluated.

The objectives of antenatal care are:

1. To predict problems on the basis of the medical, social and obstetric history and physical examination
2. To prevent or reduce the severity of problems by prophylactic measures
3. To detect and treat conditions which have harmful effects on the mother or fetus
4. To provide education, information and reassurance for the pregnant woman and her partner.

The current approach to routine antenatal care ideally involves:

1. Prepregnancy counselling (see Ch. 19)
2. Booking visit
3. Routine antenatal visits
4. Antenatal education classes
5. Inpatient care if required.

BOOKING VISIT

Assessment

The booking visit is the most important visit in most women's antenatal care. At this visit, risk factors are assessed and future antenatal care and place of delivery decided. Pregnant women are usually seen by a midwife initially and a history is taken, special investigations are performed or ordered, information on maternity benefits and antenatal education classes is given and a date is made for a further appointment. At the next visit the woman sees a member of the medical staff, by which time results of initial investigations are available to assist in further decisions. This process may also be completed at a single visit.

Timing

Ideally the woman should be seen as early as possible to confirm pregnancy and to deal with any early requirements, e.g. chorionic villus sampling at 10–12 weeks. At the latest, the woman should be seen by 16–18 weeks' gestation to allow for accurate assessment of gestational age and exclusion of structural anomalies by ultrasound, and by amniocentesis if necessary.

History

The booking history should include:

1. Identification details
2. Social history
3. Menstrual/contraceptive history
4. Past obstetric history
5. Medical conditions
6. Factors associated with genetic risk
7. General condition.

Identification details. These should include the woman's full name, address, next of kin and race. In addition, her general practitioner's name, address and whether he or she wishes to undertake shared care should be recorded.

Social history. Details of the woman's occupation, marital status and social circumstances should be noted. The social history should include her attitude to the pregnancy and that of her partner. Her partner's race, occupation and level of support should be recorded. Details of housing are important as these may need to be changed during pregnancy and eligibility for benefits assessed.

A full drug history should be obtained including prescribed and illicit drugs, alcohol and tobacco. All women should be encouraged to give up the latter three and prescribed medications may need to be modified in pregnancy.

Menstrual/contraceptive history. The date (and degree of certainty) of the last menstrual period (LMP) must be established along with the regularity and length of the menstrual cycle. If the LMP was abnormal the last normal menstrual period should be recorded with a note of any subsequent bleeding. If the woman was using the combined oral contraceptive then it should be determined whether the LMP was a withdrawal bleed. In some cases, such as pregnancy after a period of amenorrhoea or after previous pregnancy, the menstrual history is unhelpful. Duration and treatment of previous infertility should be noted.

If an intrauterine device is still present (and the strings are visible on examination) this should be removed to reduce the possibility of later septic abortion. As in all women of reproductive age who present with amenorrhoea, ectopic pregnancy should be excluded.

Past obstetric history. This is the most important part of the history in terms of identifying risk factors for the current pregnancy. Details of all previous pregnancies including miscarriages, terminations of pregnancy and ectopic pregnancies should be recorded. The gestations of previous pregnancies, complications and details of delivery, and postnatal complications should be noted. The paternity of all previous pregnancies should also be determined. Previous stillbirth or intrauterine growth restriction are indications for increased monitoring of pregnancy in the third trimester. A history of recurrent, painless mid-trimester abortion suggests cervical incompetence that requires a cervical suture. A previous baby delivered spontaneously and prematurely is the best predictor of preterm delivery in the current pregnancy. If a previous baby was delivered by caesarean section, the indications for operation and the woman's attitude to the operation must be carefully determined to assess whether a trial of labour is suitable. This may require communication with a previous hospital. Any problems in the third stage of labour will necessitate the presence of an obstetrician at subsequent deliveries. A previous baby with a congenital abnormality or other neonatal problems may be an indication for prenatal testing.

Medical conditions. Any medical condition in the woman should be noted. A brief series of direct questions to exclude major disease should include:

1. Diabetes (gestational or pre-existing)
2. Epilepsy
3. Thromboembolic disease
4. Anaemia
5. Chest disease
6. Hypertension
7. Cardiac disease (congenital or acquired)
8. Renal disease
9. Endocrine disease (thyroid, adrenal)
10. Sexually transmitted disease
11. Rubella.

All of these conditions affect, or are affected by, pregnancy to a greater or lesser extent.

Previous operations, particularly those with relevance to the pregnancy, e.g. previous cone biopsy (risk of cervical incompetence) or bladder surgery (risk of weakening repair) should be recorded. Any psychiatric history increases the risk of postpartum psychiatric problems and should be specifically elicited as many women wish to avoid discussing this. Any allergies should be prominently recorded in the hospital notes and any record the woman keeps.

All women should be asked the date and result of their last cervical smear and this should be repeated if it has not been done in the previous 2 years or was previously abnormal.

Genetic risk.   Individuals at increased risk of fetal abnormality include:

1. Maternal age greater than 35 years—risk of chromosomal abnormality
2. Afro-Caribbean women—risk of sickle cell disease
3. Mediterranean or Asian women—risk of thalassaemia
4. Ashkenazi Jews—risk of Tay–Sachs disease
5. Previous child with abnormality
6. Family history of fetal abnormality, inherited diseases, e.g. haemophilia.

Prenatal diagnosis should be discussed with these women and appropriate action taken (see Ch. 19).

General condition.   The woman should be asked if she has any complaints currently including vaginal bleeding or discharge, vomiting or concern over the pregnancy. Any questions the woman has about antenatal care or her health should be answered at this stage.

Examination

The woman should be weighed and her height and blood pressure measured. The cardiovascular and respiratory systems should be examined and the breasts checked for masses or inverted nipples. Abdominal examination is performed to confirm the presence of a pelvic mass (after 12 weeks' gestation) or, later in pregnancy, fetal growth, presentation and lie.

The fundus reaches the umbilicus at 20–24 weeks' gestation and the xiphisternum at 36–38 weeks. The presence of the fetal heart is confirmed with a Pinard fetal stethoscope (after 28 weeks' gestation) or a sonicaid (after 12–14 weeks). The lie is readily determined after 28–30 weeks.

Pelvic examination confirms gestation, excludes pelvic pathology and permits a cervical smear to be taken. However, unless a cervical smear is required, the value of a routine pelvic examination is debatable in a setting where routine ultrasound is performed.

Investigations

Blood tests

The blood tests routinely performed at booking are:

1. FBC
2. Blood group and antibody screen
3. Serology for hepatitis B, syphilis, rubella, HIV
4. Triple test screening (may be offered).

Also in at-risk groups:

1. Sickle test
2. Haemoglobin electrophoresis.

The most common form of anaemia detected is due to iron deficiency. The lower limit of normal in pregnancy is reduced because of the haemodilution that occurs (10.5 or 11 g/dL). If the hepatitis serology is positive (HBsAg), then further testing for HBeAg and HBsAb is carried out. Routine testing for syphilis usually includes Venereal Diseases Research Laboratory (VDRL) and *Treponema pallidum* haemagglutination assay (TPHA) and, if these are positive, testing for current infection is carried out. Rubella immunity is assessed by screening for IgG unless there has been a possible recent contact, in which case the IgM levels are measured and repeated in 2 weeks to look for a rise in titre (indicating recent infection). If the IgG is negative and there is no prenatal infection, vaccination is performed after delivery.

Nuchal translucency scan and serum test
This is carried out at 11–13 weeks (see Ch. 19).

Triple test for Down syndrome
This is performed at 16–18 weeks; amniocentesis is indicated if there is increased risk (see Ch. 19).

Routine ultrasound scan (see Figs 20.1 and 20.2)
In most units this is carried out at 18–20 weeks for the following reasons:

1. Accurate assessment of gestation. Even in those women with certain dates, ultrasound has been demonstrated to be more accurate. It is also important for interpretation of the triple test for Down syndrome.
2. Detection of multiple pregnancy.
3. Detection of congenital abnormalities in the fetus.

Fig. 20.1   Ultrasound scan in which the spine is seen in its entirety.

Fig. 20.2 Ultrasound scan. The defect in the spine (spina bifida) is clearly seen.

4. Determination of the placental site. Although the placental site can usually be detected accurately at this gestation, many units do not routinely rescan those women with a low-lying placenta because the vast majority will resolve as the lower segment forms at 28–34 weeks.
5. Reassurance for mother and partner.

There is no evidence that ultrasound in the prenatal period is dangerous for the fetus (or the mother).

Assessment of risk

Many lists of risk factors have been published and one is included in Appendix II. Failing to identify risk factors or to take appropriate action when they are known to be present is a common error in antenatal care. Pregnant women can be classified as being of low, moderate or high risk and their pregnancy managed accordingly. Risk based on factors in the history is assessed at the booking visit but the development of problems in pregnancy may necessitate reappraisal.

Type of antenatal care

For most women this involves a choice between full hospital care shared between general practitioner and hospital or total midwifery care. For low-risk women, shared care is usually more convenient and reduces waiting times in hospital antenatal clinics. High-risk women are usually seen exclusively at the hospital while the care of those with moderate risk should be decided on an individual basis.

Place of delivery

Only 1% of women now deliver at home. If the woman wishes to do so, then she should be of low risk and supervised by a registered domiciliary midwife and doctor. Ideally, these women should be seen at the hospital for a booking visit and at least one visit later in pregnancy although, in practice, women who opt for home delivery often avoid hospitals. Low-risk women suitable for home delivery must:

1. Be healthy women aged 19–34 years
2. Be para one or two
3. Have no major contraindications.

Major contraindications include:

1. Previous complicated obstetric/medical history
2. Major gynaecological surgery or condition (including infertility)
3. Under 152 cm (5 ft) in height
4. Excessive weight
5. Abnormality in current pregnancy
6. Postmaturity in current pregnancy
7. Significant social problems
8. No telephone available/difficult access to home.

An alternative to home delivery offered in most delivery units is 'domino' (domiciliary in and out) care. Women in labour of low or moderate risk are cared for in the delivery unit by domiciliary midwives and, provided all is normal, discharged 6–12 hours after delivery. If there are problems in labour, then care can be safely and efficiently transferred to the hospital.

SUBSEQUENT VISITS

The timing of routine antenatal visits is variable but is traditionally every 4 weeks until 28 weeks, fortnightly until 36 weeks and weekly thereafter. If the woman is receiving shared care then the same routine should be followed but hospital visits should be at 32 weeks, and 40 or 41 weeks. Reducing the frequency of visits has not been shown to compromise fetal or maternal outcomes but may make women less satisfied with their antenatal care.

There is wide variation between hospitals on the timing of these visits. If an abnormality is detected then the frequency of visits is increased and care may be transferred completely to the hospital.

Examination

As most antenatal visits will reveal no abnormality, it is important to avoid complacency and to maintain a high degree of alertness for potential problems. At each visit, the woman's blood pressure is measured and a urine sample tested for protein and glucose.

The blood pressure usually falls in the second trimester and should be considered abnormal if it is more than 140/90 mmHg on two separate occasions 24 hours apart.

Proteinuria may be due to contamination of the specimen by vaginal discharge. If present on a midstream urine sample early in pregnancy, it is usually due to infection or chronic renal disease and these should be investigated. Its appearance later in pregnancy suggests infection or pre-eclampsia and, in the presence of even mildly elevated blood pressure, warrants admission for further assessment.

Glycosuria on more than one occasion is an indication for an oral glucose tolerance test to exclude diabetes, although it is commonly due to the lowered renal threshold for glucose excretion in pregnancy.

Abdominal examination is performed to assess fetal growth and the symphysiofundal height. There is debate over the relative merits of the tape measure versus the hand, but candidates should be able to use a tape measure to assess fundal height whatever their clinical practice. The liquor volume is assessed and presentation checked from 32 weeks. After 36 weeks persistent breech presentation should be managed appropriately (see Ch. 29). The fetal head often engages from 36–38 weeks in nulliparous women but in at least 40% of parous women, engagement does not occur until labour begins. Abnormal causes of an unengaged head are:

1. Pelvic mass—placenta praevia, fibroid
2. Large presenting diameter—hydrocephalus, malpresentation, malposition
3. Large uterus—polyhydramnios, multiple pregnancy, multiparity
4. Small pelvis—cephalopelvic disproportion, abnormal pelvis.

The ease with which the head enters the pelvis can be determined by gently pressing the head into the pelvis with the woman semiseated. A pelvic examination may be performed to exclude major bony abnormality, and many obstetricians will repeat the ultrasound scan if the head remains high after 38 weeks. The efficacy of these measures has not been determined.

Investigations

Routine screening tests have been described. The haemoglobin concentration and antibody titres in Rhesus-negative women are measured at 30 and 36 weeks unless they are abnormal.

The most common causes of anaemia in pregnancy are iron and folate deficiency. These can be avoided by the administration of combined iron/folate preparations but many women find them difficult to take. Opinion on their routine use varies, but anaemia, if associated with microcytosis, should be treated with oral iron. Women should be seen weekly and compliance checked by asking the woman the colour of her stools and by measuring the haemoglobin concentration and reticulocyte count. Iron infusion is dangerous and it is better to admit the woman to ensure compliance with oral iron.

In some centres, Rhesus-negative women are routinely given anti-D immunoglobulin at 28 and 34 weeks to reduce the incidence of sensitization prior to delivery. It is now common to perform a screening test for abnormal glucose tolerance between 28 and 32 weeks. This usually comprises a 50 or 75 g oral glucose load with a blood glucose level 1 hour later. Normal values vary widely depending on the load given and the criteria adopted by each hospital.

Assessment of fetal growth

One of the major reasons for antenatal care is the detection of reduced fetal growth and yet failure to do so is common (50% undetected). The means of monitoring fetal growth are:

1. Clinical assessment at antenatal visits/symphysiofundal height
2. Fetal movements
3. Fetal heart rate recordings
4. Ultrasound assessment
5. Biophysical profile of the fetus
6. Doppler investigation of fetoplacental circulation
7. Cordocentesis.

The use of tests representing placental synthetic function, e.g. urinary oestriol, human placental lactogen (HPL), has largely been superseded by other measures. This is principally because these tests do not specifically measure fetal well-being and may be unreliable.

Clinical assessment

The importance of vigilance during routine antenatal clinics has been stressed.

Fetal movements

Every pregnant woman attending for antenatal care should be questioned regarding fetal movements over the preceding few days. A significant decrease in movements warrants further investigation, i.e. ultrasound scan and fetal heart rate recording and subsequent closer surveillance.

Most women report that their babies move less towards term and it is often difficult to assess. It is better to be overcautious in this respect. The efficacy of fetal movement charts is debated but they do make women more aware of fetal activity.

Ultrasound assessment

Ultrasound will only assess fetal growth if used in a serial manner. Although a single scan may suggest growth restriction, i.e. disproportionately low overall fetal measurements (symmetrical growth restriction), reduced abdominal circumference (asymmetrical growth restriction) or reduced liquor volume, a follow-up scan is usually necessary to assess growth. The routine scan at 18–20 weeks is vital to confirm that gestation is correct.

Biophysical profile

A fetal heart rate monitor and ultrasound machine are used simultaneously to assess in the fetus:

1. Limb and body movements
2. Breathing movements
3. Tone
4. Amniotic fluid volume
5. Heart rate variability.

Each of these variables is scored to make up the profile. Of these parameters, amniotic fluid volume is probably the most important.

Fetal heart rate recording

This gives an indication of the current status of the fetus. A normal pattern with accelerations in response to fetal movements is a good indication of normal fetal well-being. However, its ability to predict future fetal health is uncertain.

The significance of some patterns can be difficult to interpret, particularly in very preterm fetuses. The presence of decelerations when the woman is not in labour usually indicates that delivery is required.

Fetoplacental blood flow

The use of the Doppler principle to measure blood flow velocity in the uterine and umbilical arteries, together with the fetal arterial system, is helpful in the assessment of high-risk pregnancies. Perinatal outcome has been shown to be improved using this technique. Studies in low-risk pregnancies as a screening test for detecting fetal compromise have shown no benefit.

Reduced, absent or even reverse flow in the umbilical artery during diastole is an indication of increased placental resistance and probably impaired fetal oxygenation. Used in conjunction with other tests this investigation may be helpful in judging when to deliver preterm fetuses.

Cordocentesis

Rarely cordocentesis is used to monitor the condition of the severely compromised fetus, usually in the second trimester when a karyotype may also be required. The measurement of fetal arterial pH, acid–base status and oxygenation may give information about a severely compromised fetus at one time point, but unfortunately cannot give predictive information. As the risks of serial sampling are not insignificant, non-invasive assessment is preferred.

General advice in pregnancy

Pregnancy is a stressful time for both partners (and other children). Antenatal visits should provide the opportunity for women to ask about minor problems as well as ensuring that all screening tests and routine assessment are carried out. Most hospital clinics provide mothers with an easily readable information booklet.

Diet

Although pregnancy increases the mother's dietary requirements, a balanced diet is sufficient to provide all the calories, protein, minerals and vitamins required. The only exception is iron. If iron is not given in pregnancy, iron stores will decline. However, provided that these were adequate initially this is not a problem. Women who are already anaemic, have depleted iron stores (grand multipara, recent pregnancy) or who have a multiple pregnancy should have combined iron and folate supplementation.

Exercise

The amount of exercise desirable in pregnancy has never been determined. It seems prudent not to begin vigorous exercise when pregnant and similarly safe to continue routine exercise as long as it is not causing serious discomfort.

Sexual activity

There is no evidence that coitus is harmful in pregnancy. Most obstetricians advise against coitus in the first trimester in women who have had recurrent miscarriages, but there is no evidence to support this view. Some women lose their inclination for sex as pregnancy advances because of their increasing awkwardness and feelings of not being attractive. Couples should be encouraged to communicate these feelings. Sexual techniques may need to be modified as pregnancy advances.

Rest and sleep

Most women are more easily fatigued in pregnancy and there is some evidence that regular resting improves fetal outcome. Resting should therefore be encouraged.

Sleep patterns tend to become less regular with more frequent waking as pregnancy continues and women may need daytime naps to catch up.

Employment

The evidence regarding the effect of work on pregnancy is difficult to assess. Jobs involving a lot of standing may lead to reduced fetal growth but other variables are important, such as the number of children the pregnant woman cares for at home. It seems sensible to advise each woman individually depending on her wishes, type of work and demands of her home life.

Heavy manual labour should be avoided and pregnant women must be allowed to rest if necessary. Noxious fumes, extremes of temperature and working to exhaustion should be avoided.

Clothing

A supportive brassiere and comfortable clothes are the basic requirements. Most women find flat-heeled shoes more comfortable in later pregnancy.

Preparation for lactation

All participants in antenatal care should strongly encourage breast-feeding. In the antenatal period it is important to ensure that the woman understands the advantages of breast-feeding and the normal events in milk production after delivery.

There is no need to encourage frequent handling of the nipples to prepare them for feeding. Inverted nipples usually correct themselves during pregnancy and can be made to protrude with gentle manipulation. If these measures are unsuccessful then nipple shields are used and kept in place by the brassiere.

Antenatal education

Classes are usually available in hospital clinics. A wide range of matters need to be covered including changes in late pregnancy, when to come in to the delivery suite, choice of methods for delivery position and pain relief, what clothes the baby will need and when to buy them, how to cope with a new baby and discussion on how the baby is likely to affect the couple.

Most classes take prospective parents on a tour of the labour and postnatal wards. Birth plans are encouraged at most hospitals but it is important to emphasize that labour and delivery can be unpredictable and that all women (and their partners) need to retain an open mind. Questioning should be encouraged and all answers should be given in terms which can be easily understood.

Follow-up

One of the most important aspects of antenatal care is that follow-up should occur so that the woman and her partner have the opportunity to discuss their labour and management. Much of this discussion occurs on the postnatal ward and with the visits of the domiciliary midwife after discharge from hospital. This information is important in ensuring that misunderstandings are corrected and negative experiences discussed. Where the pregnancy and, particularly, the delivery have been difficult, follow-up with an obstetrician to discuss these matters may be helpful.

21   Minor disorders of pregnancy

Gregory Davis

Expectations of the examiners

As these disorders are not usually disabling they are often managed by general practitioners. The examiners will therefore expect candidates to have a sound understanding of, and a common sense approach to, their management.

Nausea and vomiting

The majority of women experience some nausea in early pregnancy and 50% will vomit. Although classically worse in the mornings, nausea may occur throughout the day and is often made worse by the odours associated with preparing food. If severe, multiple pregnancy and hydatidiform mole need to be excluded. Symptoms usually improve after 14–16 weeks although many women continue to experience nausea, and sometimes vomiting, more frequently than when not pregnant.

Management

In most instances, symptoms can be controlled by dietary measures. Greasy or highly spiced foods should be avoided and frequent small meals usually improve the nausea. A rearrangement of housekeeping duties may be required if the woman is responsible for these. Reassurance, practical help in coping with the symptoms and the knowledge that the problem usually improves, are important aspects of the medical care. Supplementation with multivitamin preparations has been shown to reduce nausea in early pregnancy significantly.

Admission to hospital is required if the woman is becoming dehydrated (ketones in urine), if there is significant weight loss or if the social situation is getting out of control. In hospital, fluids are given intravenously (with potassium supplementation), antiemetics are used (initially metoclopramide then prochlorperazine if this is ineffective) and no oral intake is permitted. The condition usually improves by 24–36 hours and dry biscuits can usually be introduced by 48 hours. If there is no improvement, then intravenous alimentation may be required. Early discharge from hospital should be discouraged as it is often followed by prompt readmission.

Heartburn

This is also common in pregnancy and results from gastric reflux due to relaxation of the lower oesophageal sphincter and pressure from the enlarging uterus later in pregnancy.

It should be treated by discouraging smoking (increases sphincter relaxation), recommending frequent, light, bland meals, avoiding a late meal, and raising the head of the bed by about 20 cm. Antacid preparations, e.g. magnesium trisilicate, may also be helpful but those that are likely to cause constipation should be avoided (aluminium-containing).

Constipation/bloating

It is thought that these symptoms are due to decreased bowel motility because of high levels of progesterone. Normal measures should be used to combat constipation: dietary fibre and fluid intake should increase, sugar intake should decrease and a bulk laxative, e.g. ispaghula husk, used if necessary. Bloating seems to occur independently and is difficult to treat effectively. It is more of a problem in early pregnancy.

Haemorrhoids

These occur more frequently in pregnancy due to progesterone-induced venodilatation, obstruction of venous return from the lower body by the enlarging uterus, and increased bearing down because of constipation or at delivery.

Prolapse is best treated with ice packs and replacement if possible. Bleeding is common and a rectal examination should be performed in this instance. For mild symptoms, a soothing preparation with a mild astringent action is usually sufficient. Rarely surgical intervention may be necessary.

Epistaxis

This occurs as a result of increased peripheral vascularity. Normal first aid measures usually suffice and definitive treatment is rarely necessary.

Varicose veins

Varicosities occur mostly in the legs but also in the vulva and vagina and cause aching and tiredness. Thrombophlebitis is the commonest complication and deep venous thrombosis may also occur, although this is more common in the puerperium.

For leg varicosities, the best treatment is a combination of elevation and the use of full-length support tights. Surgical management is best reserved for at least 2–3 months postpartum when the veins will have returned to normal after pregnancy.

Backache

This is a common symptom and results from increased joint laxity in the lumbar spine and the exaggerated lordosis which occurs in pregnancy. Sacroiliac joint laxity may also cause pain. Management is conservative: rest, analgesia and improvement in posture.

Breast soreness

This is commonest in early pregnancy as the breasts increase in size. Reassurance and symptomatic relief with a brassiere that provides adequate support are all that is needed.

Fatigue

This is a common symptom early in pregnancy when the cause is unclear. and late in pregnancy when it is due to the increased physical effort required for everyday life and often a disturbed sleep pattern. The only treatment is frequent rest and reassurance that fatigue is normal.

Peripheral paraesthesiae

Numbness and tingling occur due to compression of peripheral nerves because of fluid retention; most commonly the median nerve is involved (carpal tunnel syndrome). Other nerves may be affected such as the lateral cutaneous nerve of the thigh which supplies the lateral aspect of the thigh. No treatment is usually required when the cause has been explained to the patient although wrist splints at night may be helpful in disabling carpal tunnel syndrome.

Headache

This is usually a typical tension headache and is best treated by rest and mild analgesia. Migraine often improves but may deteriorate, stay the same or occur de novo in pregnancy. The use in pregnancy of agents normally used in the treatment of migraine is not associated with adverse fetal outcome but doses should be kept to the minimum required.

Postural hypotension

This is more likely to occur in pregnancy because of venous pooling in the lower limbs (see 'Haemorrhoids' above). It is best prevented by avoiding precipitating factors: standing up quickly, hot baths and standing in hot weather.

Pruritus

Itching in pregnancy may be localized or generalized. Local causes are usually infectious (e.g. thrush). Generalized itching (pruritus gravidarum) usually begins in the third trimester. If there is no rash it is usually associated with some degree of biliary obstruction. Liver function tests should be carried out and fasting bile acids measured. Frank jaundice is rare but cholestasis of pregnancy must be distinguished from other causes of liver disease in pregnancy and non-pregnancy.

Cholestasis in pregnancy used to be considered a benign condition. However, more recent evidence suggests an increased perinatal mortality. For this reason, most obstetricians would induce labour at 36–38 weeks depending on the severity of the cholestasis. The use of synthetic bile salt analogues is very effective in relieving the itch and correcting the biochemical abnormalities in bile acids and liver function tests. Anecdotally the fetal outcomes also appear improved. Treatment with skin lubrication and topical anti-pruritics may be sufficient and antihistamines are of limited benefit.

The pruritus disappears shortly after delivery but recurs in 50% of subsequent pregnancies.

Frequency of micturition

Again this is a symptom of early pregnancy when it is due to increased renal filtration, and of late pregnancy when it is due to pressure from the enlarged uterus. There is no treatment for this symptom except delivery. Urinary tract infection is also common in pregnancy and needs to be excluded.

Insomnia

Disturbed sleep is often a result of normal anxiety about being pregnant and, later, discomfort from the increased size of breasts and abdomen. Sedatives should be avoided unless the woman is exhausted and should then be used for a very brief period, e.g. 2–3 nights. Relaxation exercises to relieve anxiety may be of benefit.

SUMMARY

Minor disorders of pregnancy are very common but serious conditions need to be excluded, e.g. imminent eclampsia causing headache, viral hepatitis causing pruritus. Education and reassurance together with simple, practical remedies are the basis for treatment of most of these conditions.

22 Infections in pregnancy

Adam Rodin

Expectations of the examiners

An understanding of the effects on the mother and the fetus of significant infections in pregnancy is needed.

Interesting facts

Maternal infections during pregnancy are common and usually insignificant but may result in congenital infection and handicap. The incidence of death or handicap as a result of intrauterine infection is estimated to be 0.4 in 1000 live births. The incidence of many congenital infections shows marked regional variation, e.g. toxoplasmosis is commoner in France than in the UK. In some cases, congenital infections can be prevented and/or treated. The role of ascending infection in the causation of preterm labour is currently being evaluated.

Pathogenesis

Infections may reach the fetus by four main routes:

1. Transplacental spread from the maternal bloodstream
2. Ascending infection from the genital tract after rupture of membranes
3. Infection acquired during passage of the fetus through the birth canal
4. Rarely, infection following invasive intra-amniotic procedures, e.g. amniocentesis and fetoscopy.

The effects on the fetus depend on the nature of the infective organism, the gestation at which infection occurs and the immune status of the mother. Following maternal infection there may be no spread to the fetus; however, it may reach the placenta and infect the fetus in utero. Fetal infection may manifest itself by abortion or stillbirth. If the pregnancy continues, the infant may be born with a variety of abnormalities (TORCH syndrome, see below) and it may develop acute neonatal illness. An infant of an infected mother who appears normal at birth may develop late effects and should be followed up.

The infectious agents causing the TORCH syndrome are:

1. Toxoplasmosis
2. Rubella
3. Cytomegalovirus
4. Herpes simplex.

These cause a mild, non-specific maternal illness and similar patterns of fetal damage. Features of the TORCH syndrome include:

1. Low birth weight
2. Microcephaly
3. Congenital heart disease
4. Eye lesions
5. Jaundice
6. Hepatosplenomegaly
7. Petechiae/purpura
8. Late effects
   a. Visual defects
   b. Deafness
   c. Developmental delay
   d. Mental retardation.

RUBELLA

The association between maternal rubella infection in pregnancy and congenital heart disease and cataracts in the neonate was first described in 1941. Rubella is an RNA virus and is spread by droplet infection.

Maternal illness
There is a mild febrile illness with a macular rash and lymphadenopathy; many infections are subclinical. One infection confers a high degree of immunity and congenital infection usually follows primary maternal infection.

Fetal effects
The risk of congenital defects depends on the gestation at which infection occurs; infection in the first trimester carries a high risk of major defects and infection between 12 and 16 weeks may cause sensorineural deafness.

Hearing impairment is the most frequent defect associated with rubella.

Screening
All women are screened for rubella antibody (IgG) at booking. Susceptible women who develop a rash or come into contact with rubella have blood taken to check rubella IgG. If this is positive, IgM is measured to confirm recent infection.

Immunization
A live attenuated virus vaccine was introduced in 1970 and this was given to prepubertal girls and non-immune women.

Ninety-eight per cent of women in the UK attending antenatal clinics are now immune to rubella.

In 1988, MMR (measles, mumps and rubella) vaccination was introduced and this is given to all male and female infants between 1 and 2 years of age in an attempt to eradicate rubella. Vaccination of prepubertal girls and non-immune women will continue until sufficient numbers have received it.

Vaccination should not be administered during pregnancy and conception within 3 months should be avoided.

CYTOMEGALOVIRUS

Cytomegalovirus (CMV) is the most common congenital infection and approximately 3 in 1000 live births are infected in England and Wales each year. CMV is a DNA virus of the herpes group and it is spread venereally by the oropharyngeal route or by blood transfusion.

Maternal illness
CMV infection is usually symptomless; therefore diagnosis is retrospective following discovery of a congenitally infected infant. Fifty per cent of adults have antibodies to CMV. Fetal infection may follow primary maternal infection or reactivation of maternal infection.

Fetal effects
Diagnosis is made by isolation of the virus from urine or a throat swab in the first few weeks of life.

Defects may follow infection at any gestation and 10% of infected infants have significant handicaps. Sensorineural deafness is the most common sequel. Acute neonatal illness (cytomegalic inclusion disease) occurs in 5% of infected infants and is associated with a high mortality.

Screening
This is not useful because congenital infection may follow reactivation of an old infection and defects may follow exposure at any gestation. Most cases of maternal CMV infection are asymptomatic.

Immunization
Immunization is not available.

TOXOPLASMOSIS

This is an infection with the protozoon parasite *Toxoplasma gondii*. Oocysts from this organism are found in raw meat and cat faeces. The incidence of infection in the UK is estimated to be 2 per 1000 pregnancies. Congenital infection is rare in this country and approximately 1 in 100 000 live births are infected.

Maternal illness
The infection is asymptomatic in 60–70% of cases. When symptoms are present they are usually mild and non-specific. Ten per cent of affected women have fever and lymphadenopathy.

About 80% of women are seronegative. If infection is suspected maternal serum is sent to the reference laboratory.

Fetal effects
Fetal infection is generally only seen after primary infection in the mother; however, congenital toxoplasmosis has been reported following reactivation of latent infection in immunocompromised mothers. The risk of transmission increases as gestation advances, with an average risk of 40%. The earlier the infection occurs, the more severe the effects. Classic manifestations are hydrocephaly, retinochoroiditis and intracranial calcification. Stillbirth, neonatal death or severe handicap occurs in 5% of these infants.

Fetal infection is confirmed by amniocentesis and polymerase chain reaction (PCR).

Management
Spiramycin is the drug of choice for treatment of the mother with confirmed acute infection in pregnancy. Treatment is continued until delivery. This drug reduces the risk of congenital infection by 60–70%.

Screening
There is no antenatal screening programme in the UK. Women thought to be at risk may request a blood test for *Toxoplasma* IgG antibody. As most women are seronegative at booking, there is a possibility of seroconversion during pregnancy. Maternal screening will not identify fetal infection.

HERPES SIMPLEX

Herpes simplex virus (HSV) is a DNA virus and is widespread in human populations. Most perinatal infections are caused by HSV type II. Transplacental infection is rare and infection usually occurs during delivery. Primary genital herpes acquired at or near the time of delivery is associated with a significant risk of transmission to the neonate estimated at 40%.

Maternal illness
Primary infection with HSV type II is classically associated with genital ulceration but may be asymptomatic or undetected. It may be difficult to distinguish between primary and recurrent genital herpes in pregnancy. Recurrent genital herpes is associated with a very low risk of neonatal herpes.

Fetal effects

Neonatal herpes is rare in the UK with approximately 10 new cases reported per year. The incidence is 1.65/100 000 live births. In the USA the incidence is higher at 1 in 7500 live births. It causes a systemic viral infection with severe neonatal morbidity. Infected infants may develop meningitis or encephalitis, with mental retardation in survivors. Approximately 75% of neonatal infections are due to HSV type II and 25% due to HSV type I.

Management

Women with primary genital herpes presenting in pregnancy should be referred to a genitourinary physician. Aciclovir is prescribed. It appears to be safe in pregnancy with no evidence of fetal or maternal ill effects. Delivery by caesarean section is recommended for all women who develop primary genital herpes near term. Recurrent genital herpes is not considered an indication for delivery by caesarean section.

Screening

There is no screening programme for herpes in pregnancy. Due to the low incidence of neonatal herpes, screening is unlikely to be cost-effective. The practice of taking viral swabs to detect recurrent herpes at the end of pregnancy is no longer recommended.

CHICKENPOX (VARICELLA)

Chickenpox or primary herpes zoster is unusual during pregnancy as most adults are infected in childhood and 90% of the antenatal population are seropositive for varicella zoster virus IgG antibody. Varicella zoster virus is a DNA virus from the herpes group. It is highly contagious and is spread by droplets or contact with vesicular fluid.

Maternal illness

Chickenpox is a febrile illness with a characteristic pruritic rash. Incubation period is 21 days. It is infectious 48 hours before the rash appears and until vesicles crust over.

After primary infection the virus remains dormant in the sensory nerve root ganglia. It can be reactivated to form a painful skin rash known as shingles. This does not cause fetal complications.

Varicella infection in adults is associated with higher morbidity than in children. Complications include pneumonia, hepatitis and encephalitis. Pneumonia occurs in 10% of pregnant women with chickenpox and its severity increases with advancing gestation. Maternal death has been reported.

Fetal effects

Maternal infection in the first half of pregnancy may be complicated by fetal varicella syndrome in 1–2% of cases. This is characterized by skin scarring, eye defects, limb hypoplasia and neurological abnormalities.

Infection between 20 and 36 weeks is not detrimental to the fetus. Later infection may result in varicella infection of the newborn (previously known as congenital varicella). Severe neonatal chickenpox is likely if birth is within 7 days of the onset of the mother's rash.

Management

If there is a history of significant contact with chickenpox the susceptibility of the woman should be ascertained. If there is a definite history of chickenpox it is safe to assume that she is immune. If there is a doubt serum should be taken to check varicella zoster virus IgG. If it is present within days of contact she can be reassured that she is immune. Non-immune women should be given varicella zoster immune globulin (VZIG) as soon as possible.

Pregnant women (> 20 weeks) with chickenpox should be prescribed oral aciclovir if they present within 24 hours of development of the rash. VZIG is of no benefit.

If the mother develops chickenpox within 5 days of delivery, the neonate should be given VZIG and observed for any signs of lesions.

LISTERIA

Listeriosis is caused by *Listeria monocytogenes*. This is a Gram-positive bacillus which is widely distributed in the environment. It has been found in soft cheeses and prepacked foods. Listeriosis occurs in 1 in 7000 pregnancies.

Maternal effects

There is a non-specific febrile illness.

Fetal effects

Listeriosis is associated with spontaneous abortion, stillbirth and neonatal death.

Management

Ampicillin is used.

PARVOVIRUS B19

This is a DNA virus which is spread by respiratory droplets. In children it causes fifth disease, which is a febrile illness characterized by a rash producing a 'slapped cheek' appearance. It has an incubation period of 4–14 days and is no longer infectious by the time the rash appears.

Maternal illness
There is a non-specific illness with arthralgia, lymphadenopathy, fatigue and depression. Following maternal viraemia, transmission of virus to the fetus occurs in 30% of cases.

Fetal effects
Fetal infection is associated with non-immune hydrops fetalis due to profound haemolytic anaemia. It may also be associated with intrauterine growth retardation. No specific teratogenic effect has been identified. Stillbirth may occur 1–12 weeks after infection.

Management
If maternal infection is suspected serology is used to confirm. Symptomatic treatment is given to the mother. Weekly scans are performed to watch for development of hydrops. If hydrops develops fetal blood transfusion may be necessary.

OTHER INFECTIONS IN PREGNANCY

Urinary tract infections
Urinary tract infections are common and range in severity from asymptomatic bacteriuria to pyelonephritis. *E. coli* is responsible for up to 90% of urinary tract infections during pregnancy. Bacteriuria (> 100 000 bacteria/ml urine) may be asymptomatic and is found in 5% of women on routine screening. Acute pyelonephritis complicates up to 2% of pregnancies and is associated with an increased incidence of preterm labour. Patients are admitted to hospital and treated initially with intravenous antibiotics.

See also Chapter 39, 'Sexually transmitted infections in women'.

23 Major complications of pregnancy

PART 1
PRETERM LABOUR   *Adam Rodin*

Expectations of the examiners

A clear understanding of this subject is essential and the candidate is expected to be able to discuss the areas of controversy in its management.

Definitions

Prematurity is defined as delivery prior to 37 completed weeks of pregnancy (WHO definition). In practical terms, most complications occur at gestations less than 34 weeks and most obstetricians would allow delivery beyond this gestation. Low birth weight infants weigh less than 2500 g at delivery and they may be preterm, growth-restricted or both. Very low birth weight infants weigh less than 1500 g at delivery.

Interesting facts

Preterm labour complicates 5–10% of pregnancies and it is the major factor contributing to perinatal mortality and morbidity. Preterm delivery is responsible for 75% of all perinatal deaths and 85% of neonatal deaths not due to congenital abnormality. The diagnosis of preterm labour is difficult and up to 50% of women who complain of painful uterine contractions prior to 37 weeks do not proceed to delivery.

The survival rate of preterm infants has increased in recent years and this is mainly due to advances in neonatal care. After 32 weeks, survival is almost equivalent to that of infants born at term, and in most centres, survival of infants weighing > 1000 g is 70%. Preterm delivery may be associated with long-term handicap.

Pathophysiology

The mechanism of normal and preterm labour remains unknown and therefore the pathophysiology of this process remains uncertain. In about 60% of cases a cause can be identified but the remainder are idiopathic.

Causes of preterm labour
1. Maternal
   a. Pre-eclampsia
   b. Antepartum haemorrhage
   c. Chorioamnionitis
   d. Other infections, e.g. pyelonephritis
   e. Uterine abnormalities, e.g. congenital septa, cervical incompetence
   f. Polyhydramnios
2. Fetal
   a. Multiple pregnancy
   b. Intrauterine death
   c. Congenital abnormality
   d. Growth retardation.

In addition, a number of risk factors have been identified which are thought to increase the chances of preterm labour and delivery in an individual:

Risk factors for preterm labour
1. General
   a. Low socioeconomic class
   b. Multiparity
   c. Maternal age < 20 years
   d. Low prepregnancy weight
   e. Smoking
2. Past obstetric factors
   a. Previous preterm labour
   b. Previous low birth weight infant
   c. Previous antepartum haemorrhage
3. Current pregnancy
   a. Threatened miscarriage
   b. Unexplained elevated AFP
   c. Antepartum haemorrhage

Attempts to devise scoring systems to predict the risk of preterm delivery have been unsuccessful and the best predictor is a previous preterm delivery.

The role of infection as a cause of preterm labour is being evaluated. Vaginal colonization with *Gardnerella vaginalis*, *Mycoplasma hominis*, *Ureaplasma urealyticum*, *Trichomonas vaginalis*, Bacteroides and group B streptococcus all increase the risk of preterm labour and delivery. Bacterial vaginosis is most closely associated with preterm labour and delivery.

Assessment
It is essential to make an accurate diagnosis of preterm labour before any intervention is initiated. A history is taken and questions are directed at finding a cause for preterm labour. Gestational age is checked. General examination is performed and the state of the cervix is assessed noting whether membranes are ruptured or intact.

Cardiotocography is used to assess fetal condition and to confirm regular uterine activity. Ultrasound examination can be used to confirm fetal presentation, to exclude major fetal abnormalities, and to obtain an estimate of fetal weight.

The presence or absence of fetal breathing movements (FBMs) has been suggested as an indicator of the outcome of preterm labour. It has been shown that in patients in preterm labour who show no FBMs over a 45-minute period, delivery in the next 48 hours is almost inevitable. The presence of FBMs indicates that the pregnancy is likely to continue.

The decision to attempt to stop preterm labour depends on a number of factors:

1. Gestational age
2. Cause of preterm labour
3. State of cervix and membranes
4. Maternal condition
5. Fetal condition
6. Local paediatric facilities.

Management
The use of tocolytics
Tocolytics act by inhibiting smooth muscle contractility. The most commonly used agents are the β sympathomimetics (salbutamol, ritodrine etc.) which have the effect of reducing the concentration of free calcium ions within the myometrial cells and preventing contraction. These drugs have important maternal side-effects, including tachycardia and impaired glucose tolerance, and their use should be avoided in women with cardiac disease and type 1 diabetes mellitus. Acute pulmonary oedema is a rare complication and is usually associated with fluid overload. An oxytocin antagonist is now available which does not cause these side-effects.

Other agents which have been used include alcohol, prostaglandin synthetase inhibitors and calcium antagonists. Tocolytics have been shown to prolong pregnancy; however, they have not yet been shown to improve perinatal mortality. They may be used in the short term to permit prenatal transfer or in the longer term to allow steroid-induced maturation of the fetal lungs. There is no evidence to support the use of oral sympathomimetics as prophylaxis for preterm labour.

The use of glucocorticoids
Antepartum administration of glucocorticoids reduces the incidence of respiratory distress syndrome (RDS) and mortality from RDS in infants between 28 and 32 weeks' gestation. (Steroids may be effective at gestations < 28 weeks but evidence is lacking.) For optimum effect, delivery should take place more than 24 hours and less than 7 days after the start of treatment. A suitable regimen is betamethasone 12 mg—two doses are given intramuscularly 12 hours apart. The use of steroids in the presence of ruptured membranes is controversial because of the theoretically increased risk of intrauterine infection.

Delivery

If local neonatal intensive care facilities are inadequate, consider transfer of the patient. In utero transfer is preferred to neonatal transfer.

The mode of delivery of premature infants is controversial. Generally, infants presenting by the vertex are delivered vaginally. The routine use of forceps in these cases confers no benefit and may contribute to morbidity. Elective episiotomy is generally used. There is no consensus about the safest route of delivery for preterm infants presenting by the breech.

Prevention of preterm labour

There is much interest currently in strategies aimed at preventing preterm labour and delivery. Advice about smoking and nutrition is given routinely. Specific measures can be taken in the minority of cases when there is an identifiable cause, e.g. antibiotics to treat a vaginal 'infection' or cervical cerclage in cases of cervical incompetence. Screening techniques to identify those at risk of preterm labour are undergoing evaluation. Fetal fibronectin has been proposed as a biochemical marker for preterm delivery. This glycoprotein is found in amniotic fluid and placental tissue. Its presence in cervicovaginal secretions during the second and third trimesters identifies a group of women who will deliver preterm.

PRETERM PREMATURE RUPTURE OF MEMBRANES (PPROM)

Definition

PPROM is defined as rupture of the membranes before the onset of labour and before completion of the 37th week of pregnancy.

Interesting facts

PPROM occurs in up to 40% of all labours.

Assessment

On admission, a history is taken and a sterile speculum examination is performed to confirm the presence of ruptured membranes. An endocervical swab is taken for microbiological examination.

Management

The risks of maternal and fetal infection must be balanced against the risks of prematurity and, in the presence of group B streptococci or active genital herpes, delivery must be expedited regardless of gestation.

If gestation is 34 weeks or more, there is little to be gained by delay and labour should be induced if spontaneous contractions do not commence within a reasonable period of time. At earlier gestations, management is conservative and both mother and fetus are carefully monitored for signs of intrauterine infection:

1. Maternal pyrexia > 37.2 °C
2. Maternal leukocytosis
3. Uterine tenderness
4. Offensive liquor
5. Fetal tachycardia
6. Raised C reactive protein.

If contractions occur, intrauterine infection must be excluded before tocolytics and steroids are administered.

SUMMARY

Preterm delivery is a major cause of perinatal morbidity and mortality. In about 40% of cases, the cause is unknown. The use of risk factors to identify at-risk pregnancies is generally unsuccessful. The risks to the mother and fetus through continuing the pregnancy must be balanced against the risks to the fetus of preterm delivery.

PART 2
HYPERTENSIVE DISORDERS   *Janice Rymer*

Expectations of the examiners
As pre-eclampsia is one of the commonest complications of pregnancy, the examiners will expect a thorough knowledge of all aspects of the subject. They will expect you to know how to classify 'hypertension' in pregnancy.

Definition
Hypertension may be defined as:

1. Mild—two diastolic blood pressure (DBP) recordings of 90 mmHg or more 4 hours apart or a diastolic blood pressure of 110 mmHg or more on one occasion
2. Severe—two DBP recordings of 110 mmHg or more 4 hours apart, or DBP of 120 mmHg or more on one occasion.

Classification (WHO, RCOG)
Gestational hypertension.   Hypertension after 20 weeks, during labour or the puerperium.
Pre-eclampsia.   Proteinuric (> 0.3 g/24 hours) hypertension after 20 weeks' gestation.
Chronic hypertension.   Hypertension before 20 weeks/pre-existing.
Chronic renal disease.   Proteinuric hypertension before 20 weeks.
Unclassified.   No recording before 20 weeks.

PRE-ECLAMPSIA

Definition
Pre-eclampsia is a pregnancy-specific syndrome that is characterized by raised blood pressure with proteinuria that develops after 20 weeks' gestation and may terminate in eclampsia.

Interesting facts
Pre-eclampsia is the most important cause of intrauterine growth restriction (IUGR) in singletons with no malformations.

Cerebral haemorrhage is the major cause of maternal death in pre-eclampsia.

Pathophysiology
The aetiology is unknown, but there is thought to be an abnormality of the trophoblast or of the maternal response to the trophoblast. In normal pregnancy, sensitivity to angiotensin is lost, but in pre-eclampsia this does not occur.

High blood pressure is caused by vasoconstriction associated with decreased circulating plasma volume. The fundamental pathophysiological process affects all maternal organs with specific effects on placenta, cardiovascular, renal, clotting and nervous systems, and the liver.

Assessment
Symptoms are usually absent in pre-eclampsia. However, if it is severe, the patient may complain of headache, blurred vision and epigastric pain.

On examination the woman may have high blood pressure, vasoconstriction, hyperreflexia, vomiting, tender liver, oliguria, spontaneous bleeding, bruising and signs of raised intracranial pressure. (Oedema is a normal phenomenon of pregnancy but may be gross in pre-eclampsia.)

Investigations
FBC and platelets
As mentioned above, pre-eclamptic women have a reduced plasma volume so the haemoglobin concentration will be elevated, as will the packed cell volume. With severe disease, platelet consumption occurs, and the platelet level drops. Disseminated intravascular coagulation can develop so clotting tests must be performed.

Urea, creatinine, urate
When the renal system becomes involved there is reduced uric acid clearance, thus elevating the plasma uric acid. With worsening disease the urea and creatinine levels will also rise and renal failure may develop in severe cases.

Urine

Screening relies on dipsticks but may give false-positive results if the urine is alkaline, and false negatives if the urine is highly dilute or contains proteins other than albumin. Any positive result (+1 or more) necessitates an MSU to exclude infection. The amount of proteinuria should be determined in a 24-hour collection.

Liver function tests

In the presence of proteinuria or a reduced platelet count, liver enzymes should be measured (e.g. plasma aspartate transaminase).

Ultrasound scan

As the uteroplacental circulation is impaired the fetus is at risk. Perinatal mortality increases once proteinuria is established. IUGR is more common with early onset disease.

Management

Mild disease

Admit for 48 hours for assessment or see daily in a day assessment unit.

1. Monitor mother
   a. 4-hourly BP
   b. Full blood count and platelets, and clotting function
   c. 24-hour urine for protein estimation
   d. Serum urate, urea and creatinine
   e. Liver function tests
2. Monitor fetus
   a. Movement chart
   b. Ultrasound scan.

If the blood pressure settles, cases of mild disease can be managed on an outpatient basis with daily midwife visits to check the blood pressure and the urine for protein.

Moderate disease

Manage as for mild disease, but inpatient rather than outpatient care is advised. The place for drug treatment in pre-eclampsia is to gain control of the blood pressure to protect the cerebral vessels. It is a temporary inpatient measure as delivery is the definitive treatment. If antihypertensive medication is commenced it must be remembered that one of the major signs of worsening disease is masked.

Severe disease

Admit and deliver.
   Do baseline investigations as above including clotting studies.

Commence antihypertensives. It is difficult to know which patients should be commenced on anticonvulsants. Hyperreflexia can be used as an indicator but is unreliable. Clonus indicates that eclampsia is imminent especially if there are more than two beats. Assess general well-being, as a woman who feels well is unlikely to have an eclamptic fit.

The mode of delivery depends on the gestation, the presentation of the fetus, and the state of the cervix.

After delivery the patient is still at risk of an eclamptic fit for at least 48 hours. The clotting factors and the urine output must be watched carefully. Fluid management is difficult as the patient may be oliguric and haemoconcentrated, so a central venous pressure line is advisable.

If a clotting disorder has developed and the platelet count is $< 100 \times 10^9/1$, an epidural is contraindicated.

Antihypertensives

Labetalol. Labetalol is an α- and β-adrenergic blocker that causes vasodilatation and bradycardia, and reduces myometrial activity. Commence with 100 mg b.d. and increase up to 2.6 g daily.

Methyldopa. Methyldopa acts centrally, decreasing the sympathetic outflow from the brain. An initial dose of 500 mg is given and then 250 mg 6-hourly to a maximum of 750 mg 6-hourly.

Hydralazine. Hydralazine is a non-specific vasodilator that causes a reflex tachycardia and sometimes headache. It is useful for the acute reduction of blood pressure, where it can be given intravenously, e.g. 5 mg boluses given every 5 minutes titrated against the blood pressure (maximum of 20 mg).

Nifedipine. Nifedipine is a calcium channel blocker and vasodilator. It is useful for treating the acute rises in blood pressure, 10 mg orally, and may cause headache. Slow release formulations are preferred for maintenance therapy, up to 30 mg retard b.d.

Anticonvulsants

It is difficult to identify the patients who need anticonvulsants. If there are symptoms or signs of imminent eclampsia then anticonvulsants are advisable. The purpose of anticonvulsants is to prevent fitting rather than to sedate the patient.

Magnesium sulphate is significantly more effective then phenytoin or diazepam in preventing convulsions. It is given as an i.v. infusion and the respiratory rate and patellar reflexes must be checked regularly. Reduced patellar reflexes usually precede respiratory depression. If one measures $MgSO_4$ the desirable levels are between 2.0 and 3.5 mmol/l, and should be checked at 1 and 4 hours and then 6-hourly.

ECLAMPSIA

This is a serious complication of pre-eclampsia because it is associated with increased maternal and fetal morbidity and mortality.

Aetiology

Fitting is a result of brain hypoxia due to ischaemia secondary to oedema and intense vasospasm.

Management

It is not known whether all women with severe pre-eclampsia should be commenced on anticonvulsant therapy and the MAGPIE study is currently investigating this issue. If fits occur, basic measures are needed to establish an airway, and maintain breathing and circulation. The fit should be stopped with either intravenous diazepam or magnesium sulphate, the blood pressure controlled, and anticonvulsants commenced. If the fetus is still in utero, delivery must be expedited. Monitoring should be continued for at least 48 hours, including BP, urine output, clotting and liver function tests.

HELLP SYNDROME

HELLP is an acronym for haemolysis, elevated liver enzymes and low platelets. It is a variant of pre-eclampsia affecting 4–12% of those with pre-eclampsia/ eclampsia and is commoner in multigravidae. There may be acute renal failure and disseminated intravascular coagulation, and there is an increased incidence of abruption. Management is as for severe pre-eclampsia.

ESSENTIAL HYPERTENSION

In essential hypertension, the prepregnancy blood pressure is elevated and there is an absent mid-trimester drop. Essential hypertension is one of the major predisposing factors to pre-eclampsia (five times the risk). The majority of hypertensive women who do not develop pre-eclampsia can expect a normal perinatal outcome. The control of moderate chronic hypertension in early pregnancy does not lessen the eventual incidence of superimposed pre-eclampsia.

The general aims of antenatal care are to keep the blood pressure at a safe level and to monitor maternal renal function. Growth of the fetus should be assessed regularly by serial ultrasound.

Adam Rodin

Expectations of the examiners

The candidate should have a knowledge of the pathophysiology of this uncommon complication, and the importance of anti-D prophylaxis should be understood.

Interesting facts

The incidence of Rhesus isoimmunization has fallen dramatically since the introduction of anti-D prophylaxis in the late 1960s, and Rhesus disease is no longer a major cause of perinatal mortality and morbidity. The few cases that occur are mainly due to a failure of prophylaxis or to haemolytic disease occurring in the Rhesus-positive mother with other maternal alloantibodies.

Pathophysiology

The Rhesus gene is made up of three parts which may be C or c, D or d, and E or e, respectively. Rhesus-negative women constitute 15% of the population and they are homozygous for d. Maternal anti-D antibodies (IgG) may form when Rhesus-positive fetal cells enter the circulation of a Rhesus-negative mother. This commonly occurs at delivery, but fetomaternal haemorrhage may follow other complications and procedures.

Causes of fetomaternal haemorrhage

1. Spontaneous abortion
2. Termination of pregnancy
3. Ectopic pregnancy
4. Antepartum haemorrhage
5. External cephalic version
6. Amniocentesis/chorionic villus sampling
7. Delivery
8. Manual removal of placenta.

As immunization usually occurs at the end of the woman's first pregnancy, it is the second and subsequent pregnancies which are affected by haemolytic disease. If the fetus is Rhesus-positive in the next pregnancy there is a rise in maternal anti-D IgG which crosses the placenta and causes haemolysis of fetal red cells. This results in anaemia and, in severe cases, hydrops fetalis.

Destruction of fetal red cells leads to a rise in unconjugated bilirubin which crosses the placenta to reach the maternal circulation and liver. Some of the unconjugated bilirubin enters the amniotic fluid where levels can be measured. After delivery, haemolysis continues and levels of unconjugated bilirubin continue to rise with a risk of kernicterus. (Free unconjugated bilirubin is toxic to cells of the central nervous system and this may be a fatal condition; surviving infants may have cerebral palsy, mental retardation and deafness.)

Assessment

Assessment of the sensitized woman is aimed at determining whether treatment is necessary and when treatment should be initiated.

Past obstetric history

Severity of disease increases in successive pregnancies and this helps to plan management of the current pregnancy.

Serology

If antibodies are detected, the partner's genotype is checked; if he is Rhesus-negative, further action may be unnecessary if paternity is certain. If the antibody titre exceeds 4 IU/ml, amniocentesis is indicated.

Amniocentesis

Amniotic fluid bilirubin concentrations correlate with the severity of haemolysis. Spectrophotometry at an optical density of 450 nm produces a peak which is directly proportional to the amount of bilirubin in the liquor. Timing depends on past history and maternal antibody levels. Action-line analysis charts are used to interpret the result and plan future management.

Fetal blood sampling

Cordocentesis provides a means of directly assessing the haematological state of the fetus.

Management

At booking, screening for irregular antibodies is performed on all women. An ultrasound scan to confirm gestation is particularly important. Early referral to a regional unit is indicated for women who have had previous affected pregnancies.

In non-sensitized Rhesus-negative women, screening is repeated at 28, 32 and 36 weeks. If antibodies are detected and the partner's genotype is Rhesus-positive, the woman is referred to a regional unit for care. Maternal antibody levels are monitored. Further management is guided by the results of amniocentesis and/or fetal blood sampling. Premature delivery may be necessary.

Treatment

1. Plasmapheresis. This has been used to reduce the maternal circulating antibody level before intraperitoneal transfusion can be performed (< 20 weeks). This technique continues to be controversial.
2. Intrauterine transfusion
   a. Intraperitoneal
   b. Intravascular.

Blood tests at delivery

1. Maternal—Kleihauer test (see below)
2. Fetal—haemoglobin, blood grouping, Coombs test, bilirubin.

Prevention of Rhesus isoimmunization

The administration of anti-D IgG to the mother within 72 hours of a fetomaternal haemorrhage will prevent isoimmunization provided it is given in sufficient quantity. The size of fetomaternal transfusion can be assessed by performing a Kleihauer test. A film of maternal blood is treated with acid and maternal cells become ghosted because of the denaturation of haemoglobin; fetal haemoglobin is resistant and so fetal and maternal red cells may be distinguished. The finding of five fetal cells per 50 high power fields corresponds with a fetomaternal transfusion of 2.5 ml. 500 IU of anti-D IgG will neutralize 4–5 ml of fetal blood. This dose is given to all unsensitized Rhesus-negative mothers delivering at > 20 weeks' gestation. In pregnancies which terminate before this gestation 250 IU are sufficient.

Failure of prophylaxis may be due to failure to give any or sufficient anti-D. It may also follow silent immunization during the antenatal period. Antenatal administration of anti-D has been suggested to counter this.

SUMMARY

Rhesus isoimmunization is now an uncommon complication following the introduction of prophylactic anti-D IgG. Affected pregnancies should be supervised at regional centres.

PART 4
INTRAUTERINE GROWTH RESTRICTION *Adam Rodin*

Expectations of the examiners

An understanding of the two patterns of growth restriction is needed. The candidate will be expected to know how this condition may be detected clinically and how the diagnosis is confirmed.

Definition

Intrauterine growth restriction (IUGR) is defined as fetal weight less than the tenth percentile for gestational age.

Interesting facts

Before the introduction of ultrasonography, IUGR could only be diagnosed at birth when the infant was found to be small for gestational age, although it may have been suspected antenatally on clinical grounds. The diagnosis of IUGR relies on accurate dating and this has been facilitated by the use of ultrasound in early pregnancy. Ethnic variations in birth weight must be considered. Growth-retarded infants have a higher perinatal mortality rate and a higher incidence of neonatal morbidity, and long-term cognitive performance may be impaired when compared to normal-sized infants.

Pathophysiology

The pathophysiology of IUGR differs according to its aetiology but there are two main mechanisms:

1. *Asymmetrical growth restriction.* The supply of nutrients to the fetus is inadequate to support growth and this usually results from 'placental insufficiency'. This type of IUGR usually presents in later pregnancy when fetal needs are increasing. The vital organs are protected and there is sparing of head growth initially.
2. *Symmetrical growth restriction.* This occurs when the growth potential of the fetus is reduced, e.g. it may be due to chromosomal abnormalities or intrauterine infection. This type of IUGR usually appears early in pregnancy.

IUGR may be associated with oligohydramnios.

Aetiology

1. Maternal
   a. Pre-eclampsia/hypertension
   b. Placental abruption
   c. Diabetes mellitus
   d. Renal disease
   e. Smoking
   f. Alcohol
   g. Infections
2. Fetal
   a. Chromosomal abnormalities
   b. Sickle cell disease
   c. Achondroplasia
   d. Potter's syndrome
   e. Anencephaly
   f. Multiple pregnancy.

IUGR may be idiopathic. It is associated with low socioeconomic class and may recur in subsequent pregnancies.

Assessment

An ultrasound scan is performed routinely at 18–20 weeks to confirm gestation. Some women will be in a high-risk group because of pre-existing medical disease or a past history of IUGR. Fetal growth in this group should be checked by serial ultrasound scans. In others, detection of IUGR depends on a high index of clinical suspicion. Maternal weight gain is a poor indicator of fetal growth.

On examination the uterus may be small for dates and there may be oligo-hydramnios. Measurement of symphysiofundal height is a sensitive test for IUGR and when this is abnormal an ultrasound scan should be arranged.

The parameters used in ultrasound growth assessment are biparietal diameter (BPD) (see Fig. 23.1), head circumference (HC), abdominal circumference (AC) (see Fig. 23.2) and femur length (FL) (see Fig. 23.3). In addition, liquor volume should be noted. In symmetrical IUGR, growth in all measured parameters is uniformly decreased. In asymmetrical IUGR (see Fig. 23.4), rate of growth of the fetal abdomen is slowed while head growth remains normal. The role of Doppler flow studies in the assessment of the growth-retarded fetus is being evaluated.

Investigations

In symmetrical IUGR a TORCH screen should be performed and fetal karyotyping may be indicated.

Management

Once the diagnosis of IUGR has been made, hospital admission is arranged so that the condition of both mother and fetus can be monitored. History should be reviewed and a physical examination should be performed.

Growth scans are repeated every 2 weeks. Fetal well-being is assessed by monitoring of fetal movements and cardiotocography. Biochemical tests of placental function are no longer used routinely. In the future, Doppler flow studies and blood gas analysis of fetal blood obtained by cordocentesis may contribute to the management of these cases. Timing of delivery is usually determined by fetal well-being. In some cases, delivery is prompted by a deterioration in maternal condition.

Fig. 23.1 The biparietal diameter must be measured when the head is in the occipitotransverse position, i.e. with the midline echo from the fetal brain at right angles to the ultrasound beam.

Fig. 23.2   The abdominal circumference.

SUMMARY

IUGR is associated with increased perinatal morbidity and mortality. Suspected cases should be assessed by ultrasound scan. Once IUGR has been confirmed, fetal well-being should be monitored and the timing of delivery depends on fetal condition and subsequent growth.

Fig. 23.3   Femur length is visualized on ultrasound scan and then measured.

(a)   Normal growth

Fig. 23.4 Ultrasound measurements plotted on fetal growth charts. a, Normal growth; b, asymmetrical intrauterine growth restriction.

PART 5
ANTEPARTUM HAEMORRHAGE

Adam Rodin

Expectations of the examiners

The topic of antepartum haemorrhage (APH) is particularly favoured by examiners and a clear understanding of the management of this condition is essential.

(b)   Asymmetrical IUGR

Definition

APH is bleeding from or into the genital tract after the 24th week of pregnancy and before delivery. The previous definition was after 28 weeks but as the definition of fetal viability has changed, 24 weeks is more useful.

Interesting facts

APH complicates 3% of all pregnancies and is associated with morbidity and mortality for both mother and fetus. The risk of APH rises with increasing maternal age, increasing parity and cigarette smoking.

Causes of antepartum haemorrhage
1. Bleeding from the placenta
    a. Placental abruption
    b. Placenta praevia
    c. Bleeding from placental margin
2. Bleeding from other sites
    a. Local causes, e.g. cervical polyp, cervical ectropion, cervical carcinoma
    b. Vasa praevia (rare)
    c. Unknown.

PLACENTAL ABRUPTION

Bleeding occurs due to separation of the placenta before delivery of the infant. This can vary in severity from a minor separation to complete placental detachment. The amount of vaginal bleeding does not correlate with the degree of placental separation and there may be total separation with no revealed bleeding.

Pathophysiology
Rupture of one or more maternal spiral arterioles occurs in the decidua basalis. The bleeding may be limited with the formation of a decidual haematoma. If bleeding continues, any or all of the following may occur:

1. Blood may track under the placenta extending the degree of placental separation and compromising the fetus.
2. Blood may dissect under the membranes to reach the cervix and vagina.
3. Blood may enter the amniotic cavity or infiltrate between the fibres of the myometrium. This causes an intense inflammatory response in the myometrium and may trigger uterine contractions. Extravasation of blood may lead to discoloration of the uterus (Couvelaire uterus). Minor separation of the placental edge may occur but presentation is less dramatic than frank abruption.

Following major placental abruption there is release of thromboplastin into the maternal circulation which may trigger disseminated intravascular coagulation (DIC). Maternal death following abruption is usually associated with DIC.

Aetiology
The aetiology of placental abruption is unknown. It may occur following trauma or after sudden uterine decompression which may follow rupture of membranes in a case of polyhydramnios. Abruption is associated with low socioeconomic class, hypertension, pre-eclampsia and previous abruption. The risk of placental abruption is increased in women who smoke during pregnancy.

Assessment

The clinical picture is determined by the extent of the abruption. Abdominal pain is the most constant feature and is usually of sudden onset. Abruption may precipitate labour. Vaginal bleeding may occur. The patient may be shocked and the uterus is tender and tense on palpation. It may be difficult to feel fetal parts and the fetal heart sounds may be absent. The differential diagnosis includes other causes of pain and bleeding in pregnancy.

Placental abruption is diagnosed clinically. Investigations are aimed at monitoring fetal and maternal well-being. Ultrasonography may reveal a retro-placental haematoma but the absence of this finding does not exclude the diagnosis of placental abruption.

Management (see also 'General management of antepartum haemorrhage' below)

When a firm diagnosis of abruption is made, delivery is indicated. The diagnosis is sometimes difficult, particularly prior to 34 weeks' gestation. If the woman is in labour and there is no evidence of fetal or maternal compromise then the membranes should be ruptured; otherwise caesarean section is usually indicated.

PLACENTA PRAEVIA

The placenta is low-lying in 20% of pregnancies at the end of the second trimester but the incidence falls with advancing gestation as the lower segment forms. Placenta praevia complicates approximately 0.5% of pregnancies at term; however, a significant proportion deliver before this. Abruption may occur in placenta praevia.

Aetiology

The aetiology of placenta praevia is unknown but previous myometrial damage (e.g. following curettage) has been implicated. Placenta praevia is commoner in pregnancies after caesarean section and if it occurs the possibility of pathological adherence of the placenta must be anticipated. There is an association with multiple pregnancy and Rhesus disease where the placental area is larger.

Assessment

Painless recurrent vaginal bleeding is the characteristic symptom of placenta praevia; however, in some cases bleeding does not occur until the onset of labour. On examination, the uterus is not tender and there may be a breech presentation, or an abnormal lie, or the presenting part may be high. These findings should raise the suspicion of placenta praevia even in the absence of vaginal bleeding. *Vaginal examination should not be performed if placenta praevia is suspected.*

Investigations

Placental localization is performed by ultrasound. This technique is usually accurate but is not infallible. There are four grades of placenta praevia:

Grade 1   Lower margin of placenta encroaches on the lower segment.
Grade 2   Lower margin of placenta reaches the internal os.
Grade 3   Placenta partially covers the internal os.
Grade 4   Placenta completely covers the internal os.

Placenta praevia is more simply classified into major and minor degrees. A minor degree of placenta praevia is equivalent to grade 1 or 2, and a major degree corresponds with grades 3 and 4.

Management

If a low-lying placenta is detected by routine scan in early pregnancy no action is necessary, but the placental site is checked again at 32 weeks' gestation. If a major degree of placenta praevia persists the patient is admitted to hospital because of the risk of haemorrhage. Cross-matched blood is kept continuously available and ultrasound scans are repeated at 2-week intervals to monitor placental position and fetal growth.

If a major degree of placenta praevia persists at 38 weeks, delivery is by elective caesarean section. This should be performed by a senior obstetrician and general anaesthesia is advised. Women with minor degrees of placenta praevia would usually be allowed to labour spontaneously. Examination under anaesthesia is rarely indicated.

Other causes of antepartum haemorrhage

Vasa praevia is a rare condition and can occur when there is a velamentous cord insertion. The cord inserts in the membranes and the vessels course across the membranes to reach the placenta. When membranes rupture, the vessels may be torn and fetal exsanguination may occur. Facilities should be available to test for fetal haemoglobin, most commonly in the form of the NaOH test.

General management of antepartum haemorrhage

Management depends primarily on the severity of the clinical situation. It is obligatory to assume that bleeding is placental in origin until proven otherwise.

Minor haemorrhage

At home.
1. Refer patient to hospital.
2. *Do not perform a vaginal examination.*

In hospital.
1. Take a history and examine the patient.
2. *Do not perform a digital vaginal examination.*
3. Gentle speculum examination may be performed after the placental site is known.
4. Assess fetal well-being—cardiotocography.
5. Consider siting an intravenous line.
6. Take blood to check haemoglobin and platelets, and group and save serum.
7. Admit to hospital for rest and observation.
8. Arrange ultrasound scan.
9. Give anti-D to Rhesus-negative mothers.

It is common practice to advise women to remain in hospital for 48 hours after bleeding has stopped as there is a risk of the antepartum haemorrhage precipitating premature labour.

Major haemorrhage
At home
1. Arrange urgent admission to hospital/call obstetric flying squad.
2. Insert intravenous line and commence resuscitation.
3. *Do not perform a vaginal examination.*

In hospital
1. Call for assistance.
2. Insert wide-bore cannula and commence intravenous infusion; two lines may be necessary.
3. Request 6 units of cross-matched blood urgently.
4. Send blood to check haemoglobin, platelets and clotting screen.
5. Insert CVP line.
6. Insert urinary catheter; monitor fluid balance.
7. *Do not perform a vaginal examination.*
8. If the fetus is alive, deliver by emergency caesarean section.

Complications of antepartum haemorrhage
1. Maternal/fetal death
2. Postpartum haemorrhage
3. DIC (particularly following abruption)
4. Renal failure
5. Preterm delivery.

SUMMARY

Placental abruption and placenta praevia are the important causes of antepartum haemorrhage. Assessment in hospital is essential in all cases of antepartum haemorrhage and management is determined by the clinical situation.

PART 6
MATERNAL SYSTEMIC DISORDERS   *Adam Rodin*

Expectations of the examiners

The candidate is expected to have a knowledge of the common medical disorders which occur in pregnancy. The candidate should be able to discuss the role of the general practitioner in their management.

ANAEMIA

Interesting facts

Anaemia is one of the commonest medical complications of pregnancy.

Pathophysiology

Plasma volume increases steadily through pregnancy and reaches a plateau after 32 weeks. The magnitude of the increase is related to fetal size and the effect is exaggerated in multiple pregnancy. There is a concomitant increase in red cell mass and total haemoglobin but because of the larger rise in plasma volume, the haemoglobin concentration and packed cell volume (PCV) fall.

IRON DEFICIENCY ANAEMIA

Demands for iron increase during pregnancy due to the rise in red cell mass and fetal demands. Total iron requirement through pregnancy is 700–1400 mg with a daily requirement of 4 mg rising to 7 mg in later pregnancy. A reduction in haemoglobin concentration is a relatively late sign of iron deficiency. This is preceded by depletion in iron stores and a fall in serum iron levels.

Assessment

Iron deficiency can be detected before anaemia develops by measuring serum ferritin which gives a reflection of iron stores. Serum iron and total iron binding capacity are also useful markers.

The red cell indices suggestive of iron deficiency are reduced mean cell volume (MCV) and a reduced mean cell haemoglobin concentration (MCHC).

Management

Oral iron supplements are usually adequate for prophylaxis. Standard preprations contain between 100 and 200 mg of elemental iron often in combination with folic acid.

Treatment of established iron deficiency depends on the severity of the anaemia and the gestation. Treatment options include:

1. Oral iron supplementation
2. Parenteral iron/dextran (i.v./i.m.) ⎫
3. Blood transfusion. ⎭ Rarely needed

Adequate treatment should increase the haemoglobin concentration at the rate of 1 mg/dl/week and a reticulocyte count 2 weeks later should confirm a response to iron therapy.

MEGALOBLASTIC ANAEMIA

A deficiency in folic acid is the usual cause of this type of anaemia in pregnancy. Folate is needed for cell growth and division and requirements increase as pregnancy progresses. Folate deficiency anaemia affects 5% of pregnant women in the UK and much larger numbers in developing countries. The daily requirement of folate in pregnancy is 100 μg.

Assessment
The red cell indices show a raised MCV and macrocytes are seen on the blood film.

Management
Oral folate supplements, 5 mg daily for documented folate deficiency, are often combined with iron supplements. Prophylactic dose is 200–500 μg of folate.

SICKLE CELL ANAEMIA

Sickle cell disease is one of the most important haemoglobinopathies. It is due to a single amino acid substitution on the β chain of haemoglobin. The haemoglobin formed (HbS) is insoluble when reduced and this results in distortion of erythrocytes and subsequent blockage of small blood vessels. Sickle cell disease is common amongst AfroCarribean populations and in some Mediterranean groups. Heterozygotes for this abnormal gene have sickle cell trait (HbAS). Complications in pregnancy are rare. Homozygotes (HbSS) have sickle cell disease and may suffer from recurrent sickling crises. They develop a chronic haemolytic anaemia.

Assessment
Sickle cell disease and other haemoglobinopathies are detected by haemoglobin electrophoresis which should be carried out in at-risk women

at booking. The partner's blood should also be tested to assess the risks of fetal disease.

Management

Women with sickle cell trait pose few special management problems. Haemoglobin electrophoresis should be performed on the baby's father to assess the risk of the infant being affected.

Women with sickle cell disease should be managed in specialist centres and further discussion is beyond the scope of this book.

CARDIAC DISEASE

Interesting facts

Less than 1% of all pregnancies in the UK are complicated by heart disease; however, it remains an important cause of maternal mortality. Greater numbers of women with congenital heart disease are now reaching adulthood due to paediatric cardiac surgery and many of these women are becoming pregnant. The numbers of women with acquired (mainly rheumatic) heart disease complicating pregnancy are falling.

Pathophysiology

During normal pregnancy the cardiovascular system undergoes a number of adaptations. During the first trimester cardiac output increases by 40% due to raised stroke volume and a small increment in heart rate. Blood volume also increases by about 40% in early pregnancy and this is maintained until term. A fall in peripheral resistance occurs due to general relaxation in arterial and venous tone. An ejection systolic murmur is audible in up to 90% of normal pregnant women. At delivery, contraction of the uterus expresses about 500 ml of blood into the circulation. The normal woman can cope with these haemodynamic alterations but in a woman with heart disease they may precipitate cardiac failure.

Classification of heart disease

1. Congenital heart disease
2. Rheumatic heart disease
3. Other
   a. Cardiomyopathy
   b. Myocardial infarction.

Maternal mortality is most likely in those conditions where pulmonary blood flow cannot be increased, e.g. Eisenmenger syndrome and primary pulmonary hypertension. Fetal outcome in patients with rheumatic heart disease and acyanotic congenital heart disease is usually good. Mothers with cyanotic congenital heart disease tend to have growth-restricted infants.

Although rheumatic heart disease is becoming rare in the UK it is the commonest form of heart disease complicating pregnancy worldwide. The most important lesion is mitral stenosis and these women are particularly likely to develop heart failure during pregnancy.

Women with artificial heart valves should receive anticoagulation through pregnancy and the puerperium.

Management

Prepregnancy
Avoidance or termination of pregnancy may be recommended in certain conditions (e.g. Eisenmenger syndrome).

Antenatal
1. There should be hospital care with regular visits to obstetrician and cardiologist.
2. Avoid cardiac failure
   a. Treat infections promptly.
   b. Treat hypertension.
   c. Avoid anaemia.
3. Treat cardiac failure.
4. Monitor fetal growth with serial ultrasound scans.

In labour
1. Antibiotic cover may be indicated.
2. Aim for vaginal delivery.
3. Assure adequate analgesia—epidural analgesia can be used in most cases but should be avoided in women with Eisenmenger syndrome and hypertrophic cardiomyopathy (i.e. fixed output states).
4. Control intravenous fluids strictly.
5. The second stage is short.
6. Do not give ergometrine.

DIABETES MELLITUS

Interesting facts
Diabetes affects about 3% of the obstetric population and before the introduction of insulin, diabetic pregnancy had a very high maternal and fetal mortality.

Pathophysiology
Hormonal changes during pregnancy have profound effects on carbohydrate metabolism. Insulin resistance develops as pregnancy advances and it is most marked in the last trimester. In normal pregnancy, increased insulin production counters the rise in insulin resistance and blood glucose levels are

maintained within a narrow range. Glucose crosses the placenta freely by facilitated diffusion and maternal homeostatic mechanisms regulate fetal glucose levels in the normal situation. In the diabetic pregnancy, fetal hyperglycaemia stimulates fetal insulin production.

Glycosuria is common during normal pregnancy. This is due to an increased glomerular filtration rate and reduced tubular reabsorption of glucose.

There are three main clinical types of diabetes in pregnancy:

1. Type 1 (insulin-dependent) diabetes
2. Type 2 (non-insulin dependent) diabetes
3. Gestational diabetes.

Gestational diabetes is the term applied when women become diabetic during pregnancy. Many will revert to normal after pregnancy, but a proportion do not.

Effects of diabetes on the pregnancy
Fetal effects
1. Increased perinatal mortality due to
   a. Congenital abnormalities: increased risk of sacral agenesis and cardiac abnormalities due to hyperglycaemia during organogenesis
   b. Respiratory distress syndrome
   c. Birth trauma associated with macrosomia (birth weight > 4000 g)
   d. Intrauterine growth retardation
   e. Prematurity
2. Increased neonatal morbidity
   a. Birth asphyxia/trauma
   b. Hypoglycaemia
   c. Polycythaemia
   d. Jaundice
   e. Respiratory distress syndrome.

Maternal effects
1. Pre-eclampsia: increased incidence in diabetic pregnancy
2. Polyhydramnios
3. Preterm labour.

Good diabetic control reduces the incidence of these complications but the raised incidence of congenital abnormalities persists.

Assessment
Risk factors should be identified antenatally and these women should be offered a glucose tolerance test.

Risk factors for gestational diabetes are:

1. Glycosuria on two or more occasions
2. Maternal obesity (> 20% of ideal weight)
3. Family history of diabetes in first-degree relative

4. Previous congenital abnormality, neonatal death, unexplained stillbirth, macrosomic infant
5. Polyhydramnios in current pregnancy
6. Previous gestational diabetes
7. History of polycystic ovarian syndrome.

Routine antenatal screening is recommended by some because about 30% of gestational diabetics have none of these risk factors.

The diagnosis of diabetes is made by the finding of a fasting blood glucose level of 8 mmol/l or more, or 11 mmol/l or more after food. A fasting glucose level of < 6 mmol/l excludes the diagnosis. A glucose tolerance test (GTT) with a 75 g glucose load distinguishes between diabetes, impaired glucose tolerance (IGT) and normality. The significance of IGT to the pregnancy is uncertain but some women with IGT will develop gestational diabetes later in the pregnancy.

Management

Medical management of diabetes is by diet alone or diet and insulin depending on the type of maternal diabetes. Oral hypoglycaemic agents are not used. Insulin is given at least twice daily using a mixture of short-acting and medium-acting preparations. Continuous subcutaneous insulin administration has been used with good effect.

Prepregnancy

Established diabetics should be assessed before pregnancy to achieve optimal blood glucose control before conception. Women with diabetic retinopathy and nephropathy require careful assessment.

Antenatal

1. Early booking.
2. Hospital care at joint obstetric/diabetic clinic.
3. Optimize blood glucose control
   a. Dietary advice.
   b. Home blood glucose monitoring.
   c. Regular urinalysis.
   d. Regular HbA_1 and fructosamine monitoring.
4. Monitor fetal well-being
   a. Check maternal serum AFP between 16 and 18 weeks.
   b. Anomaly scan at 18 weeks.
   c. Serial ultrasound scans to monitor fetal growth.
5. Do not allow pregnancy to proceed past 40 weeks.

In labour

1. Vaginal delivery if possible.
2. Continuous intravenous infusion of insulin and 5% dextrose with regular monitoring of blood glucose
3. Continuous fetal monitoring
4. Adequate analgesia.

After delivery, insulin requirements fall rapidly and careful monitoring is essential.

EPILEPSY

Interesting facts
Pregnancy does not trigger epilepsy or cause an exacerbation of pre-existing epilepsy. Untreated epileptics have an increased risk of congenital abnormalities which is poorly understood. The incidence of congenital malformations is increased two- or threefold in infants of women on anticonvulsants. Phenytoin is associated with an increased risk of cleft lip/palate, congenital heart disease and hypoplasia of the nails and digits. Sodium valproate is associated with an increased incidence of neural tube defects.

Management
Prepregnancy
1. Check that fits are well controlled.
2. Emphasize the importance of good drug compliance during pregnancy.

Antenatal
1. Continue on the usual anticonvulsant at the prepregnancy dose unless fits occur, then levels should be checked and the dose adjusted accordingly.
2. Women taking anticonvulsants may become folate deficient and 5 mg daily should be given throughout pregnancy.
3. Carry out maternal serum AFP estimation at 16–18 weeks.
4. Perform fetal anomaly scan at 18 weeks.
5. Anticonvulsants may cause depression of vitamin K-dependent clotting factors in the mother and fetus; vitamin K should be given from 36 weeks until delivery and the neonate should be given vitamin K intramuscularly. All antiepileptic drugs are excreted in low concentrations in breast milk. Mothers taking antiepileptic drugs other than phenobarbital should be permitted to breast-feed.

THROMBOEMBOLIC DISEASE

Interesting facts
Thromboembolic disease is an important cause of maternal mortality. The risk of thromboembolism during pregnancy and the puerperium is six times higher than in the non-pregnant state.

Pathophysiology
Pregnancy is accompanied by changes in normal haemostatic mechanisms which decrease the risk of haemorrhage at delivery. These changes include an

increase in clotting factors and a dampening of fibrinolysis, favouring thrombosis. Risk factors for thromboembolism in pregnancy include:

1. High maternal age
2. Multiparity
3. Obesity
4. Immobility
5. Previous history of thromboembolism
6. Operative delivery
7. Blood disorders (rare)
8. Use of diethylstilbestrol to suppress lactation.

Blood group O appears to confer some protection against thromboembolism. The recurrence rate of deep venous thrombosis (DVT) or pulmonary embolus (PE) in women who have had thromboembolic disease in previous pregnancies is 5–10%.

Assessment
Women with a history of thromboembolism should be identified in the booking clinic. Suspected thromboembolism occurring during pregnancy or the puerperium should be actively investigated to reach a definitive diagnosis. Clinical diagnosis of DVT is unreliable and venography or ultrasonography should be arranged. Clinical suspicion of PE should be confirmed by a ventilation-perfusion scan of the lungs. Chest X-ray, ECG and arterial blood gas measurement may also be helpful. Anticoagulation should be commenced when thromboembolism is suspected without waiting for confirmation.

Management
PE/DVT during pregnancy
1. Commence intravenous infusion of heparin 40 000 IU/day; continue for 5–7 days.
2. Change to subcutaneous heparin 10 000 IU b.d. and continue until the end of the puerperium.

History of previous DVT/PE
Prophylactic anticoagulation should be considered because of risk of recurrence. There is no consensus about who to treat and which regimen to follow and the benefits of anticoagulation should be balanced against the risks of fetal and maternal side-effects (see below). Regimens which have been used include:

1. Continuous subcutaneous heparin through pregnancy and the puerperium
2. Subcutaneous heparin until 13 weeks; warfarin between 13 and 36 weeks; subcutaneous heparin from 36 weeks until the end of the puerperium
3. Dextran 70 in labour followed by heparin (subcutaneous) or warfarin during the puerperium.

Anticoagulation with either heparin or warfarin is associated with risks for both mother and fetus. Heparin does not cross the placenta and it has a short half-life. Its actions are readily reversible by protamine sulphate. However, it is associated with maternal thrombocytopenia and prolonged administration causes bone demineralization. Warfarin crosses the placenta and can cause chondrodysplasia punctata, microcephaly and optic atrophy in the fetus. Later in pregnancy it can cause fetal intracranial haemorrhage. Therefore warfarin is avoided in the first trimester and from 36 weeks onwards. Warfarin has a long half-life and its effects cannot be rapidly reversed in the event of a complication such as antepartum haemorrhage. Breast-feeding is not contraindicated in women taking heparin or warfarin.

THYROID DISEASE

Interesting facts
Thyroid disease has been estimated to complicate 0.5% of all pregnancies. It is usually pre-existing but may appear for the first time in pregnancy.

HYPOTHYROIDISM

The main causes of hypothyroidism are idiopathic, Hashimoto's thyroiditis and postablative hypothyroidism.

Assessment
The clinical diagnosis of hypothyroidism may be difficult during pregnancy but may be suggested by inappropriate weight gain, cold intolerance or skin changes. There may be a goitre and reflexes may be sluggish. Laboratory investigations show a low free thyroxine (T4) level and a raised thyroid stimulating hormone (TSH) level. Total serum T4 is low for pregnancy but may be within the normal range for the non-pregnant woman.

Management
Thyroxine should be given as a single daily dose. Thyroid function should be checked as the pregnancy progresses. Breast-feeding is not contraindicated.

HYPERTHYROIDISM

Hyperthyroidism in pregnancy is usually due to Graves' disease. Untreated hyperthyroidism is associated with an increased incidence of preterm labour and low birth weight and a raised perinatal mortality rate. Women who have had surgery for Graves' disease may still have thyroid stimulating autoantibodies which can cross the placenta and cause neonatal thyrotoxicosis.

Assessment

The symptoms of hyperthyroidism may mimic the normal changes of pregnancy and include heat intolerance, palpitations, emotional instability and fatigue. A goitre may be present. TSH is undetectable while free T3 and T4 are elevated.

Management

The aim of management is to control maternal hyperthyroidism while allowing the development of normal thyroid function in the fetus. Both drug therapy and surgery have been used. The thiourea derivatives, carbimazole and propylthiouracil, are in common use and their main action is to inhibit synthesis of T3 and T4. These drugs cross the placenta and may affect the fetal thyroid causing transient hypothyroidism at delivery. There is no contraindication to breast-feeding.

24 Labour—first stage

Janice Rymer

Expectations of the examiners

The candidate is expected to understand the mechanism of labour and the management of normal and abnormal labour. The principles of active management of labour are essential to modern obstetrics.

Definition

Labour is defined as the process by which the fetus, placenta and membranes are expelled from the birth canal. The first stage of labour commences when regular uterine contractions are associated with cervical change, and concludes with full dilatation of the cervix.

Interesting facts

Previously labour was said to be normal when spontaneous delivery occurred within 24 hours of the onset of spontaneous regular contractions. However, as the complications of labour are directly related to its duration, labour is now deemed normal if spontaneous delivery occurs within 12 hours; with the use of epidurals labour may be prolonged, but is deemed 'normal' if adequate progress is occurring.

Physiology

In pregnancy, the uterus is in a relaxed state and must expand to accommodate the growing fetus. However, when labour commences, it must contract regularly and forcibly so that the cervix progressively effaces and dilates allowing the fetus to descend through the birth canal.

In labour, the myometrial smooth muscle contracts at regular intervals, resulting in intrauterine pressures of 50–75 mmHg. The wave of excitation, and hence the resulting contraction, normally passes downwards from the fundus of the uterus. As the muscle contracts, it also retracts (the muscle does not relax to its original length, but stays at a shorter length). Successful parturition involves regular and effective uterine contractions and a responsive cervix. Cervical ripening is characterized by softening, effacement and dilatation, but the hormonal control of this process is still not understood. Prior to term, the release of prostaglandins causes an increase in the water content of the cervix and breakdown of cervical collagen. PGE_2 has a marked effect on cervical ripening. During labour, prostaglandins and oxytocin interact in the generation of uterine contractions.

Mechanism of normal labour
Descent. Significant descent of the head into the pelvis occurs in most primigravidae in the later weeks of pregnancy. In multigravidae descent may not occur until the onset of labour.

Engagement. This occurs when the maximum diameter of the head has passed through the pelvic brim. It may occur before labour commences, and the head usually engages in the occipitotransverse.

Flexion. This is a continuous process during labour. With full flexion the posterior fontanelle is easily palpable on vaginal examination through the dilated cervix, and the most favourable diameter presents.

Internal rotation. This is rotation of the head inside the pelvis, and it occurs because of the shape of the birth canal, the position of the head, and the inclination of the levator ani. Usually the rotation is anterior, so that the denominator (the occiput) swings from left occipitotransverse (LOT) to direct occipitoanterior (OA).

Extension. The head remains flexed until the vertex reaches the perineum. As the head 'crowns' it extends, following the axis of the birth canal.

External rotation (restitution). The head reverts to the position it previously held before internal rotation occurred (occipitotransverse).

Lateral flexion. The anterior shoulder appears, followed by the posterior shoulder. Delivery of the trunk is then achieved by lateral flexion.

Assessment
The diagnosis of labour is made when regular uterine contractions are associated with cervical change. As the cervix effaces, the operculum (mucus plug in the cervix) is released (a 'show'). Each obstetric unit should be clear on its criteria for the diagnosis of labour, and the delivery suite should be reserved for women in active labour.

History
Specific questioning should involve:

1. Contractions
   a. Time of onset
   b. Frequency
   c. Duration
2. Presence of a show
3. Rupture of the membranes.

Examination
1. Abdominal palpation is performed to assess
   a. Gestation
   b. Lie of the fetus

c. Presentation
d. Descent of the head (see Fig. 24.1)
2. Vaginal examination
   a. Speculum examination if there is any question as to whether liquor is draining; nitrazene reaction has been used to indicate the presence of liquor but is unreliable
   b. Digital examination to assess the softness, length and dilatation of the cervix, and the station (relative to the ischial spines) of the presenting part

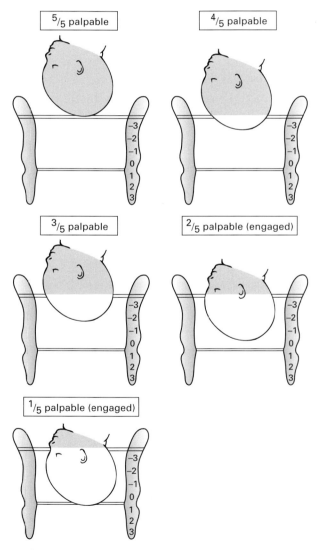

Fig. 24.1 The abdominal palpation of the fetal head can be described in 'fifths' of the head palpable above the brim.

3. Fetal well-being
   a. Fetal movements
   b. Fetal heart rate (no evidence for efficacy of 'admission test' cardiotocograph)
   c. Presence of meconium in the liquor.

Management

Once the diagnosis of 'labour' is made then the best way to record progress is to use a partogram, i.e. a visual representation of progress in labour. This should include a record of:

1. The date and time of admission.
2. Cervical dilatation. This is marked in centimetres at zero time (on admission) and at subsequent examinations.
3. Descent of the head. This is determined by abdominal palpation of the number of 'fifths' of the head palpable above the brim and by vaginal assessment of the relationship of the presenting part to the ischial spines (station).
4. Contractions
   a. Frequency
   b. Duration
   c. Strength: assessment of strength of contractions by palpation is unreliable.
5. Fetal heart rate.
6. Colour of the liquor and time and manner of membrane rupture.
7. The use of oxytocin.
8. Maternal status
   a. Blood pressure
   b. Pulse
   c. Temperature
   d. Urinalysis
   e. Medication.

Progress in labour

The regular assessment of progress is the key to good management. In primigravidae, delivery should be achieved within 12 hours. The minimum rate of cervical dilatation acceptable in primiparous women is 1 cm/hour. Delay in progress may be due to:

Inefficient uterine action (primary dysfunctional labour). In primiparous women this is common. The earlier the diagnosis is made, the more chance there is of correcting it and achieving a normal delivery. Once diagnosed, an oxytocin infusion should be commenced and progress assessed regularly. (See Appendix VI for partograms.)

Secondary arrest. If the fetal head is partially extended it does not fit into the lower uterine pole well and this is more common in primiparous women, especially with an occipitoposterior position. These women generally have a bad start to labour, and may present with inefficient uterine action. Premature rupture of membranes is common. The head remains high and deflexed and there may be severe backache. The sinciput reaches the pelvic floor first and therefore rotates anteriorly, i.e. the occiput is posterior. The larger occipito-frontal diameter of the head presents (10 cm), making its passage through the pelvis more difficult.

Cephalopelvic disproportion (see Ch. 25.) In multiparous women, labour is more rapid and inefficient uterine action is rare. Delay in a multiparous woman may be due to obstruction, with subsequent uterine rupture if not recognized.

Posture during labour
The woman should adopt the most comfortable position bearing in mind that aortocaval compression must be avoided. Early in the first stage women may want to mobilize, but most adopt a recumbent position once labour is established.

Oral intake
Women in labour have delayed gastric emptying and this will be exacerbated by narcotics and fatigue. It is advisable to allow clear fluids and no food. H_2 antagonists should be given 6-hourly, if food has been taken.

Support during labour
Labour is a stressful event and a woman requires support from a person known to her and a midwife who ideally remains with her throughout her labour.

Active management of labour
The aim of active management is to ensure that all women in their first pregnancy deliver a healthy child after a labour less than 12 hours. A woman's first experience will determine her obstetric future both emotionally and physically.

The principles of active management are:

1. Antenatal education
2. Regular assessment of progress in labour
3. Presence of a support person throughout labour (ideally, the *same* person throughout)
4. Early correction of abnormal progress
5. Provision of suitable analgesia.

If active management is correctly applied, the caesarean section rate is reduced.

25 Labour—second stage

Janice Rymer

Expectations of the examiners

The candidate will be expected to have a thorough knowledge of what is normal and abnormal in the second stage of labour. The importance of the correct timing of intervention should be appreciated.

Definition

The second stage of labour commences with full cervical dilatation and concludes with delivery of the fetus.

Interesting facts

In primigravidae the average length of the second stage is 40 minutes, and in multiparae, 20 minutes.

Physiology

The uterus continues to contract and force the fetus through the cervix. At full dilatation the cervix has retracted past the presenting part and is no longer palpable. Contractions are usually stronger but occur less frequently than in the first stage. If the normal mechanism of labour is occurring, the head rotates internally as it descends; when the pelvic floor becomes distended, the 'bearing down' reflex occurs.

Assessment

Full dilatation is diagnosed by vaginal examination. The position and station of the fetal head should be noted.

Management

When the bearing down reflex occurs the woman will want to 'push' (in the absence of an effective epidural). After breathing in, the glottis is closed, and the patient pushes down with the aid of the diaphragm and abdominal wall muscles. Two or three bearing down efforts are made with each contraction. It is essential that the woman receives constant attention during the second stage to detect signs of fetal or maternal distress.

Once anal dilatation occurs, normal delivery should follow shortly afterwards. The woman is prepared for delivery, and the accoucheur assists the delivery by ensuring that the fetal head remains flexed, and that the head is delivered in a controlled manner. If needed, an episiotomy is performed (ideally with some form of pain relief) as the head distends the perineum. Once the head is delivered the oropharynx is suctioned. The head restitutes and is then grasped and pulled downwards (towards the maternal sacrum) so that the anterior shoulder is delivered. The trunk is then laterally flexed upwards (towards the maternal umbilicus) so that the posterior shoulder is delivered, rapidly followed by the trunk. Great care of the perineum must be taken at all times.

If a spontaneous vaginal delivery has not occurred within 1 hour of full dilatation then the vaginal examination should be repeated. In primigravid women, if there has been no progress, then an oxytocin infusion should be commenced and a repeat vaginal examination should be performed in 1 hour. If there is no progress and the head is too high for an instrumental delivery, then a caesarean section is performed. If progress has occurred, then an instrumental delivery may be performed, or the second stage may be allowed to continue depending on the fetal and maternal condition. In multiparous women, it is dangerous to use oxytocin for second stage augmentation alone, due to the risk of uterine rupture.

If the position of the head is occipitoanterior and does not descend with augmentation (in primigravidae), this suggests true cephalopelvic disproportion.

If the position of the head is occipitoposterior, the station of the head will determine whether a vaginal delivery is possible. This can be performed either with a rotational delivery (vacuum extractor, manual rotation or Kjelland's forceps) (see Ch. 28), or with lift-out forceps if the head is low enough.

Cephalopelvic disproportion

In the past, slow progress in the first stage of labour was wrongly termed cephalopelvic disproportion, whereas now the most likely diagnosis is considered to be inefficient uterine action. This is treated with an oxytocin infusion.

If progress still fails to occur, then a tentative diagnosis of cephalopelvic disproportion can be entertained, provided the head is not occipitoposterior. If these strict criteria are applied to make the diagnosis, 1 in 250 primigravidae will have cephalopelvic disproportion, and if allowed to labour subsequently, 50% will deliver vaginally.

True cephalopelvic disproportion is rare, and the diagnosis can only be made in retrospect. Once this diagnosis has been made it will strongly influence the mode of delivery in subsequent pregnancies.

In parous women cephalopelvic disproportion can occur due to either a larger fetus or a reduction in pelvic capacity, or both. The uterine action in these cases will be vigorously reactive and the risk of uterine rupture is considerable, especially if oxytocin is used. The diagnosis rests on features such as delay in descent of the presenting part, exaggerated moulding and unremitting uterine activity.

SUMMARY

A prolonged second stage of labour requires sensible management if maternal and fetal trauma are to be avoided.

26 Labour—third stage

Janice Rymer

Expectations of the examiners

A thorough knowledge of the normal and abnormal third stage is essential. The candidate should appreciate that proper management of the third stage is of vital importance in reducing the incidence of postpartum haemorrhage, retained placenta and consequent maternal morbidity and mortality.

Definition

The third stage commences with the delivery of the baby and finishes with delivery of the placenta.

Interesting facts

Postpartum haemorrhage is a common cause of serious blood loss in obstetrics. It is an important cause of maternal mortality, accounting for 14% of maternal deaths from haemorrhage in England and Wales (Report on Confidential Enquiries into Maternal Deaths 1997–1999).

Physiology

The continuation of uterine contractions and the reduction of surface area of the uterine cavity cause the placenta to separate from the uterine wall. As separation occurs there is some retroplacental bleeding which contributes to the separation process.

There are two processes which help to control excessive bleeding from the placental bed:

1. Contraction and twisting of the interlacing bundles of muscle in the uterine wall compressing the vessels as the uterus decreases in size
2. Normal coagulation, i.e. release of thromboplastins, platelet aggregation and fibrin formation.

Haemostatic processes may be less efficient in the following circumstances:

1. Dysfunctional labour
2. Uterine overdistension, e.g. multiple pregnancy
3. Anaesthetic agents, e.g. halothane
4. Morbid adherence of the placenta.

Table 26.1 Risk factors for postpartum haemorrhage.

Past history of a postpartum haemorrhage	Coagulation disorders
Grand multiparity	Poor uterine contractions
Uterine overdistension (e.g. large baby, twins)	Prolonged labour
	Large placental bed (e.g. Rhesus disease)
Antepartum haemorrhage	Operative delivery

Assessment

Risk factors for a postpartum haemorrhage should be identified in the patient's previous obstetric history (see Table 26.1) or current pregnancy.

Management

The policy for management of the third stage varies between obstetric units. As the anterior shoulder is delivered an ecbolic is administered i.m. or i.v. in the form of oxytocin ± ergometrine (see Table 26.2). The placenta is usually delivered by the Brandt–Andrews technique. The cord is held with the right hand and downward traction is applied while the uterus is lifted upwards with the left hand placed suprapubically. If the placenta does not advance then it is usually still attached to the uterus. If the placenta is not delivered after 30 minutes then a manual removal is required (see 'Complications' below). Once the placenta has been delivered the fundus is briefly massaged to ensure that it contracts. The genital tract must be inspected for any lacerations and repaired appropriately. The placenta should be examined to ensure completeness and normality. An assessment of the blood loss should be recorded.

Complications

Postpartum haemorrhage

A primary postpartum haemorrhage is defined as a blood loss ≥ 500 ml within 24 hours of delivery. The incidence of postpartum haemorrhage is 5% of deliveries.

Table 26.2 Time from administration to action on the uterus for the various oxytocic drugs.

Drug	Administration	Time
Oxytocin	i.v.	30 s
Ergometrine	i.v.	40 s
Oxytocin	i.m.	2.5 min
Ergometrine + oxytocin	i.m.	2.5 min
Ergometrine	i.m.	7 min

Aetiology
1. Uterine atony
2. Local trauma to vagina or cervix
3. Retained placenta or products of conception
4. Other
    a. Uterine inversion
    b. Uterine rupture
    c. Defective coagulation.

Management. The assessment and treatment should take place simultaneously.

Examination of the fundus. If it is high and soft then uterine atony and/or retained products are the causes of the bleeding. The fundus should be massaged to expel clot and ensure maximum retraction. In severe haemorrhage, bimanual compression with the uterus compressed between a vaginal and an abdominal hand can be used. If the fundus is not palpable then uterine inversion should be suspected and an immediate vaginal examination performed. The placenta and membranes should be checked to ensure they are complete.

Resuscitation. An i.v. line of large bore (14 g or greater) should be inserted while the initial examination is taking place (two lines in severe cases). Blood should be sent for FBC and clotting studies, and 4 units of whole blood should be cross-matched. Initially, crystalloid or plasma substitute should be infused as quickly as required.

Examination of the genital tract. If the fundus is retracted and bleeding is continuing then careful speculum examination should be carried out and vaginal or cervical lacerations repaired appropriately.

Further measures. Further management depends on the findings and response to the measures already mentioned:

1. Uterine atony. In most cases this will respond to massage and the bleeding will settle. An oxytocin infusion should be commenced (40 IU oxytocin in 500 ml of crystalloid over 2–4 hours), or ergometrine 0.5 mg i.m. can be given if the patient has no history of cardiac disease or hypertension at any stage in pregnancy. If these measures are not successful, the uterine cavity should be examined under general anaesthesia (or epidural/spinal if already in situ) to remove any retained products. If bleeding continues, then prostaglandin injected directly into the myometrium is usually effective; an alternative is rectal misoprostol. If this is not effective, then surgery should be performed without delay and consideration should be given to the B-lynch suture, which contracts the uterus mechanically. Internal iliac artery ligation (or embolization) or hysterectomy should be undertaken sooner rather than later.
2. Retained products/placenta should be removed with great care under anaesthesia. It is important that maximum uterine retraction is maintained until removal and this is best accomplished by oxytocin infusion and fundal massage if necessary.

3. Uterine rupture. If an examination under anaesthesia (EUA) reveals a hole in the uterus then a laparotomy must be performed. If possible the tear is repaired, but if haemostasis cannot be achieved then a postpartum hysterectomy or internal iliac ligation (or embolization) can be performed.

Retained placenta
If the placenta is not delivered within 30 minutes then preparations should be made for a manual removal. This can be performed under spinal, epidural or general anaesthesia.

Uterine inversion
The fundus of the uterus descends through the cervix usually with the placenta still attached. This has become a rare complication with the use of oxytocics and the Brandt–Andrews technique. Management involves immediate reduction if possible. If this is ineffective, then an i.v. line must be inserted, blood cross-matched, and the hydrostatic method of reduction attempted. Sterile saline is run into the upper vagina while the forearm occludes the introitus. If this fails, then abdominal surgery is required.

Amniotic fluid embolism
The patient suddenly collapses and a severe coagulation defect develops. If the condition is recognized, the patient needs to be ventilated, given steroids, and the coagulation defect corrected. The diagnosis is usually made at post-mortem.

Causes of postpartum collapse
1. Haemorrhage
2. Pulmonary embolism
3. Amniotic fluid embolism
4. Eclampsia
5. Others.

SUMMARY

If the third stage is managed appropriately the incidence of postpartum haemorrhage will be reduced.

27 Fetal monitoring in labour

Janice Rymer

Expectations of the examiners

The candidate is expected to have an understanding of a normal cardiotocograph (CTG) and to be able to recognize abnormalities indicating fetal distress.

Interesting facts

The aim of fetal monitoring in labour is to detect fetal hypoxia so that resulting perinatal morbidity and mortality can be prevented. The reaction of the fetus to hypoxia is variable and dependent on its individual reserve. Therefore each fetus should be assessed for its relative risk of developing hypoxia in labour and surveillance during labour managed accordingly.

Methods

There are various methods of monitoring a fetus during labour:

Note the colour of the liquor.   Meconium staining may result from an episode of hypoxia which causes vagal stimulation of the gut, relaxing the anal sphincter. Thick fresh meconium is considered an ominous sign. The absence of liquor is associated with IUGR and the fetus should be treated as if the liquor is meconium-stained until proven otherwise.

Auscultation of the fetal heart using a Pinard's stethoscope.   This is an intermittent form of fetal monitoring and should be employed during and immediately after contractions to detect accelerations or decelerations in the fetal heart rate (FHR). It is useful in low-risk patients with no identifiable abnormalities.

Sonar pulse detector (sonicaid).   This is also an intermittent form of fetal monitoring and should be used in a similar way to the Pinard's stethoscope.

Continuous fetal heart rate monitoring.   This method involves either an abdominal transducer, which detects the fetal heart movements ultrasonically, or an electrode attached to the fetal scalp which records a signal from the fetal heart (see Fig. 27.1). The abdominal transducer is less accurate. Most recording instruments also record uterine activity—cardiotocograph (CTG). The CTG should always be interpreted in the light of the clinical details in each case, e.g. the colour of the liquor, the stage of labour, and the drugs administered to the mother.

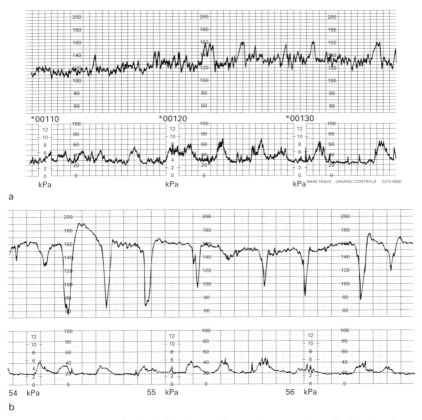

Fig. 27.1 Cardiotocographs (CTGs). a, Normal reactive trace; b, early decelerations.

Fetal heart rate patterns

Normal. The normal baseline heart rate is between 110 and 160 beats/minute. Accelerations of 10–15 beats/minute for at least 15 seconds indicate a healthy fetus. Baseline variability should be 5–25 beats/minute.

Baseline tachycardia (FHR > 160/minute.) This is associated with certain drugs, prematurity, hypoxia or maternal pyrexia.

Baseline bradycardia (FHR < 110/minute.) A rate between 90 and 110 beats/minute is only significant if there are decelerations or decreased variability. It may be due to postmaturity, hypoxia or heart block. Severe bradycardia (< 90 beats/minute) is usually associated with a preterminal condition in the fetus.

Loss of baseline variability. A normal heart rate shows irregular accelerations and if this variation is lost it may indicate hypoxia or fetal sleep rate. (95% last < 40 minutes.)

Increase in baseline variability. This can occur in high fetal activity states, and in acute or acute on chronic hypoxia.

Early decelerations (see Fig. 27.2). These decelerations begin with the onset of a contraction and return to the baseline by the end of the contraction. They

Fig. 27.2   Head compression and early deceleration (HC). (FHR = fetal heart rate)

do not drop more than 20–40 beats, are associated with compression of the fetal head and are not a sign of fetal distress.

Late decelerations (see Fig. 27.3). The low point of the deceleration occurs after the peak of the contraction and the fetal heart rate is slow to recover. The greater the lag-time between the end of the contraction and the return of the fetal heart rate to its normal baseline, the more serious the hypoxia is likely to be. Late decelerations are usually associated with fetal hypoxia and fetal blood sampling is indicated if labour is to proceed.

Variable decelerations (see Fig. 27.4). These are steep-sided and variable in shape and timing. They may be associated with cord compression. They can be identified as mild or moderate (< 60 dropped beats for < 60 seconds) or severe (> 60 dropped beats for > 60 seconds).

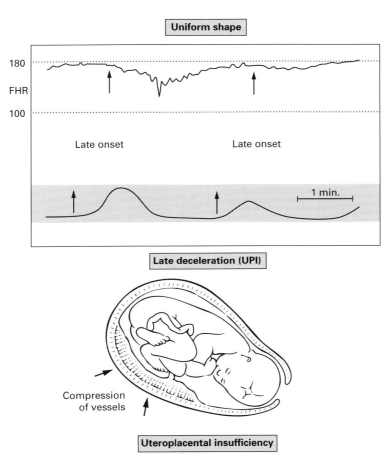

Fig. 27.3 Uteroplacental insufficiency and late deceleration (UPI).

Management

In the low-risk mother it is acceptable to use intermittent monitoring with auscultation. CTG monitoring is advised in high-risk cases. Interpreting continuous FHR recordings is difficult and the whole clinical picture must be taken into account. If the fetal heart tracing suggests fetal distress then various steps can be taken:

1. *Delivery*. For example, if a woman is in early labour with thick meconium-stained liquor and there are persistent late decelerations, then abdominal delivery is advised.
2. *Fetal blood sampling*. This should be regarded as complementary to continuous FHR recording. If the latter facility is used alone then the caesarean section rate will be higher due to false positive diagnoses (see Table 27.1). Fetal blood sampling should be repeated at least hourly as long as the CTG

Fig. 27.4 Umbilical cord compression and variable deceleration (CC).

Table 27.1 Interpretation of fetal blood sampling.

pH	Interpretation
> 7.25	Normal
	Allow labour to continue
7.20–7.25	Borderline
	If delivery is anticipated within 1–2 hours proceed but repeat pH in 1 hour
< 7.20	Abnormal
	Deliver immediately

remains abnormal. Increase the frequency of sampling if the CTG deteriorates. The rate of fall of pH between samples should be noted. A large fall (> 0.01 units/hour in first stage or > 0.02 units/hour in second stage) is significant and may indicate delivery even if both pHs are within the normal range. A fetus will attempt to maintain its pH for as long as possible but once buffering capacity is exceeded pH can fall very quickly.

3. *Resuscitation.* If the cause of acute fetal distress is due to a correctable maternal condition, then appropriate measures should be undertaken:
   a. The patient should adopt a lateral position with the foot of the bed higher than her heart.
   b. Augmentation should be discontinued and, in rare cases, uterine action should be inhibited using a tocolytic drug.
   c. Maternal hypotension should be corrected.
   d. The mother should be given oxygen.
   e. Intravenous fluids should be given for rehydration.

SUMMARY

The currently available methods for intrapartum monitoring are still unreliable; interpretation of continuous fetal heart rate patterns is difficult and must be used in conjunction with fetal blood sampling.

28 Obstetric intervention

Janice Rymer

INDUCTION OF LABOUR

Expectations of the examiners
The candidate should be familiar with the common indications and current methods of induction.

Interesting facts
Historically, induction of labour was mainly performed to ensure a small baby in cases of severe pelvic deformity. The commonest reason for induction is pregnancy persisting after 40 weeks' gestation. Routine induction between 41 and 42 weeks reduces caesarean section rates in this group of women.

Indications
Labour can be induced for numerous maternal and/or fetal reasons. When considering induction, two factors must be considered: (1) the risk to the mother or fetus if the pregnancy continues, versus (2) the risk of preterm delivery and complications of induction. The absolute contraindications are:

1. Placenta praevia
2. Abnormal lie
3. Known cephalopelvic disproportion.

Assessment
Important factors that must be considered prior to induction of labour are:

1. Gestation
2. Maternal well-being
3. Fetal well-being.

In order to determine the method of induction the maternal abdomen must be palpated to determine the presentation of the fetus and engagement of the head. A vaginal examination should be performed. The consistency, position, length and dilatation of the cervix should be documented along with the station of the presenting part (see Bishop's score in Table 28.1). If the cervix is unfavourable the chances of a good response to labour induction are low.

Table 28.1 Bishop's score (inducibility rating).

Dilatation	0	1–2	3–4	5–6
Score	0	1	2	3
Length of the cervix (cm)	3	2	1	0
Score	0	1	2	3
Station	−3	−2	−10	+1 +2
Score	0	1	2	3
Consistency	Firm	Medium	Soft	
Score	0	1	2	
Position	Posterior	Mid	Anterior	
Score	0	1	2	

Total score = 0–5 unfavourable
6–13 favourable

Method

If the presenting part is not high and artificial rupture of the membranes (ARM) is possible, then the women should be transferred to the labour ward and the membranes ruptured under aseptic conditions. This can be performed with an amnihook or Kocher's forceps; after the membranes have been ruptured, they should be swept back to induce further prostaglandin release. Some women will spontaneously commence labour if left alone, but the majority require augmentation. An oxytocin infusion is used, either immediately or after a period of time, initially at a low dose and increasing every 15 minutes until regular contractions are established. The fetal heart rate must be monitored—in most centres this is done continuously, and the cervical dilatation should be assessed regularly.

If the cervix is unfavourable, then prostaglandins can be used. In some units, even women with favourable cervices will be given prostaglandins initially. The current trend is to use intravaginal preparations, e.g. pessaries, gel or tablets. The state of the cervix is reassessed after an interval, and if possible the membranes are ruptured. If the cervix remains unfavourable, a further dose of prostaglandin can be used. The dosage and timing of prostaglandin administration are very variable. Labour will establish in 30–40% of women without any further intervention.

Complications of induction

1. Fetal distress
2. Maternal distress
3. Precipitate delivery
4. Operative delivery
5. Iatrogenic prematurity
6. Uterine rupture

7. Amniotic fluid embolism
8. Water intoxication (if high doses of oxytocin are used in conjunction with excessive fluid)
9. Diarrhoea, nausea, vomiting (systemic effects of prostaglandins).

Summary

Induced labours result in a higher proportion of operative deliveries, and the recent trend has been away from induction. Prostaglandins are being used more widely for induction of labour. The decision for induction must include a consideration of risks and benefits to both mother and fetus.

FORCEPS DELIVERIES

Expectations of the examiners

The candidate should be familiar with non-rotational forceps, e.g. Wrigley's and Neville Barnes', and be able to discuss the indications and prerequisites for forceps delivery. The candidate should also have a basic understanding of Kjelland's forceps but would not be expected to use them.

Interesting facts

A pair of forceps consists of two instruments, each a mirror image of the other. There are four components: blade, shank, lock and handle. Each blade has a cephalic and a pelvic curve (see Figs 28.1 and 28.2).

Indications for use

There must be a maternal and/or fetal reason to expedite delivery:

1. Fetal
   a. Distress
   b. Aftercoming head of breech
2. Maternal
   a. Delay in second stage
   b. Maternal disease, e.g. cardiac disease
   c. Dural tap.

Assessment

The following requirements must be satisfied before a forceps delivery can be performed:

1. Adequate analgesia
2. Bladder empty
3. No obvious cephalopelvic disproportion present
4. Cervix fully dilated
5. No head palpable above the pelvic brim
6. Membranes ruptured

a   b   c

Fig. 28.1 Forceps in common use. a, Neville Barnes' forceps; b, Kjelland's forceps; c, Wrigley's forceps.

c

b

a

Fig. 28.2 Lateral view of the forceps shown in Figure 28.1 reveals that the Wrigley's and the Neville Barnes' forceps have a much larger pelvic curve than the Kjelland's forceps (b).

7. Position of fetal head known, i.e. occipitoanterior ± 15%
8. Head at station +2 or more (for a rotational delivery the head may be higher).

229

Method

The patient is placed in the lithotomy position and cleaned and draped. The bladder is emptied, and local anaesthesia is injected at this point if it is the chosen method of analgesia. The position and station of the vertex are checked. The left blade is applied first, followed by the right; they should lock together easily if the application is correct. The direction of traction is initially forward and down, following the normal axis of delivery (only three pulls are allowed). As the perineum becomes distended, the head is extended and an episiotomy is usually performed. The forceps are removed and the delivery is conducted as normal. After delivery of the placenta, the perineum and vaginal walls are inspected and any tears appropriately repaired.

Rotational forceps

Kjelland's forceps have a cephalic curve but no pelvic curve, and a sliding lock to correct for asynclitism. They are employed when rotation of the head is required and should only be used by experienced obstetricians as they can cause significant maternal and fetal injury. Some units do not use Kjelland's forceps at all.

Complications

Fetal

Incorrect application of the forceps has been implicated in intracranial haemorrhage, and direct damage to the facial structures can occur (e.g. eye, nose, skull).

Maternal

Trauma to the birth canal is common and uterine rupture can occur. Postpartum haemorrhage is more common due to genital tract trauma and prolonged and difficult labour.

VACUUM DELIVERIES

Expectations of the examiners

The candidate is expected to be able to recognize the instrument and understand the principles behind its use.

Definition

A vacuum extractor (ventouse) is a suction cup connected to a suction device. There are a number of devices of this nature, including the original ventouse and newer hand-held variants. A vacuum is created between the cup and the fetal scalp and traction is applied in the axis of the birth canal to expedite delivery.

Indications for use

The indications are the same as for forceps deliveries, but maternal effort is needed. Therefore, in situations where maternal effort must be avoided, e.g. cardiac disease or severe hypertension, the vacuum is less useful.

An incompletely dilated cervix is not an indication for use in modern obstetrics.

Requirements for a vacuum delivery

These are the same as for a forceps delivery.

Method

The patient is prepared as for a forceps delivery. The cup is placed over the posterior fontanelle, and a vacuum of 0.8 kg/cm^2 is created. Traction is applied in the axis of the birth canal, imitating the normal mechanism of labour. Delivery must occur within three pulls, as with forceps deliveries.

Complications

These mainly involve fetal scalp injuries (which can be minimized by correct technique):

1. Cephalhaematoma—bleeding beneath the periosteum
2. Subgaleal haematoma—bleeding beneath the galea caused by emissary vein rupture
3. Intracranial haemorrhage—a rare complication related to hypoxia and prematurity.

These can be avoided if the technique is used appropriately.

Advantages

The vacuum has some advantages over the forceps:

1. It can be used with minimal or no anaesthesia.
2. It occupies no space between the fetal head and the maternal tissues.
3. There is less risk of maternal and fetal injury.

CAESAREAN SECTION

Expectations of the examiners

The examiners will assume that the candidate has assisted at caesarean sections. The indications, risks and complications of the operation should be known as well as the management in subsequent pregnancies.

Definition

A caesarean section is a surgical procedure whereby the fetus is delivered abdominally through a uterine incision.

Interesting facts

Although low, the maternal mortality following caesarean section is greater than that following vaginal delivery. A woman's obstetric future may be prejudiced by the presence of a uterine scar. The presence of a uterine scar influences management of subsequent deliveries. Rates of caesarean section are increasing for various reasons such as maternal choice, previous caesarean section and increased obstetric intervention.

Indications

There are many indications for caesarean section. The commonest are listed below:

1. Fetal
    a. Fetal distress—this can either be antenatally or intrapartum.
    b. Malpresentations and malpositions.
    c. Multiple pregnancy.
2. Maternal
    a. Failure to progress in labour.
    b. Previous caesarean section—most obstetricians would deliver a woman who had two previous caesarean sections by an elective caesarean section.
    c. Pre-eclampsia or eclampsia.
    d. Cephalopelvic disproportion.
3. Placental
    a. Praevia.
    b. Abruption.
    c. Cord prolapse.

With most of the indications listed above, other factors may need to be taken into account, e.g. gestation, stage of labour, parity.

Method

The operation can be performed under epidural, general or spinal anaesthesia. A urinary catheter is inserted into the bladder and the woman is placed with a left lateral tilt to avoid supine hypotension. The abdomen is cleaned and draped. Most caesarean sections are performed through a horizontal suprapubic skin incision (Pfannenstiel). The various layers of the abdominal wall are divided to expose the lower segment of the uterus. A transverse incision is made in the lower segment and the presenting part is then delivered manually or with forceps (if cephalic), the baby's mouth is suctioned, and the rest of the body is delivered. The cord is clamped and cut, and the placenta is removed. The wound is then repaired in layers.

A 'classic' caesarean section involves a vertical incision in the upper segment of the uterus. This leaves a significant scar on the uterus which is more prone to rupture in subsequent pregnancies. Most obstetricians would deliver a woman who had a classic caesarean with an elective caesarean section in subsequent pregnancies.

Requirements

1. Ideally the patient should be fasted and given an H_2 antagonist and an alkaline mixture prior to the operation (to neutralize the acid in the stomach).
2. The bladder must be empty.
3. An intravenous line must be in place.
4. An experienced anaesthetist must be present.
5. Blood must be available.
6. There must be adequate anaesthesia to perform the surgery.

Complications

Early

1. Anaesthetic problems, e.g. failed intubation, inadequate anaesthesia, drug overdose, hypoxia, aspiration of gastric contents
2. Haemorrhage
3. Damage to viscera
4. The original condition that caused the operation, e.g. pre-eclampsia, which may worsen postoperatively.

Late

1. Infection, e.g. uterine, wound, chest
2. Thromboembolism
3. Haemorrhage
4. Urinary tract infection
5. Wound dehiscence
6. Psychological problems.

Very late

1. Infertility (following infection)
2. Uterine rupture in a subsequent pregnancy
3. Adhesion formation.

Summary

The maternal morbidity and mortality for a caesarean section are higher when compared with a vaginal delivery.

29 Breech presentation and transverse lie

Janice Rymer

BREECH PRESENTATION

Expectations of the examiners

Although the delivery of a breech presentation is a specialist area, the examiners will expect the candidate to understand the principles of antenatal and labour management. As a general practitioner, the candidate may well have to perform a breech delivery if it has not been diagnosed prior to delivery, or if there is not enough time to call the flying squad as in preterm labour. There are several areas of controversy in the management of breech presentation, and the current trend is that all breech presentations at term (37–42 weeks) should have external cephalic version (ECV) attempted, and if this is not successful, an elective caesarean section.

Definition

The word breech means 'the buttocks'. There are three types of breech:

1. Extended leg breech—the legs are flexed at the hip and extended at the knee (frank breech) (see Fig. 29.1a).
2. Flexed leg breech—the legs are flexed at the hip and the knee (complete) (see Fig. 29.1b).
3. Footling breech—one or both feet are below the buttocks (see Fig. 29.1c).

Interesting facts

The incidence is 3–4% of all singleton pregnancies at term. The morbidity and mortality for a fetus in a breech presentation are considerably worse than for a vertex presentation. (Major contributors to this are prematurity, congenital anomalies and birth trauma.)

Aetiology

1. Maternal
   a. Grand multiparity
   b. Uterine anomalies
   c. Pelvic tumours
   d. Bony pelvic abnormality

(a) (b) (c)

Fig. 29.1 Breech presentation. a, Extended (frank); b, flexed (complete); c, footling.

2. Fetal
    a. Prematurity
    b. Multiple pregnancy
    c. Fetal abnormality
    d. Extended legs
3. Placental
    a. Cornual implantation
    b. Placenta praevia
    c. Oligohydramnios
    d. Polyhydramnios.

The frequency of breech presentation decreases as pregnancy progresses.

A breech presentation does not become a concern until 36 weeks (except in preterm labour). External cephalic version may be performed after 36 weeks to attempt to convert the breech to a cephalic presentation.

The diagnosis of a breech presentation is made on palpation of the abdomen. The presenting part is wider and the head is felt in the fundus. The fetal heart is heard above the umbilicus.

If the position of the placenta is known, then a vaginal examination should be performed to exclude pelvic masses and gross abnormalities of the pelvic bones.

Investigations

An ultrasound scan should be performed for the following reasons:

1. To confirm presentation
2. To exclude a fetal abnormality
3. To determine placental position

4. To determine whether it is a flexed or extended leg breech
5. To assess the liquor volume
6. To estimate fetal weight.

X-ray pelvimetry is no longer recommended.

Management

As mentioned above, the current recommendation is that term breeches should be delivered by caesarean section, if ECV is unsuccessful. Prior to 36 weeks unit policies vary.

However, the mother may want to consider a vaginal breech delivery, so one needs to be able to discuss this with her. The ideal weight for a vaginal breech delivery is 2500g–3500 g. Traditionally, footling and flexed leg breeches were usually delivered by caesarean section, but in multiparous women a flexed leg breech could be allowed a trial of labour. Providing there are no maternal contraindications, an extended leg breech without a fetal abnormality between 2500g and 3500g would previously have been considered favourable for a trial of vaginal delivery.

Most practitioners would not induce a breech presentation, as spontaneous onset of labour has the best prognosis. Once labour is established the membranes should be ruptured and continuous fetal monitoring should be used. An epidural anaesthetic is ideal because of the need for an operative delivery. The fetus should be monitored continuously and progress in labour assessed regularly. The use of oxytocin augmentation in a breech presentation is controversial, and slow progress in labour (< 1 cm/hour) is usually managed by a caesarean section.

Once full dilatation has occurred and the breech has descended to the perineum, then an episiotomy should be performed. As the breech continues to descend the sacrum is gently guided anteriorly, and the legs are stepped over the perineum (Pinard's manoeuvre). As the trunk descends the shoulders are delivered. If there is difficulty in delivering the shoulders then Lovset's manoeuvre must be performed. (Lovset's manoeuvre involves rotating the posterior shoulder anteriorly by rotating the trunk and then applying a downward traction. This enables the shoulders to descend below the pelvic brim and the arm usually appears spontaneously. If not, a finger can be hooked over the anterior shoulder and the arm brought down. The manoeuvre is repeated for the other arm.) The baby is allowed to hang until the nape of the neck is visible. The assistant then lifts the baby up and forceps are applied to the head to ensure a controlled delivery.

SUMMARY

Breech presentation is associated with increased perinatal morbidity and mortality, and must be considered a high-risk pregnancy. The current recommendation for term breeches is for a trial of ECV, and if this is unsuccessful, then caesarean section.

TRANSVERSE AND OBLIQUE LIE

Expectations of the examiners
The candidate should be able to detect an abnormal lie on palpation. The principles of management of a transverse and oblique lie should be known by the candidate. The management of cord prolapse is a common examination question.

Definition
The lie of the fetus is not in the longitudinal axis of the uterus.

Aetiology
1. Maternal
   a. High multiparity
   b. Uterine anomalies
   c. Pelvic tumours
   d. Pelvic contraction
2. Fetal
   a. Prematurity
   b. Multiple pregnancy
   c. Fetal abnormality
3. Placenta
   a. Placenta praevia
   b. Fundal placenta.

Assessment
On inspection the uterus appears wider than normal. The fundal height may be smaller than one would expect for the gestational age, and there is no presenting part in the pelvis. The back is lying across the maternal abdomen and the head is palpated in one or other flank. The fetal heart may be heard more laterally than normal.

As with a breech presentation, a vaginal examination should be performed (if the placental site is known) to exclude pelvic pathology.

Investigations
An ultrasound scan should be performed for the same reasons as in breech presentation.

Management
Transverse lie is uncommon. External cephalic version should not be attempted. If the transverse lie persists beyond 37 weeks, then the woman

should be admitted to hospital because of the risk of cord prolapse. If a cause for the transverse lie is found, e.g. pelvic tumour or placenta praevia, then an elective caesarean section should be performed. If no cause is found, then there are two accepted forms of management:

1. Await the onset of labour to see if the lie converts to longitudinal in labour. If it does, then the woman has a trial of labour. If it does not, then a caesarean section should be performed. If the lie converts to longitudinal prior to the onset of labour, she can be allowed home, or if the cervix is favourable, an artificial rupture of membranes (ARM) could be performed followed by oxytocin. In primiparous women this is very unlikely after 37 weeks, even when labour begins.
2. An elective caesarean section can be performed.

Cord prolapse

If a woman with a transverse lie has spontaneous rupture of membranes she must have an immediate vaginal examination to exclude cord prolapse. If the cord is felt then the woman must be put into the knee–chest position or placed on all fours. The aim of adopting these positions is to use gravity to keep the presenting part from compressing the cord against the cervix. The examining hand must remain in the vagina to elevate the presenting part until the baby is delivered. (If there is to be a long delay between the time of cord prolapse and caesarean section, then 500 ml of fluid can be infused into the bladder via a Foley catheter which is then clamped.)

Urgent arrangements must be made to deliver the baby by caesarean section.

Delivery

A transverse lie that persists must be delivered by caesarean section. These can be difficult operations, especially if the fetal back is presenting.

A general anaesthetic is preferred to ensure maximum uterine relaxation. If there is no lower segment then a vertical incision should be performed in the uterus. After the uterus is incised, a breech extraction is performed. A foot is grasped, the lie converted to longitudinal, and the feet and the remainder of the body are delivered.

A thorough inspection of the uterine cavity and the pelvis should be performed to attempt to determine a cause for the transverse lie.

SUMMARY

Transverse and oblique lie are uncommon and need specialist referral. Women should be admitted from 37 weeks onwards. Cord prolapse is more common and is an obstetric emergency.

30

Twin pregnancy

Janice Rymer

Expectations of the examiners

The candidate will be expected to be aware of the common antenatal complications of a multiple pregnancy. The overall management of multiple pregnancy should always be undertaken by a specialist unit.

Definition

A twin pregnancy is a pregnancy with two fetuses.

Interesting facts

The incidence is 1 in 80 but this is increasing due to assisted conception techniques.

Pathophysiology

Twinning can either be monozygotic or dizygotic. Monozygotic twins result from the division of one conceptus, producing identical twins. Dizygotic twins result from the fertilization of two separate ova, and the twins have a different genetic make-up. Dizygotic twins are always dichorionic and diamniotic, but monozygotic twins can vary from monochorionic and monoamniotic to dichorionic and diamniotic, depending on when division of the blastocyst occurred.

Aetiology

The frequency of monozygotic twins is constant at a rate of 1 in 250 births. However, the incidence of dizygotic twins is influenced remarkably by:

1. *Race.* In Nigeria twinning occurs in 1 in every 19 births, compared to 1 in 155 births in Japan.
2. *Heredity.* A family history of twins, especially on the mother's side, is associated with an increase in the incidence of twin pregnancy.
3. *Increasing maternal age and parity.* Both of these factors are associated with a higher rate of twin pregnancies.
4. *Assisted conception.* The overall incidence of multiple pregnancies using these techniques is 2–3%. This is due to the induction of multiple ovulations and the replacement of more than one egg or embryo.

Assessment

At the booking visit, the history may include risk factors for multiple pregnancy as outlined above. Hyperemesis gravidarum in the first trimester is more common, and on examination the uterine size may be larger than dates.

Investigations

An ultrasound scan should detect multiple pregnancies, although they can be missed.

The haemoglobin and the packed cell volume may be lower due to the exaggerated increase in plasma volume.

The α-fetoprotein levels in maternal serum are higher, making interpretation difficult.

Management

Multiple pregnancy should not be regarded as a 'normal pregnancy', and patients should be seen more regularly in the antenatal clinic.

First trimester. An early scan (< 14 weeks) should be performed for dating purposes. Severe hyperemesis warrants admission with intravenous hydration. Four-weekly visits are acceptable if there are no other complications.

Second trimester. A detailed anomaly scan should be performed at 18–20 weeks, as there is an increased incidence of fetal abnormalities.

Third trimester. After 28 weeks' gestation the patient should be seen at least every 2 weeks with regular ultrasound scans for growth assessment.

Routine admission at 28–32 weeks has not been shown to decrease the incidence of preterm labour. Admission should be offered to the patient at any stage if she is unable to rest adequately at home.

In late pregnancy the commonest presentations are vertex, vertex (45%); vertex, breech (40%); however, malpresentations are more common in multiple pregnancies.

Complications

Maternal

1. *Hyperemesis.* Severe cases require admission and intravenous hydration, but most settle by 12 weeks when the β-HCG levels begin to fall.
2. *Pre-eclampsia.* Not only does pre-eclampsia occur more often in multiple pregnancy but it tends to develop earlier and be more severe.
3. *Gestational diabetes.* The diabetogenic state of normal pregnancy is exaggerated, increasing the incidence and severity of gestational diabetes.
4. *Anaemia.* The increase in plasma volume is much greater, exaggerating the 'physiological' anaemia of pregnancy. Iron and folate deficiencies are common because of the extra demands of a twin pregnancy.
5. *General discomfort.* Having a larger uterine mass puts added strain on the musculoskeletal system.
6. *Placenta praevia.* The incidence is increased in multiple pregnancies, presumably due to the increased placental area.

Fetal

1. *Prematurity*. This is the main factor in the increased wastage associated with multiple pregnancies. More than 50% of babies of multiple pregnancies weigh less than 2.5 kg compared with 6% of singletons. There are many contributing factors to the significantly increased incidence of preterm delivery in twin pregnancies:
   a. Overdistension of the uterus
   b. Increased incidence of pregnancy-induced hypertension
   c. Increased incidence of fetal abnormalities
   d. Increased incidence of abruption
   e. Increased incidence of malpresentation.
2. *Fetal abnormality*. There is an increased incidence of fetal malformation in monozygotic twin pregnancies.
3. *IUGR*. Growth restriction is common in twin pregnancies, especially when the placenta is monochorionic. One or both twins may be affected.
4. *Twin-to-twin transfusion*. The two placental circulations may form anastomoses in monochorionic twins. One fetus may become anaemic and the other polycythaemic. The syndrome is usually diagnosed after birth, and either baby may require intensive care.
5. *Malpresentations*. These are probably more common because of prematurity, increased incidence of fetal malformations, and mechanical restrictions of the uterine cavity.

Delivery

The decision on the mode of delivery depends on the presentation of the leading twin, and the presence of maternal or fetal complications. In the majority of cases, labour occurs spontaneously around 38 weeks.

The membranes should be ruptured as soon as labour is established. An intravenous line should be inserted, and blood should be grouped and saved. Both twins should be monitored externally. If this is technically difficult then a fetal scalp electrode should be applied to the leading twin.

An epidural is the optimal form of analgesia, as an operative delivery may be required.

Progress in labour must be assessed regularly as inefficient uterine action is common.

At delivery, two obstetricians, two paediatricians, an anaesthetist and midwifery staff should be present. Following delivery of the first twin, the cord is clamped and cut. The abdomen is palpated to ensure that the lie of the remaining fetus is longitudinal. (If the lie cannot be converted to longitudinal externally, then a caesarean section should be considered.) Fundal pressure is maintained, and the membranes are ruptured during a contraction. Labour should resume, but if there are no contractions after 10 minutes, then an oxytocin infusion should be commenced. The second twin is then delivered. Breech extraction of the second twin may be necessary. The placenta is delivered, and an oxytocin infusion postpartum is advisable to prevent haemorrhage. (The ideal delivery interval between twins is ≤ 20 minutes.)

Complications

1. *Incoordinate uterine action.* This is a common occurrence in twins. There is debate as to whether labour should be augmented.
2. *Fetal distress.* The second twin is usually smaller and may not cope as well with the stress of labour.
3. *Prolapse of the umbilical cord.* The management depends on the circumstances: degree of cervical dilatation, the presence or absence of ruptured membranes, and the analgesia (see Ch. 29).
4. *Premature separation of the placenta.* If vaginal delivery can be achieved rapidly without harm to the fetus or the mother, then this should be performed. Otherwise, the fetus should be delivered by caesarean section.
5. *Locking.* This is rare but can occur when the first twin presents as a breech, and the second by the vertex. The chin of the first fetus locks in the neck and chin of the second cephalic fetus.

Postpartum

1. *Haemorrhage.* Due to the increased size of the placental bed and the overdistension of the uterus, there is an increased risk of postpartum haemorrhage.
2. *Thromboembolic disease.* Twin pregnancies have an increased risk.
3. *Anaemia.* This is due to the increased demand for iron in pregnancy and the greater blood loss.

SUMMARY

Twin pregnancies have significantly increased fetal and maternal morbidity and mortality. They are high-risk pregnancies and should be monitored carefully. The delivery should be conducted in a consultant-led unit. Only twin pregnancies have been discussed but the problems of a twin gestation are exaggerated by the presence of more fetuses. Most obstetricians would deliver pregnancies with three or more fetuses by caesarean section.

31 Obstetric analgesia and anaesthesia

Gregory Davis

Expectations of the examiners

Candidates will be expected to be able to advise women on the advantages and disadvantages of the different methods of analgesia and anaesthesia. The effects on mother and fetus, the complications and their management must be completely understood.

Definitions

Analgesia is loss of sensation to pain.
Anaesthesia is loss of all sensation including pain.

Interesting facts

There is a wide range of methods available for pain relief and the choice of a particular method will depend on a number of factors: mother's preference, severity of pain, stage in labour, methods available at the place of birth, and the presence of complications in the mother and/or fetus. Most women and their partners are anxious during labour and careful explanation and reassurance to reduce anxiety is an important aspect of the management of pain in labour. People vary widely in their tolerance of pain and their response to analgesia.

Pathophysiology

Source of the pain

Pain in labour is of two types: (1) intermittent and (2) continuous.

Intermittent pain.   This is due to uterine contractions and is probably caused by myometrial ischaemia at the peak of the contractions. The pain is most severe just prior to full dilatation (transition phase) when contractions are most intense and the cervix is dilating most rapidly. Sensation from the uterus and cervix is transmitted mainly in the sensory fibres of the T11 and T12 nerve roots, with smaller amounts in T10 and L1.

Continuous pain.   This occurs in the lower back and suprapubically and the cause of this pain is not known. Lower back pain is more prominent with occipitoposterior positions.

In the second stage of labour, pain is associated with distension of the lower vagina and perineum. The perineum is innervated principally by the pudendal nerve with fibres passing to the S2, 3 and 4 nerve roots.

Pharmacokinetics in mother and fetus

Mother. Although liver production of various proteins alters markedly in pregnancy, it is unclear whether this affects the maternal handling of anaesthetic drugs. Body fat increases by 4 kg on average during pregnancy, leading to a greater capacity to sequester lipid-soluble drugs.

Fetus. About one-seventh of the blood returning to the fetus from the placenta enters the left atrium directly. Any drugs in this blood are therefore available to affect the fetal brain. This is only likely to be significant with intravenous bolus injections. The remaining umbilical blood flow passes through the fetal liver where drugs are metabolized.

Placental transfer

Like the blood–brain barrier, the placental barrier is composed of lipoproteins so the transfer of drugs depends on lipid solubility. Most agents which affect the central nervous system will therefore cross the placenta. Highly ionized drugs, such as muscle relaxants, do not cross the placenta.

Although there has been concern that exposure of pregnant women to trace quantities of anaesthetic gases may lead to abortion or fetal malformation, the evidence for this is inconclusive. During the first half of pregnancy intra-abdominal surgery increases the risk of miscarriage, but this is probably due to uterine manipulation rather than the anaesthetic agents.

PAIN RELIEF IN LABOUR

The different components of pain relief in labour are outlined in Table 31.1.

Although in this chapter interventional management is emphasized, perhaps the most important aspect of pain relief in labour is the individual woman's attitude. The ideal approach is for women to be healthy, relaxed, supported by a labour partner, fully acquainted with the variety of methods available, free to make a choice, and with an open mind should circumstances change. It is the role of antenatal education to provide women with the opportunity to achieve such a state at the onset of labour.

Physical methods

The major advantage of these methods is that they are non-invasive and therefore not harmful to the fetus. They are useful early in labour and may act by overloading sensory inputs. Their major disadvantage is that they are often ineffective later in labour.

Table 31.1   Sources of pain relief in labour.

Education
Antenatal classes
  Information
  Demonstrations

Environment
Pleasant surroundings
Supportive helpful staff
Support of partner

Physical methods
Massage
Acupuncture
Transcutaneous electrical nerve stimulation (TENS)

Pharmacological
Analgesia
  Inhalational, e.g. nitrous oxide
  Narcotic, e.g. pethidine
  Regional analgesia: epidural, spinal, pudendal, perineal infiltration

Inhalational agents

Nitrous oxide combined with oxygen (Entonox) is the only inhalational agent now available. The advantages of inhalational agents are that they are self-administered and safe for mother and fetus. The major disadvantage is that they are commonly used incorrectly leading to failure of this method.

In active labour, although contractions last approximately 60 seconds, the first 20–30 seconds are not usually as painful as the latter part of the contractions. It takes a similar period of time, 20–30 seconds, of deep panting using nitrous oxide to achieve a blood level sufficient for analgesia. It is therefore important for the woman to begin rapid breathing with the onset of each contraction rather than waiting until the contraction is painful. Similarly, in the second stage of labour when pain is present throughout contractions, contractions must be anticipated by 30 seconds and inhalation commenced prior to the onset of the contraction if this method is to be successful.

Narcotic agents

Pethidine is the preferred narcotic for use in labour as it is less soporific than the other narcotics. Although it is a strong analgesic and easily administered, there is a high incidence of side-effects and 40% of women in labour report no relief of pain. The side-effects are:

1. Dizziness
2. Drowsiness
3. Dissociated state of consciousness
4. Nausea
5. Vomiting
6. Hypotension.

Pethidine is usually given as a bolus i.m. injection of 100 mg which may need to be repeated. It is rare for a woman in labour to require more than two doses and, if the need arises, progress in labour should be reviewed. It is unlikely to cause significant delay in the active phase of labour. The effect on the fetus is to depress heart rate variability and breathing movements and it causes respiratory depression and hypotonicity in the newborn. Respiratory depression is most likely to occur if a narcotic is given i.m. 2.5–3.5 hours prior to delivery. Respiratory depression is unlikely more than 6 hours after i.m. administration. Respiratory depression within 6 hours of narcotic administration is treated with a narcotic antagonist, most commonly naloxone 20 μg i.m., repeated if necessary.

Because nausea and vomiting are common side-effects, narcotics are often given with an antiemetic. The antiemetic chosen varies considerably but is either an antihistamine, e.g. promethazine hydrochloride, an antidopaminergic (phenothiazine), e.g. prochlorperazine, or metoclopramide. The first two have sedative and anxiolytic properties and are sometimes preferred because of these effects.

The routine use of other sedatives, e.g. diazepam or barbiturates, is not acceptable in modern obstetric practice because of their prolonged effect on the neonate.

Epidural analgesia

The epidural (or extradural) space is the potential space lying outside the dura mater and containing blood vessels, lymphatics and fat. The injection of local anaesthetics into this space produces analgesia in the spinal nerve roots to which the anaesthetic agents diffuse. Therefore, to provide effective analgesia in the first stage of labour the T10–L1 nerve roots must be blocked, while in the second stage of labour the sacral roots must be blocked. The use of epidural analgesia for caesarean section requires a more extensive block to at least T8 and sometimes even T6. There are two routes for epidural analgesia: caudal via the sacrococcygeal membrane, or lumbar between adjacent vertebral spines. In obstetrics the latter route is now used almost exclusively.

Indications
1. *Pain relief*. This is the commonest reason.
2. *Hypertensive disorders*. Blood pressure is more easily controlled when an effective epidural block is present.
3. *Maternal heart disease*. The abolition of pain reduces stress and the bearing down reflex thereby relieving strain on the heart. Care is necessary, however, if the patient has a fixed cardiac output, e.g. mitral or aortic stenosis, and cannot compensate for hypotension.
4. *Cerebrovascular disease*. This is rare in pregnancy but epidural analgesia would be indicated in the presence of an intracranial aneurysm or angioma.
5. *Twin delivery*. The presence of an effective epidural block allows intrauterine manipulation of the second twin.

Contraindications

1. Recent antepartum haemorrhage: epidural analgesia may be associated with profound hypotension in the presence of significant blood loss.
2. Coagulation disorder: a clotting defect due to anticoagulants or coagulopathy (e.g. in severe pre-eclampsia) increases the risk of haemorrhage into the epidural space.
3. Sepsis at the injection site.
4. Sensitivity to local anaesthetic agents.
5. Lack of adequately trained staff.
6. Bony disorder of the lower spine.
7. Active neurological disease.

There has been concern that the epidural analgesia may 'mask' the pain of uterine rupture in women with a scarred uterus. In most units this is no longer a contraindication to epidural analgesia.

Management

A fine plastic catheter is passed through an introducer which is inserted in the midline midway between two lumbar spinous processes—usually L2–3 or L3–4 (see Fig. 31.1). Positioning is important, with the woman lying in the left lateral position or, less commonly, sitting with her back flexed. The skin area is cleansed and the large-bore Tuohy needle (introducer) is inserted after infiltrating the skin and subcutaneous tissues with local anaesthetic.

Common local anaesthetic agents used are bupivacaine, ropivacaine and lidocaine (lignocaine). An initial test dose of 3–5 ml is given and then 5

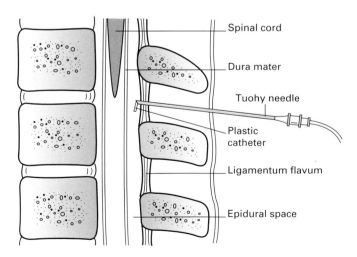

Fig. 31.1 The correct insertion of an epidural catheter. A Tuohy needle is pushed through the skin and ligamentum flavum into the epidural space. The plastic catheter is then passed through the needle and pushed a little further into the space; then the needle is removed.

minutes later the remainder is given. The purpose of giving a test dose is to ensure that the catheter has not inadvertently pierced the dura (a spinal block) or is lying in an epidural vein. Lidocaine (lignocaine) is used to provide a shorter-acting, dense block that is useful prior to assisted delivery.

Observations

Prior to insertion of the epidural catheter an i.v. line must be inserted and hypovolaemia corrected. The use of a 'preload' of 500–1000 mL crystalloid fluid is common. The fetal heart must be monitored continuously and maternal blood pressure and pulse recorded every 5 minutes for at least 15 minutes. An analgesic effect is not observed for 15–20 minutes and usually lasts 60–90 minutes. As soon as sensation begins to return the epidural catheter should be 'topped up'. Alternative methods are to give a continuous infusion of anaesthetic agent or intermittent boluses controlled by the woman (patient controlled epidural analgesia, PCEA). A low concentration of local anesthetic is infused, usually with an opioid such as fentanyl or pethidine.

Complications

1. Hypotension (drop in systolic blood pressure of > 20 mmHg) is treated by ensuring that aortocaval compression is not occurring and administering 1 litre of Hartman's solution or normal saline over 20 minutes. If these measures are ineffective or maternal or fetal distress occurs, ephedrine should be given, 5–10 mg i.v. This has an inotropic and chronotropic action on the heart and does not cause placental vasoconstriction.
2. Total spinal block occurs with injection of the local anaesthetic agent into the intrathecal space. There is rapid, progressively ascending block of motor, sensory and autonomic nerves. This is manifested by marked hypotension, bradycardia and increasing respiratory distress which may culminate in apnoea. Treatment is to provide oxygen and vasopressors initially and, if complete respiratory paralysis occurs, artificial ventilation.
3. Failure to achieve adequate analgesia can usually be treated by injecting further anaesthetic, but if this fails the epidural catheter may have to be resited.
4. Dural puncture occurs in 1–2% of cases and results in a severe headache in 70% of these cases. The headache usually starts within 48 hours of delivery and lasts for 6 days if left untreated. If it is recognized at the time of insertion the catheter is resited and good analgesia achieved. An elective forceps delivery should be performed if delivery is not speedily effected. After delivery dural puncture is treated conservatively with bed rest, analgesia and adequate fluids. If a severe headache persists after 24–36 hours a 'blood patch' is performed. To achieve a blood clot over the hole in the dura, 20 ml of the patient's blood is injected into the epidural space. The patient lies flat for 30 minutes and the headache is usually absent after this period.
5. An increased rate of assisted delivery is minimized by the aggressive use of oxytocin in the second stage of labour.

6. Local anaesthetic toxicity may develop with either accidental intravascular injection or excessive total dosage. Premonitory symptoms include a metallic taste, circumoral tingling, nervousness and nausea. If untreated, these may progress to muscle twitching and to convulsions, cardiovascular depression and cardiac arrest.
7. Other rare complications are meningitis and neurological sequelae.

The major advantage of epidural analgesia is that it is the only method of completely abolishing pain in labour (90% of patients have complete or substantial relief). The fetus is rarely affected and the woman is awake and alert. The major disadvantage is that it requires the presence of skilled personnel. Closer observation is also necessary and there is an increased incidence of operative delivery.

Caesarean section. Caesarean section under epidural anaesthesia requires a more extensive block. The advantages are that the woman and her partner can see and be involved with the infant immediately; blood loss is reduced and the incidence of postoperative complications reduced. The disadvantages are that the anaesthesia may not be sufficient necessitating general anaesthesia and, from the operator's point of view, the baby is more difficult to deliver as the patient's abdominal muscles may not be completely relaxed. Epidural infusion or PCEA with opioids may be continued for 24–36 hours for postoperative analgesia.

Spinal analgesia

Spinal block is used primarily as a single injection intrathecally in the lumbar region for instrumental delivery, caesarean section or manual removal of the placenta. A small volume of a heavy form of local anaesthetic agent usually mixed with an opioid (e.g. 2.5 ml of bupivacaine with 200 mg morphine) is injected with the patient in the sitting position to minimize the spread of the agent cephalically. The block is effective in 3–5 minutes and the patient is observed as with epidural anaesthesia. The advantage of this method is that it is rapid and gives a dense block. The disadvantages are that if it is ineffective then there is no catheter to repeat the dose, cephalic spread with consequent respiratory depression may occur and hypotension is common. Despite these drawbacks, spinal anaesthesia is becoming more widely used because of its advantages.

Pudendal block

This is a suitable method of analgesia for non-rotational forceps or vacuum extraction. The pudendal nerve is blocked by infiltrating 5–10 ml of 0.5–1% lidocaine (lignocaine) around the nerve on each side as it passes around the ischial spine. This is usually done vaginally or, rarely, through the perineum. The commonest problem is that there may be inadequate analgesia on one or both sides and perineal infiltration is often required.

GENERAL ANAESTHESIA

The major problems associated with general anaesthesia in the pregnant woman are regurgitation and aspiration of the stomach contents during induction of anaesthesia. Although this has been recognized for many years, it is still a major cause of avoidable maternal death. The reasons for the increased risk are:

1. General anaesthesia is often performed as an emergency procedure with the woman not starved.
2. There is delayed gastric emptying and relaxation of the lower oesophageal sphincter in pregnancy.
3. In labour, gastric emptying is even further delayed especially when opioids are given.
4. Oedema of the vocal cords is more common in pregnancy (due to pre-eclampsia).
5. The increase in body fat and breast size in pregnancy and the presence of an abdominal mass combine to make intubation technically more difficult.

Indications
1. Early pregnancy—abortion, termination of pregnancy, ectopic pregnancy, insertion of cervical suture
2. Caesarean section
3. Instrumental delivery—rarely necessary under general anaesthesia and should be used with great caution because of the risk of fetal trauma
4. Obstetric emergencies—cord prolapse, ruptured or inverted uterus, uncontrollable postpartum haemorrhage
5. Manual removal of the placenta.

Preoperative medication
The drugs usually given preoperatively are contraindicated in pregnancy because of the effects on the fetus. Acidity of the stomach contents is reduced by giving H_2-receptor blocking drugs orally every 6 hours in labour and prior to elective surgery in pregnancy. Ranitidine is more commonly used as it has fewer side-effects than cimetidine. An alkali mixture, e.g. 15–30 ml magnesium trisilicate or sodium citrate, is given orally immediately prior to induction of anaesthesia.

Induction of anaesthesia
The patient is placed in the left lateral position during transport to and in the anaesthetic room. Oxygen is given by mask or mouthpiece for 3–5 minutes prior to induction. This reduces the effects on mother and fetus of the apnoeic period between the onset of paralysis and the initiation of ventilation.

Following the injection of the induction agent, cricoid pressure is immediately applied and maintained until the endotracheal tube is in place and its cuff inflated. The most commonly used induction agent is thiopental (250–300 mg). This is followed immediately by suxamethonium to induce rapid paralysis to allow endotracheal intubation. Paralysis is continued throughout the operation and anaesthesia maintained with nitrous oxide in oxygen which is administered in a relatively high concentration until delivery has occurred. This mixture is supplemented with a volatile agent (e.g. halothane) in low concentrations.

Following delivery, oxytocin (5–10 IV) is given to ensure uterine contraction and the concentration of the inhalational agents is usually increased.

Complications

Because light anaesthesia is maintained prior to delivery, approximately 3% of women will experience some degree of awareness of which about one-tenth will be painful. This dilemma is difficult to resolve because of the concern over neonatal drug-induced CNS depression. The use of volatile 0.5% halothane or an equivalent dose of isoflurane or enthrane virtually abolishes awareness.

Aspiration of gastric contents (Mendelson syndrome) is the most important contributor to maternal morbidity and mortality associated with general anaesthesia. The syndrome is unlikely to occur if the pH of the gastric contents is > 3.0, stressing the importance of the prophylactic measures discussed above. Management involves bronchoscopy if solid material is aspirated, oxygen and bronchodilators, intravenous fluids, steroids and antibiotics, and artificial ventilation if necessary.

Other complications of general anaesthesia are:

1. Intraoperative
   a. Circulatory collapse
   b. Respiratory failure
   c. Cardiac failure
2. Postoperative
   a. Patient drowsy
   b. Respiratory infection
   c. Deep venous thrombosis/pulmonary embolus
   d. Gastrointestinal stasis.

32

Puerperium and breast-feeding

Gregory Davis

Expectations of the examiners

Problems arising in the puerperium are usually managed in the community and therefore by general practitioners. The examiners will expect candidates to have a good understanding of the normal course of the puerperium and practical remedies for any problems. The management of postpartum haemorrhage (PPH) is a frequent examination question as it is a life-threatening complication that is relatively common.

Definitions

The puerperium refers to the weeks following delivery in which the pregnancy-induced changes return to normal. By convention these take place over 6 weeks, although it may take longer for all the organs to return to normal.

Primary postpartum haemorrhage (PPH) is defined as blood loss from the genital tract of 500 mL or more in the first 24 hours after delivery.

Secondary PPH is defined as blood loss from the genital tract of 500 mL or more at any time in the puerperium after the first 24 hours.

Puerperal pyrexia is defined as a temperature of 38°C or greater, or 37.4°C on three successive days, within 14 days of delivery or miscarriage.

Physiology

The pelvic organs never entirely return to normal after childbirth. The uterus weighs 1000–1200 g immediately postpartum, 500 g 1 week later, and has returned to the non-pregnant weight (50–70 g) by 6 weeks. It is not normally palpable abdominally after 10–14 days. The cervix never returns to normal and is slit-like and often irregular. Mature breast milk is produced by 7 days postpartum as a result of oestrogen withdrawal.

The increased production of plasma proteins which occurs in pregnancy rapidly returns to normal after delivery and this is complete by 3 weeks postpartum. The cardiovascular and renal systems have returned to their non-pregnant state by 6 weeks, except for the renal collecting system which takes about 3 months. The cardiovascular system reverts quickly after delivery and is 50% back to normal by the third day after delivery.

Ovulation after delivery is extremely variable and affected by lactation. Of non-lactating women, 10–15% will have ovulated by 6 weeks but in lactating women, ovulation is rare before 10 weeks. Menstruation often occurs prior to initial ovulation.

PRIMARY POSTPARTUM HAEMORRHAGE

See 'Labour—third stage' (Ch. 26).

SECONDARY POSTPARTUM HAEMORRHAGE

Blood loss in secondary PPH is not usually as great as in primary PPH but can be very frightening for the woman.

Aetiology
1. Infection
2. Retained products of conception.

Assessment
1. History
   a. Amount of blood loss—as most cases occur at home this is often difficult to assess.
   b. Method of delivery.
   c. Completeness of placenta at delivery.
   d. Fever.
   e. Offensive lochia.
2. Examination
   a. Temperature, other vital signs.
   b. Height and tenderness of fundus.
   c. State of cervical os.
3. Investigations
   a. Ultrasound scan will demonstrate retained products of conception, although cervical dilatation is usually obvious.
   b. FBC, cross-match.
   c. Cervical swabs.
   d. Blood cultures and other investigations as required if the patient is septicaemic.

Treatment
In most cases the diagnosis is clear. If the cervical os is open then evacuation of the uterus will be necessary. If the woman is febrile and/or toxic then 12–24 hours of intravenous antibiotics are required prior to the evacuation. A tender

well-retracted uterus with a closed cervical os in an otherwise well woman should be treated with oral antibiotics, amoxicillin and metronidazole (200 mg t.d.s. in breast-feeding women).

PUERPERAL INFECTION

Interesting facts
This was the largest cause of maternal mortality until the 1930s when aseptic techniques and then antibiotics were introduced. Puerperal fever was caused by the spread of group A streptococcus from woman to woman in hospitals. Anaemia increases the susceptibility of women to infection postnatally.

Pathophysiology
Although infection may occur at any site, the puerperal woman is particularly susceptible to wound infection and infection of the reproductive, urinary and respiratory tracts, and the breasts.

1. The reproductive tract has usually been traumatized and there may be retained products or blood clot. In practice, the severity of infection is varied and may be complicated by pelvic vein thrombosis
   a. Mild infection confined to the vagina, cervix, and uterus.
   b. Moderate infection with spread to the pelvic organs to give salpingitis and pelvic peritonitis.
   c. Severe cases where generalized peritonitis and septicaemia develop.
2. The urinary collecting system is still dilated and the woman may have been catheterized during delivery.
3. General anaesthesia predisposes the woman to postnatal chest infection.
4. The nipples may crack in the first few days after delivery, allowing bacterial contamination and infection.
5. The presence of an abdominal wound after caesarean section is a focus for infection.

Bacteriology
1. Reproductive tract
   a. Endogenous organisms
      i.   Coliforms
      ii. *Streptococcus faecalis*
      iii. Anaerobic streptococci
      iv. *Clostridium welchii*
   b. Exogenous organisms
      i. Haemolytic streptococcus (group A)
      ii. *Staphylococcus aureus*
2. Urinary tract
   a. *Escherichia coli* (90%)

b. Others
  i. *Proteus*
  ii. *Klebsiella*
3. Breasts
  a. *Staphylococcus aureus* (> 90%).

Assessment

Women with puerperal pyrexia need a careful history and examination, diagnosis of the site of infection, and appropriate treatment. Deep venous thrombosis (DVT) is more common in the postnatal period and may cause pyrexia. The pelvic veins may be involved, particularly if sepsis is present.

History
1. Method of delivery
2. History of trauma to birth canal
3. Time of onset of fever (infections in the birth canal usually giving a rise in temperature 12–24 hours after delivery)
4. Site of pain
5. Any other symptoms suggesting incidental infection, e.g. sore throat.

Examination
A full physical examination should be made with particular attention to:

1. Signs of septicaemia
  a. Temperature.
  b. Rapid, weak pulse.
  c. Hypotension.
  d. Pallor.
  e. Altered consciousness.
2. Chest—signs of infection.
3. Abdomen
  a. The fundus may be tender and high if endometritis is present.
  b. More widespread tenderness or peritonism is associated with severe puerperal sepsis.
  c. The abdominal wound is the commonest site of infection after caesarean section.
4. Vagina
  a. The perineum should be inspected.
  b. If the cervical os is dilated then retained products are likely.
5. Lower limbs.

Investigations
1. Midstream specimen of urine
2. High vaginal/endocervical swabs for culture
3. Blood cultures if temperature > 38°C
4. Other investigations if septicaemic
5. Doppler flow study of lower limbs if suspicion of DVT

6. Ventilation/perfusion scan of lungs if pulmonary embolus is suspected.
7. Sputum if chest infection is suspected
8. Wound swab if abdominal delivery.

Treatment

1. *Reproductive tract.* Evacuation of retained products should be performed after 12–24 hours of i.v. antibiotics. Septicaemia will need appropriate circulatory support and these women may need to be nursed in an intensive care unit. Treatment should begin before the infecting agent or its sensitivities are known, but after appropriate swabs have been taken.
   a. Mild
      i. Amoxicillin (oral).
      ii. Metronidazole (oral).
      iii. Amoxicillin/clavulanic acid (oral).
   b. Moderate
      i. Ampicillin (i.v.).
      ii. Metronidazole (i.v.).
   c. Severe
      i. Cephalosporin (i.v.).
      ii. Gentamicin (i.v.).
      iii. Metronidazole (i.v.).
2. *Urinary tract*
   a. Amoxicillin, or
   b. Nitrofurantoin—this is more effective than amoxicillin but there is a small risk of haemolysis in patients with glucose-6-phosphate dehydrogenase deficiency.
   c. Pyelonephritis requires i.v. cephalosporin or ampicillin.
3. *Breast infection.* See 'Breast-feeding' below.
4. *Chest infection*
   a. Amoxicillin, or
   b. Erythromycin.
   c. Other antibiotics as appropriate.

OTHER PROBLEMS

Thrombosis

There is an increased risk of thrombosis in the puerperium because of the hypercoagulable state of the blood (oestrogen effect) and other predisposing factors: pelvic trauma during delivery, bed rest, varicose veins. If there is any suspicion of DVT or pulmonary embolus, full heparin anticoagulation is indicated with urgent definitive investigation. Warfarin passes into breast milk but in such small quantities that breast-feeding is not contraindicated.

Haemorrhoids

The venodilatation that occurs in pregnancy is exacerbated by the woman's expulsive efforts in labour, and haemorrhoids are a common problem in the first few days postpartum. The treatment is conservative with the use of salt baths and proprietary soothing agents. Advice on a high fibre and fluid diet should be given. Prolapsed haemorrhoids should be replaced after each bowel movement. Surgery, except in extreme cases, should only be performed when the problem still persists 3 months after delivery.

Psychiatric complications

The 'blues' begin on day 2–3 after delivery in 50% of women. Clinical depression occurs in 5% and frank puerperal psychosis in 0.3%. The cause of these disturbances is unknown but the high incidence suggests a metabolic cause, e.g. oestrogen deficiency. Risk factors are:

1. Previous postpartum psychiatric disorder
2. Previous psychiatric history
3. Previous stillbirth or early neonatal death
4. Ambivalence about motherhood or relationship with her partner
5. Lack of social contacts
6. Major problem in the pregnancy or puerperium.

Features of the blues are lability of mood, anxiety, tiredness and insomnia. They are best treated by education, support, and night sedation if sleeping is a problem. Any sign of more severe psychiatric disturbance should precipitate early referral to psychiatric services. Depression may become evident at any time up to 3–4 months postnatally and is recognized by tiredness, insomnia, psychomotor slowing, loss of confidence and a withdrawal from relationships with partner and/or baby. Treatment involves restructuring the woman's daily life so that she has adequate rest, and counselling and specialist referral may be required.

Psychosis is rare, is usually depressive in nature and usually occurs rapidly after delivery. It can be life-threatening to mother, baby or both. Urgent psychiatric referral and care are required and the best results are achieved if mother and baby remain together. Recent reports have suggested that oestrogen replacement therapy may be beneficial in some women.

BREAST-FEEDING

Physiology

The principal hormone involved in milk biosynthesis is prolactin but complete development of the terminal areolar cells of the breast into active milk-secreting units also requires insulin, cortisol, oestrogen and progesterone. During pregnancy, prolactin, which is secreted by the anterior pituitary, increases from 8 weeks to reach its maximum at term. Human placental lactogen (HPL) is secreted by the placenta in huge amounts and may have some lactogenic effect but its major role in pregnancy is in the regulation of lipolysis. Full lactation in pregnancy is prevented by high levels of progesterone which interfere with the binding of prolactin to its receptors in the glandular tissue of the breast.

During pregnancy and for the first 3–4 days after delivery, only colostrum is produced, consisting of desquamated, epithelial cells and a transudate from maternal serum. The trigger for full milk secretion is the rapid clearance of oestrogen and progesterone which occurs after delivery. Prolactin levels also fall but more slowly. Suckling initiates milk 'let-down' by stimulating tactile sensors in the areolae which cause oxytocin release from the posterior pituitary. The blood-borne oxytocin causes the myoepithelial cells in the breast ductal system to contract and eject stored milk. Suckling also stimulates prolactin secretion which is necessary for the ongoing synthesis of milk. Optimal milk production depends on the availability of thyroxine, insulin and cortisol, dietary intake of nutrients and fluid, frequent feeding and a supportive environment. As a general principle, 1% of any drug administered to the mother will cross to the infant.

Composition

Colostrum is a yellow fluid with a high content of antibodies, particularly secretory IgA. It contains more protein (desquamated cells) but less carbohydrate and fat than normal breast milk. Most of the protein is lactalbumin and casein with the lactalbumin providing the essential amino acids (see Table 32.1).

In extreme circumstances, the high levels of sodium and phosphorus in cows' milk may lead, respectively, to hypernatraemia in infants with diarrhoea, and low calcium and convulsions. Preterm babies need larger amounts of sodium, calcium and phosphorus.

Table 32.1 Composition of milk. (From T E Oppe 1974 Present day practice of infant feeding. DHSS Report on Health and Social Subjects. London, HMSO.)

	Human	Cow
Protein	1.0 g/dL	3.3 g/dL
Fat	3.8 g/dL	3.7 g/dL
Carbohydrate	7 g/dL	4.8 g/dL
Sodium	15 g/dL	58 g/dL
Calcium	33 g/dL	125 g/dL
Phosphorus	15 g/dL	96 g/dL
Energy	67 g/dL	66 g/dL

Management
Antenatal
Women should be encouraged to breast-feed, and general health and diet should be maintained. Nipple shields may be of some value to women with inverted nipples. Daily stimulation of the nipples is probably not of great benefit.

Postpartum
The mother and infant should have learned how to breast-feed by 3–4 days postpartum when normal milk production begins. It can be a stressful time for both partners so gentle reassurance, supervision and education by an experienced person is helpful. Mother and infant should be comfortable and the mother should have washed her hands. The nipple (including part of the areola) is fed into the baby's mouth and the nose is kept clear by the mother pressing a finger on the breast just above the baby's nose. The 'let-down reflex' occurs in the first 3 minutes and the infant obtains 90% of its feed in the first 3–5 minutes. When the infant is finished, the nipple is gently withdrawn and the baby is 'winded'. Feeding is most effective if the infant is fed when hungry rather than to a schedule.

Problems
Engorgement
This is due to the sudden secretion of milk on the third or fourth day and is best avoided by frequent feeding under supervision. Treatment is to use heat in the form of a shower or bath, analgesia, a firm, supportive brassiere and reassurance. Sometimes expression of a small amount of milk relieves tension in the breast sufficiently for the infant to fix on the nipple adequately.

Infection
Mastitis. This usually occurs as a result of a cracked nipple and a blocked duct. There is a tender, inflamed wedge of breast tissue and fever. *Staphylococcus aureus* is the cause of 95% of mastitis, and it should be treated with flucloxacillin or erythromycin. Breast-feeding should continue unless this is too painful, in which case milk should be expressed from the affected breast.
Abscess. Abscesses develop if mastitis is not treated promptly or correctly. Fluctuance may be difficult to elicit but an abscess should be suspected if mastitis does not resolve with antibiotics. The treatment of the abscess is to stop breast-feeding from the infected side, continue expressing the milk, and incision and drainage.

Nipples
Problems with nipples are one of the major reasons for women giving up breast-feeding and therefore should be treated assiduously.
Pain. Pain is experienced by 80% of women 2–4 days after delivery. This is usually associated with engorgement and is treated by more frequent, brief feeds, keeping the nipples clean and exposing them to air and sunlight.

Cracked nipples. Superficial cracks are treated as above, but with deep cracks the baby should be temporarily removed and the breast gently expressed by hand until it heals. Antiseptic sprays or creams are not useful.

Contraception

If breast-feeding is used exclusively and menstruation does not appear, ovulation usually does not occur before the 11th week postpartum. Menstruation resumes in 40–75% of women while still breast-feeding and ovulation occurs shortly after. The contraceptive effectiveness of lactation depends on the frequency of suckling, the use of supplemental feeding and the level of maternal nutrition (if low, the contraceptive effectiveness is greater). As oestrogens inhibit prolactin release their use in the postpartum period is contraindicated, although many women will continue to breast-feed normally if commenced on the combined oral contraceptive once breast-feeding is well established.

The other options for contraception are progestogens (the progestogen-only pill (POP) or Depo-Provera), barrier methods or IUDs. Most women opt for the POP which should be started in the first postpartum week. Its commonest complications are irregular bleeding and a higher failure rate compared to the combined pill or Depo-Provera.

Suppression of lactation

In most cases, this is achieved by not stimulating the breasts (no suckling), a firm supportive brassiere and analgesia if required. By 5–6 days postpartum the discomfort improves. Complete suppression of lactation may be indicated in perinatal death, adoption of the infant, severe breast problems, or active maternal tuberculosis. This can be achieved with the use of cabergoline, an ergot derivative, given as a single dose of 1 mg (two tablets) on the first day postpartum. This has replaced bromocriptine, which was reported to be associated with hypertension, stroke and myocardial infarction when used in the postpartum period.

OTHER PUERPERAL CONSIDERATIONS

Contraception

Contraception in breast-feeding women is discussed above. In women who are not breast-feeding, a small proportion will ovulate prior to the 6-week postnatal check, so contraception should be instituted in the first 3 weeks after delivery. In the non-lactating woman the choices are similar to those for the non-puerperal woman.

Vaccinations

All women lacking rubella antibodies should be vaccinated after delivery providing contraception can be assured for the ensuing 3 months. All Rhesus-negative women delivering Rhesus-positive babies should be given anti-D prophylaxis (not strictly a vaccination) within 72 hours of delivery.

Postnatal examination

This is traditionally performed at 6 weeks postpartum as most of the pregnancy-induced changes in maternal physiology have returned to normal and it is an appropriate time for assessing the mother–infant interaction.

As mentioned above, contraception in the non-lactating woman should have been initiated prior to this visit. At the visit a brief history should be taken focusing on the maternal reproductive tract and breasts, and the infant's feeding, behaviour and health. Maternal blood pressure should be checked, particularly if this has been a problem in pregnancy, and the breasts and lower genital tract examined. A smear should be performed if necessary.

33

Obstetric and gynaecological emergencies

Janice Rymer

Expectations of the examiners

Emergencies are a common theme in examination questions and the candidate must be familiar with their immediate management, particularly as regards shoulder dystocia and postpartum haemorrhage.

CORD PROLAPSE

Definition

After membrane rupture the umbilical cord prolapses into the vagina and may even protrude past the introitus. Cord presentation is when the cord is presenting and the membranes are still intact.

Interesting facts

If cord prolapse occurs in hospital the prognosis for the fetus is much better than if the event occurs in the community.

Aetiology

The presenting part is usually high allowing the cord to descend below it. Most cord prolapses occur with a malpresentation but they can occur with a cephalic presentation. They can occur with artificial (ARM) or spontaneous rupture of membranes but the prognosis is much better if it occurs with ARM, as the diagnosis is instantly made and management can be instituted without delay.

Management

Once the cord is felt in the vagina the woman should be turned into the all-fours position with her head down and buttocks elevated (or any other position that allows gravity to pull the head away from the cervix) so that the cord is not compressed between the cervix and the presenting part. The examining hand remains in the vagina to continue elevating the head away from the cervix, taking care to handle the cord as little as possible thus avoiding spasm of the cord vessels. Immediate help must be summoned to arrange a caesarean section. The hand remains in the vagina until the uterus is opened.

If a patient needs to be transported and there will be considerable delay, a Foley catheter can be inserted into the bladder and 500 ml of normal saline can be infused into the bladder to keep the presenting part out of the pelvis, thus alleviating compression of the cord.

Prognosis
If cord prolapse occurs in hospital and is rapidly diagnosed and dealt with appropriately then the outcome is usually good.

SHOULDER DYSTOCIA

Definition
As the fetus is delivering, the shoulders are in the anteroposterior position and the anterior shoulder becomes impacted on the symphysis pubis.

Interesting facts
Time is of the essence as the fetus is unable to breathe while the thorax is compressed so management must be immediate.

Management
Shoulder dystocia tends to occur with large babies. If it is anticipated then senior staff should be present at delivery. The diagnosis is made when the head is delivering but there is delay in the delivery of the chin and it appears to recede. Without delay the woman should be put into the MacRobert's (knees to shoulders) position, or her legs elevated in such a fashion as to cause flexion of the sacrum. A large episiotomy should be performed and suprapubic pressure exerted by an assistant aiming to push the anterior shoulder forwards . The majority of shoulder dystocias will be corrected with these procedures. If the shoulders are still impacted then an attempt is made to deliver the posterior shoulder by rotating the shoulders so that they go from an anteroposterior position to a diagonal position in the pelvis, as the diagonal diameters are wider. The posterior arm is delivered and the shoulders are then rotated to deliver the next arm posteriorly. If this cannot be achieved then the clavicles can be broken by snapping them between the accoucheur's second and third fingers. If the shoulders are still firmly impacted one can resort to symphysiotomy by infiltrating above the symphysis with local anaesthesia (not needed if an epidural is already sited and working adequately) and inserting a Foley catheter into the urethra. The catheter is then pulled to one side (to avoid urethral damage) and an incision is made over the symphysis downwards until the ligament is divided. The pelvis will immediately widen and

delivery will follow. Zvenelli's manoeuvre can also be used instead of symphysiotomy. The head is pushed upwards and a caesarean section is performed.

Prognosis

This is entirely dependent upon the time delay between shoulder dystocia occurring and delivery of the baby. Trauma to the baby is common, e.g. Erb's palsy.

ANTEPARTUM HAEMORRHAGE (see Ch. 23)

Definition

Antepartum haemorrhage is defined as bleeding from the genital tract after the 24th week of pregnancy and before the delivery of the baby.

Interesting facts

Placenta praevia and placental abruption must always be considered as the diagnosis.

Management

This will depend on the amount of bleeding and the gestation. Assuming significant bleeding, the management is as with any haemorrhage—resuscitate the mother ensuring an airway, breathing and circulation. Once the mother is stable one needs to:

1. Assess the amount of blood that has been lost and is being lost (remembering that with an abruption the blood loss may be concealed).
2. Assess the status of the fetus.

If active bleeding is continuing then delivery must be considered. The mode of delivery will depend on diagnosis, gestation and fetal status. For example, if there is active bleeding with a major placenta praevia at 32 weeks then an emergency caesarean section must be performed; however, if there is active bleeding with a placental abruption at 32 weeks and the baby is dead, then an ARM and oxytocin would be appropriate.

Prognosis

Disseminated intravascular coagulation (DIC) can develop with placental abruption or with any severe haemorrhage. After delivery in all cases of antepartum haemorrhage, the woman is at risk of postpartum haemorrhage and oxytocin (or ergometrine maleate if no raised BP) must be given with the delivery of the anterior shoulder and then a 40 IU oxytocin infusion for 2–4 hours after delivery.

Fluid management in these women can be very difficult, so insertion of a CVP line in the early stage is helpful.

UTERINE RUPTURE

Definition

The uterus ruptures either as a primary rupture where there has been no previous uterine surgery or trauma, or as a scar dehiscence. The latter can vary from rupture of the peritoneum to the endometrium, or the peritoneum may remain intact but the underlying uterine tissue ruptures.

Interesting facts

Placental abruption and uterine rupture can present with similar symptoms and signs. When maternal collapse in labour occurs, one must consider uterine rupture.

Aetiology

Most cases are associated with a previous caesarean section scar, especially a classic scar. A primary rupture is usually associated with obstructed labour, injudicious use of oxytocin in a multiparous woman or where there has been a previous perforation at evacuation of uterus. Uterine rupture can also occur from traumatic instrumental deliveries and intrauterine manipulations. Cervical stenosis can obstruct labour, and if not recognized can cause the uterus to rupture.

Management

The main symptom of uterine rupture is usually pain (abdominal or shoulder-tip) and the signs include fetal distress, signs of shock, alteration in uterine shape or fetal presentation, vaginal bleeding, haematuria and cessation of contractions. If the peritoneum overlying the previous scar is intact the signs may be subtle.

Resuscitation must be immediate and is followed by a laparotomy. After delivery of the baby the uterus is then repaired or a hysterectomy is performed and this will depend on the site and extent of the rupture, and the woman's condition, age and parity.

Summary

Uterine rupture is an obstetric emergency which requires immediate resuscitation of the mother and urgent laparotomy and delivery of the baby.

UTERINE INVERSION (see Ch. 26)

Definition

The fundus of the uterus is inverted as the placenta is being pulled in a downward direction by cord traction.

Interesting facts

If correct management of the third stage is employed, uterine inversion should not occur.

Aetiology

Uterine inversion is usually due to premature attempts to deliver the placenta without a hand placed suprapubically to provide countertraction to the uterus. It can be associated with morbid adherence of the placenta or a very short umbilical cord.

Management

The fundus should be immediately replaced to its original anatomical position and no attempt to remove the placenta should be made. The longer the delay, the more chance there is that manual replacement will not be possible. When attempting immediate replacement, a fist is preferable to fingers to avoid uterine perforation. If replacement does not occur then the hydrostatic method is used. This involves filling the vagina with warm fluid maintaining a seal with a hand and a pack at the introitus. The pressure of the fluid should push the uterus back to its original position. Once the uterus is in place, then the placenta can be removed manually. An oxytocin infusion should be instituted for at least 4 hours post-inversion.

Summary

Uterine inversion must be corrected immediately and the placenta should not be removed until the fundus has returned to its anatomical position.

AMNIOTIC FLUID EMBOLISM

Definition

Amniotic fluid escapes into the systemic circulation, the thromboplastin causes an anaphylactic type reaction and a severe coagulation defect develops.

Interesting facts

The diagnosis is usually made at post-mortem.

Aetiology

Amniotic fluid embolism is usually associated with high parity, women > 35 years, precipitate labour, intense uterine stimulation, overdistension of the uterus, uterine rupture and DIC.

Management

The patient may present with acute dyspnoea and signs of cardiovascular collapse. The event is usually undiagnosed and fatal, but if it is recognized the patient must be given oxygen by a facial mask initially and then intubated and ventilated and given high-dose steroids. An attempt should be made to correct the coagulation defect. A massive postpartum haemorrhage may occur.

POSTPARTUM HAEMORRHAGE

See Chapter 26.

PULMONARY EMBOLISM

Definition
A thrombosis (usually from the legs or pelvis) embolizes to the lungs causing complete or partial obstruction of the pulmonary arterial blood flow to the distal lung.

Interesting facts
Pregnant women have an increased risk of thromboembolic disease and this is exaggerated in the presence of twins, polyhydramnios, an operative delivery, advanced maternal age, obesity and thrombophilia.

Clinical presentation
The presentation will depend on the size and location of the embolus. Severe cases will present with acute collapse which may be accompanied by chest pain and shortness of breath.

Management
Women at high risk of pulmonary emboli should be given TED stockings and, depending on the history, prophylactic anticoagulation.

Basic resuscitation principles are followed, namely: establish an airway, ventilate and give fluids. Once the patient is stable then she should be fully heparinized. A positive diagnosis must be made on a ventilation/perfusion (VQ) scan.

Prognosis
This will depend on the immediate management and the size and location of the embolus.

RUPTURED ECTOPIC PREGNANCY

Definition
The ectopic gestation has ruptured through the structure it is within, i.e. fallopian tube, cornu of the uterus or ovary.

Clinical presentation

The woman may present in hypovolaemic shock due to the intraperitoneal haemorrhage. If she is cardiovascularly stable she may complain of symptoms of pregnancy, severe constant abdominal pain which was sudden in onset, and feeling faint on sitting or standing.

On examination she may be tachycardiac and hypotensive (or demonstrate postural hypotension) with a rigid abdomen.

Management

If shocked the patient needs resuscitation and then an immediate laparotomy. Blood should be taken for FBC and 4 units cross-matched. Decompensation may occur on entering the peritoneal cavity as the blood in the peritoneal cavity is often compressing the bleeding vessel(s). The site of bleeding must be found immediately and controlled. This can vary from oversewing the tube to total salpingectomy. (The current RCOG guidelines are to remove the tube if the other tube appears normal.) Depending on the amount of blood loss and the condition of the patient, blood may need to be transfused.

Prognosis

Ectopic pregnancy is a cause of maternal mortality. In the latest triennial report (1997–99) deaths in early pregnancy are the second leading cause of direct deaths. The largest number of these are due to ectopic pregnancy and the rate was 11.1/1000 estimated pregnancies, of whom 0.4/1000 died. However, as ectopic pregnancies occur in women in the reproductive age group they tend to do well. There is a 10% risk of recurrence in the next pregnancy.

CERVICAL SHOCK

Definition

Cervical shock is defined as a vasovagal reaction caused by distension of the cervix producing bradycardia and hypotension.

Clinical presentation

Cervical shock can occur during insertion of an IUD, endometrial sampling or hysteroscopy. If a woman is miscarrying either clots or products of conception can distend the cervix.

Management

The products of conception (or whatever is distending the cervix) must be removed immediately and the patient will instantly recover. This should be done before setting up an intravenous line and the usual resuscitation techniques. An urgent evacuation of the products should be arranged. If it occurs during IUD insertion, atropine either i.v. or i.m. should be administered.

TORSION OF AN OVARIAN MASS

Definition
The ovarian mass torts on its pedicle thus compromising its blood supply.

Interesting facts
Ovaries are as important and as vulnerable as testes and a torted ovarian mass should be managed with the same urgency as a testicular torsion.

Assessment
The patient may give a history of previous intermittent pelvic pain, urinary frequency and other symptoms of a pelvic mass. When torsion occurs the presentation is that of severe colicky pain. On abdominal examination the patient is tender and may have rebound and guarding. Vaginal examination is exquisitely tender. An ultrasound examination may confirm the diagnosis.

Management
Depending on the size of the mass laparoscopic management may be possible; the mass is untwisted and then removed laparoscopically. If not, a laparotomy may be performed.

OVARIAN HYPERSTIMULATION

Definition
The ovaries are overstimulated leading to a syndrome resulting from many large ovarian follicles.

Clinical presentation
The situation usually occurs as a result of parenteral gonadotrophins. The patient may complain of lower abdominal pain, swelling of the abdomen or shortness of breath, depending on the severity of the disease and whether or not ascites and pulmonary oedema have developed.

Management
The aim is supportive therapy until the condition resolves but some severe cases require ventilation and intensive intravascular fluid management.

34   Home deliveries

Ian Page

Expectations of the examiners

The candidate will be expected to be aware of the arrangements needed for home deliveries, and to appreciate under which circumstances women initially suitable for home delivery should be transferred to specialist care. In addition, the candidate should be able to perform a normal delivery, to recognize abnormalities that may occur in labour, and to resuscitate a mother or baby.

Epidemiology

The place of delivery was first recorded nationally in 1927, when 85% of births took place at home. Successive government committees advocated increasing the proportion of hospital deliveries so that by 1965 only 26% of women delivered at home. The hospital delivery rate continued to rise, so that by 1987 less than 1% of women gave birth at home.

The many advantages that were claimed for hospital delivery are now being reassessed, and it is acknowledged that there is no evidence to support the claim that the safest policy is for all women to give birth in hospital. The proportion of home births is now slowly increasing.

Assessment

Every woman has the right to have her baby at home, and health authorities are required (without exception) to ensure that a midwifery service for home births is provided. General practitioners are not required to provide care for women who wish to have a home delivery, but should attend if summoned in an emergency.

An antagonistic approach to the woman's request for a home delivery by her GP or hospital staff is unhelpful, as it will make her less likely to accept transfer to hospital delivery if problems do arise.

The assessment of suitability for a home delivery covers two aspects:

1. The anticipated 'normality' of the delivery for the mother and baby
2. The adequacy of facilities in the home.

Home facilities

These are usually assessed by the midwife who will be undertaking the delivery. The birth room should be capable of being heated to, and maintained at, about 22°C. It should be clean and well-lit, with a work-top of some form for the midwife's equipment. If the woman intends to give birth on her bed, the mattress should be firm enough to allow the midwife access to the woman's perineum.

Ideally, a telephone should be present in the house to enable the midwife to summon help immediately if it is required. A neighbour's telephone is acceptable, providing there is easy access to it. Nowadays the midwife herself may carry a radio or cell-phone.

Hot water should be available, as should some means of warming the blankets and clothes the baby will wear (a hot water bottle is adequate).

Obstetric assessment

Guidelines regarding the place of delivery were laid down by the Maternity Services (Cranbrook) Committee in 1959 and are still broadly applicable. Their aim is to try to avoid transfer of the mother and baby during labour, as this may worsen the outcome. However, early transfer due to delay in labour is unlikely to do this.

Where there is an apparent medical or obstetric contraindication to home delivery, the midwife and GP should encourage the woman to have a consultant's opinion. Ultimately, if the woman decides to have the baby at home, the midwife *must* attend. She can call on *any* GP to attend in an emergency, or she can request the assistance of the local obstetric (or paediatric) flying squad (see Appendix VII).

Height. Women under 152 cm (5 ft 0 in) have a higher perinatal mortality rate (PNMR), and a higher incidence of caesarean section in labour.

Age. Nulliparae under 18 years or over 35 years are known to have an increased perinatal mortality rate (PNMR), as do parous women over 40 years.

Parity. Nulliparae are known to have an increased incidence of prolonged labour which makes intrapartum transfer more likely. They are also more likely to develop pre-eclampsia, and to require induction of labour for prolonged pregnancy.

'Grand multiparae' have an increased risk of multiple pregnancy, placenta praevia, fetal malpresentation and unstable lie. There is an increased risk of disproportion, which may present as uterine rupture or shoulder dystocia. Paradoxically, the uterus tends to relax more in the third stage, giving rise to an increased risk of postpartum haemorrhage.

Weight. Obese women are more difficult to assess as 'normal' in pregnancy and labour, and often have large babies. It is more difficult to treat them if problems arise.

Maternal disease. Any coexisting disease, such as hypertension or diabetes mellitus, is a contraindication to home delivery.

Previous uterine surgery. A scar in the uterus (previous caesarean section, hysterotomy or myomectomy) is at risk of dehiscence which may require urgent major surgery.

Obstetric history. Any woman who has suffered a previous perinatal loss is usually advised against home delivery. Similarly, previous low birth weight babies (when due to growth retardation) or difficult deliveries are contra-indications to home delivery, as are problems in the third stage (PPH, retained placenta) which have an increased risk of recurrence.

Current pregnancy. If the pregnancy becomes abnormal then care should be transferred to the hospital antenatally. Abnormalities can occur at any stage of pregnancy, and examples include isoimmunization, pre-eclampsia, antepartum haemorrhage, malpresentation (after 37 weeks), multiple pregnancy and fetal growth retardation.

Clinical assessment summary

A healthy woman, over 152 cm tall, who has had a normal pregnancy and has no current medical or obstetric problems can be defined as 'low-risk' and home delivery viewed as acceptable. Where such a woman goes into spontaneous labour at term she can expect a normal, safe outcome to her labour.

Advantages

Many of the claimed advantages for home delivery are difficult, if not impossible, to quantify as they refer to the way the mother feels about the birth. It is certainly true to say that being treated as an individual is more likely at home, as most hospitals have policies of management which have been designed to cope with the abnormal and do not need to be applied to low-risk cases. Some studies have shown there is a greater risk of medical intervention simply by being booked for hospital delivery, and this would be avoided by home delivery.

Disadvantages

The incidence of serious, unexpected emergencies that can harm the mother or her baby is about 7%, even in low-risk cases. They include shoulder dystocia, neonatal apnoea, postpartum haemorrhage and retained placenta. Most of them can, however, be managed safely by the attending midwife or general practitioner. Specific training courses for the management of such emergencies (such as Advanced Life Support in Obstetrics) now exist and may help improve their outcomes.

The major problems arise in those few cases where more specialized medical assistance and skill are required. In these cases there may be some considerable delay awaiting the arrival of the local flying squad (if it exists), during which time the condition of the mother or baby may markedly deteriorate.

SUMMARY

Home delivery is now a relatively rare event in the United Kingdom. Recent evidence shows it is safe for 'low-risk' mothers providing the attending midwife makes adequate arrangements for assistance in an emergency. A supportive approach from the woman's general practitioner (and obstetrician) will also be of value. In addition, the woman and her partner should have a full understanding of the risks and benefits of a home delivery.

35 Stillbirths

Marie McDonald

Expectations of the examiners

The examiners will expect the candidate to understand the causes of stillbirth, and to know how to manage the event appropriately and arrange follow-up.

Definition

'Stillborn child' means a child which has 'issued forth from its mother after the 24th week of pregnancy and which did not at any time after being completely expelled from its mother breathe or show any other signs of life, and the expression 'stillbirth' shall be used accordingly' (section 41; Stillbirth (Definition) Act 1992, HMSO).

Interesting facts

Due to the advances in neonatal medicine and obstetric management the legal age of viability was reduced from 28 to 24 weeks by an Act before Parliament in 1992.

Perinatal mortality rate equals stillbirths plus early neonatal deaths (up to 7 days) per 1000 births. The current rate is 8.9/1000.

A Confidential Enquiry into Stillbirths and Deaths in Infancy (CESDI) was established in 1992 and conducted along similar lines to the Confidential Enquiry into Maternal Mortality. All fetal and baby deaths in the CESDI range are reported for England, Wales and Northern Ireland. Since April 1996 responsibility for the enquiry rests with a consortium drawn from the Royal College of Obstetricians and Gynaecologists, the British Paediatric Association, the Royal College of Pathologists and the Royal College of Midwives.

Risk factors

1. Maternal
   a. Age—adolescent and advanced maternal age
   b. Obstetric history—previous stillbirth
   c. Existing medical conditions, e.g. diabetes, renal disease
   d. Smoking
   e. Alcohol
   f. Narcotics abuse
   g. Diet—inadequate nutrition

h. Infection, e.g. syphilis, parvovirus, listeria
i. Rhesus incompatibility
2. Fetal
    a. Sex
    b. Multiple pregnancy
    c. Birth weight
    d. Fetal anomaly
    e. Chromosome abnormality
3. Socioeconomic
    a. Ethnicity
    b. Education
    c. Income
    d. Marital status
    e. Occupation.

Assessment

The death of the baby can occur during the pregnancy or in labour. An intra-uterine death in pregnancy may be detected at a routine antenatal check-up. The clinician may find that the fetal size is not consistent with gestational size. There may be absence of the fetal heart sounds. The woman may present with a history of diminished or absent fetal movements. Unfortunately, some women delay reporting the latter through a mistaken belief that the baby's movements slow down significantly at the end of pregnancy due to lack of space.

Investigations

1. Maternal
    a. An ultrasound scan to determine the following:
        i.   Confirmation of clinical diagnosis of intrauterine death.
        ii. Confirmation of the presenting part; in the case of a multiple pregnancy, confirmation of the well-being of the other fetuses.
    A second medical opinion on ultrasound may be obtained to support the original diagnosis.
    b. Blood samples are required for:
        i.   Full infection screen—TORCH.
        ii. Prothrombin time.
        iii. Kleihauer test.
        iv. Screen for antiphospholipid syndrome if appropriate, e.g. second trimester loss.
        v.   Coagulation screen.
    c. Swab from the lower vagina to detect the presence of group B β-haemolytic streptococci.
2. Baby
    a. Surface swabs for detection of group B β-haemolytic streptococci.
    b. Birth weight.
    c. A full post-mortem examination (prior to a pathological post-mortem examination).

d. Full skeletal X-ray even if parents are unwilling to have a post-mortem. Additional tests may be requested by the pathologist or obstetrician, e.g. axilla skin sample for karyotyping, or specific blood specimens.
3. Placenta
   a. Weight.
   b. Swabs for full infection screen.

Treatment
Intrauterine death

Intrauterine death is the death of a fetus after 24 weeks of pregnancy and prior to the onset of labour. This allows some degree of preparation for the parents.

Confirmation of the diagnosis needs to be presented in a manner which encourages the woman (and her partner if possible) to ask questions. If the maternal condition permits, she may choose the time of induction of labour, allowing her to return home and make suitable arrangements for other children and to collect her belongings for hospital confinement. In the mean time the delivery suite will be informed of the planned induction.

The local policy for the induction of labour is followed, with particular reference to guidelines on artificial rupture of the membranes. Many units delay this until the woman is established in labour because of the risk of infection.

Adequate information about her progress should enable the woman to participate in her care appropriately and to make informed choices where necessary. Interpreters should be utilized for non-English-speaking women. Where possible, continuity of carers should be maintained, as this will enhance the quality of care and reduce the feeling of loss of control which many women experience at this time. Care of the partner or companions should include the location of refreshments, the telephone and overnight accommodation.

Progress of labour is assessed by vaginal examination. If the onset of labour has been spontaneous it may still be necessary to augment further if delay occurs. Throughout labour adequate analgesia needs to be provided. Sedatives may be prescribed to assist with the emotional pain.

If possible the midwife or doctor should try to prepare the woman for the appearance of the baby, particularly if the fetus is likely to be macerated. Work undertaken by bereavement counsellors and support groups has revealed that women do appreciate seeing their baby, even with gross abnormalities. Many recount stories of how their imagination was much worse than the reality, of how they visited libraries to learn more. Gentle encouragement and sensitive handling of the situation can ensure that the experience assists them in remembering their dead child. Focusing on the details of the baby can help the parents enormously, such as the colour of the hair, the tiny hands with their fingernails, and so on.

The birth may be very traumatic for the woman as the reality of the situation can no longer be denied. The delivery is conducted as any labour. The placenta is saved for transfer to the mortuary with the baby.

Intrapartum death

Intrapartum death is a fetal death which occurs in labour, either during the first stage or at delivery. Fetal distress will indicate the potential danger to the fetus and appropriate action to relieve the situation may already have been taken; this can result in a stillborn baby delivered by caesarean section. The loss of a baby during labour not only affects the parents but can traumatize the midwives and doctors involved in providing the immediate care. Possible errors of management should be reviewed at a later date but the primary responsibility is to ensure that the mother is not in danger and to assist her through the remainder of the labour. A paediatrician may be present for the delivery to perform resuscitation if at all possible.

The parents should be informed immediately of the outcome of the birth. They are likely to be shocked and may not comprehend the events straight-away. The situation needs to be explained to them as far as possible at this time.

Management following delivery

The baby should be given to the parents to hold and examine for themselves. Photographs should be taken of the baby and other mementos such as a lock of hair or a footprint given to the couple. They may wish other family members to see the baby and be involved and this should be arranged. They should have the opportunity to spend as much time as they wish with the baby prior to transfer to the mortuary.

The practical arrangements following the birth include the completion of a stillbirth certificate. At an appropriate time when the woman has rested the doctor should discuss the post-mortem examination and obtain consent. The parents may have questions about the procedure and wish to see the baby afterwards. In most hospitals this would not be a problem, but the doctor should be aware of local policy, particularly if the body will be sent to another hospital for specialist post-mortem. Many pathologists now use Strong glue or dental floss to repair the body, enabling the parents to view the baby afterwards.

Completion of clinical details is essential for the pathologist. When the baby is transferred to the mortuary, all clothing and sheets should be removed as they will speed up the rate of autolysis.

The decision about disposal of the body generally rests with the parents and the doctor should be aware of the options available locally. This will be a hospital burial or cremation, or may be arranged privately by the couple. In order to make the choice the mother and her partner need to appreciate that if arrangements are made by the hospital a shared, unmarked grave may be used although the baby will be in an individual casket, and there is unlikely to be a funeral service. A private funeral can be arranged according to the parents' wishes but they may need assistance in knowing who to approach locally. If cremation is chosen the doctor must complete the necessary form.

Discharge

The mother should decide her own time of discharge in consultation with medical and midwifery staff. Cabergoline may be prescribed to suppress lactation. The GP and community midwife should be informed of the outcome of the pregnancy and the care to date. A follow-up appointment with the consultant obstetrician should be given for 6 weeks' time. In some units joint perinatal loss clinics have been established which provide an opportunity for the woman to return and meet with the obstetrician and a neonatologist. Appointment times need to recognize that there may be a number of questions to answer and explanations to give and the appointment provides an opportunity to go over the post-mortem findings in person.

SUMMARY

The management of stillbirth involves close liaison with other disciplines, including midwifery and social workers. Groups such as the Stillbirth and Neonatal Death Society (SANDS) provide a network of support for the parents who can access this via telephone links or group meetings at an appropriate time for themselves. For the staff left behind, the key issue is what lessons have been learnt from the experience: 'Could we have done something differently which would have had a better outcome?' The answer lies in regular auditing of perinatal loss, and perinatal mortality and morbidity meetings have a significant role to play in responding to this question. Reporting accurate information to CESDI will enable national audit findings to be published. Finally, staff should also remember that delivery of a stillbirth can be a distressing event for doctors and midwives, and preparation in handling sensitive situations of this nature should begin as early as possible.

36

Maternity benefits

Ian Page

Expectations of the examiners
The candidate will be expected to be aware of the various benefits which are available to pregnant women and mothers.

Accuracy
Details of the benefits change with the Chancellor's budget each year. The details below follow the April 2001 Budget. Details of current benefits can be found at *www.dwp.gov.uk*.

DURING PREGNANCY

Dental treatment
Details are set out in leaflet D11-NHS 'Dental treatment'. Free dental treatment is available during pregnancy and for 12 months after delivery. It is also available for anyone receiving income support or income-based jobseeker's allowance (see below). Form F1D, available from the dental surgery, should be completed even if the woman is receiving either family credit or income support to ensure that she can receive free treatment for the full period if she should stop being eligible for the benefit.

Prescription charges
Details are set out in leaflet P11-NHS 'prescriptions'. A prescription charge exemption certificate is available during pregnancy and for 12 months afterwards. Form FW8, which is available from GP surgeries or midwives, should be completed even if the woman is receiving family credit or income support (as with dental treatment).

Hospital fares
Although these do not strictly constitute a maternity benefit, women receiving family credit or income support can claim public transport fares, petrol costs or occasionally taxi fares for their antenatal (and postnatal) visits. Details are set out in leaflet HC11 'Are you entitled to help with health costs?' The

claim is paid at the hospital on production of the benefit order book. If the woman has a low income she can apply to the benefits agency using form AGI 'Help with NHS costs' and a certificate of entitlement may be issued.

'Sure start' maternity grant

Details are set out in leaflets FB8 'Babies and benefits' and FB27 'Bringing up children?' The grant is intended to help with expenses for the new baby, and can only be made to women receiving income support, income-based job-seeker's allowance, working families tax credit or disabled person's tax credit. The amount is £300.00 for each baby expected, adopted or born but is reduced if the claimant or her partner hold over £500 in savings. Form SF100 'Sure start', available from antenatal clinics or benefits agency offices, should be completed between 11 weeks before and 13 weeks after delivery.

Statutory maternity pay (SMP)

Details are set out in leaflets FB8 'Babies and benefits' and NI17A 'A guide to maternity benefits'. Maternity pay is provided by the woman's employer.

To qualify, the woman must work for her employer for the 26 weeks up to the 15th week before her estimated date of delivery (EDD) and work one day of that week, and also earn enough (£72 per week – April 2001) during the last 8 weeks to pay class 1 national insurance (NI) contributions.

If she is dismissed before the 15th week before her EDD because of problems in the pregnancy or premature delivery she may still be eligible for SMP.

SMP is paid for up to 18 weeks, starting any time after 11 weeks before her EDD. It is not paid while the woman is working, but she can now work right up to her delivery without losing any of her benefit.

To claim SMP the woman must:

1. Inform her employer in writing, at least 3 weeks before stopping work, that she intends to stop work because of pregnancy and intends to claim SMP
2. Send her maternity certificate (form Mat B1 available from her midwife or doctor after 26 weeks of pregnancy) to her employer before the end of the third week in which she claims SMP.

SMP is paid at two rates. To qualify for the higher rate (6 weeks at 90% of earnings, then 12 weeks at the standard rate) a woman must have worked more than 2 years full-time or 5 years part-time. The standard rate is paid for the whole 18 weeks to women who have worked between 6 months and 2 years, and is £62.20 per week. Income tax and NI contributions may have to be paid on SMP.

Maternity allowance (MA)

Details are set out in leaflets FB8 'Babies and benefits' and NI17A 'A guide to maternity benefits'. This allowance is paid by the benefits agency.

It is payable to women who have recently changed or given up their jobs, or have recently been self-employed, and who cannot obtain SMP.

To qualify a woman must have paid class 1 or 2 NI contributions for at least 26 of the 66 weeks ending in the week before her EDD. As with SMP, the maternity allowance is not paid if the woman is working.

To claim MA, the woman must complete form MA1, available from her antenatal clinic or benefits agency office, and send it with her form Mat B1 to the Social Security office.

STILLBIRTHS

If the baby is stillborn (by definition after the 24th week of pregnancy) entitlement to the following benefits is not affected:

1. Free NHS dental treatment
2. Free NHS prescriptions
3. 'Sure start' maternity grant
4. Statutory maternity pay
5. Maternity allowance.

AFTER DELIVERY

Child benefit
Details are set out in leaflets CH2INT 'Claiming child benefit'. It is payable for every child under 16 (19 if in full-time education) living with the claimant.

Payment is usually by a book of orders which can be cashed at the post office every 4 weeks.

The claim form is available from Social Security offices and should be accompanied by the child's birth certificate.

Child benefit is £15.50 per week for the eldest qualifying child and £10.35 for each of any other children.

Widowed parent's allowance
Details are set out in leaflet NP45 'A guide to bereavement benefits'. It can be paid from the time of the spouse's death for children for whom the parent receives child benefit, or from the time of delivery if she is widowed while pregnant.

The claim form (form BBI) is available from benefits agency offices. The allowance is £72.50 per week with an extra £9.70 per week for the first and £11.35 for each subsequent child.

OTHER BENEFITS

As income support and working families tax credit have been mentioned in relation to most of the benefits payable during pregnancy, they are briefly described here. They are general, not maternity, benefits.

Income support

Details are set out in leaflet IS1 'Income support', available from post and benefits agency offices.

Income suppport is a taxable benefit for people who do not have enough money on which to live, and who work less than 16 hours per week. The amount varies with individual circumstances, and is reduced if the claimants have capital or savings over £3000.

If income support is paid, the family are automatically entitled to the same benefits as those on working families tax credit (see below).

Working families tax credit

Details are set out in leaflet CTC/FS1 'Working families tax credit', available from Inland Revenue offices.

This is a tax-free benefit for anyone bringing up one child (or more) and working at least 16 hours per week. The amount varies with income, and is reduced by savings or capital over £3000. Once the rate has been assessed it remains constant for 26 weeks, regardless of changes in circumstances.

If this benefit is paid the family are automatically entitled to:

1. Free NHS dental treatment
2. Vouchers for spectacles
3. Free NHS prescriptions
4. Refund of hospital fares
5. 'Sure start' maternity grant.

37

Statistics

Ian Page

Expectations of the examiners

The candidate will be expected to have an understanding of the epidemiology of perinatal and maternal morbidity and mortality as well as ethnic variations, and to understand the importance of accurate obstetric records in clinical audit. The candidate should also be aware of the Confidential Enquiry into Stillbirths and Deaths in Infancy (CESDI) and the Confidential Enquiries into Maternal Deaths in the United Kingdom. Further details can be found at *www.statistics.gov.uk, www.cesdi.com, www.doh.gov.uk, www.official-documents.co.uk/ document/doh/wmd/wmd-hm.htm*.

BIRTH RATE

Definition
Total live and stillbirths per year per thousand women aged 15–44 years.

Interesting facts
The birth rate is currently about 60 in the UK, and has remained at this level since 1980. All births are registered by a midwife (or doctor) with the local health authority within 36 hours, and the parents must notify the local registrar of births and deaths within 42 days of the birth. The rate for women aged 20–29 has decreased for the past 30 years, but increased for women aged 30 and over.

ABORTION

This comprises spontaneous abortions (usually referred to as miscarriages) and induced (legal) abortions.

Definition
Termination of a pregnancy before 24 weeks' gestation with the expulsion of a dead fetus.

Interesting facts

The miscarriage rate is estimated to be about 15% of conceptions. The induced abortion rate in 1999 was 15.4 per year per thousand women aged 14–44 years in the UK. Induced abortion may only be performed on premises approved by the Secretary of State under the 1967 Abortion Act. The NHS carried out 74% of induced abortions in 1999. Over 80% of induced abortions are now performed within the first trimester of pregnancy.

STILLBIRTH RATE

Definition

Number of infants born with no signs of life after 24 weeks' gestation per thousand total births. (Prior to October 1992 it was 28 weeks.)

Interesting facts

The stillbirth rate in 2000 in the UK was 5.3.

NEONATAL DEATH RATE

Definition

Number of deaths, within 28 days of birth, of all live-born infants (regardless of gestation) per thousand live births.

PERINATAL MORTALITY RATE (PNMR)

Definition

Number of stillbirths and first-week neonatal deaths per thousand total births.

Interesting facts

The PNMR has been recorded since 1930 in England and Wales and in 2001 was 8.0. It is showing a downward trend.

Epidemiology

Age

PNMR is lowest in the age group 20–24 years. The higher rate in the under-20s is thought to reflect the greater number of primigravidae and unmarried mothers and a lower uptake of antenatal care. The increase in PNMR with maternal age reflects the greater incidence of maternal disease (such as diabetes and hypertension) and increased parity.

Parity

A similar 'j-shaped' curve is seen when comparing PNMR with parity, with the lowest PNMR occurring in women in their second pregnancy.

Race

Asians (Indians and Pakistanis) have an increased PNMR reflecting a higher incidence of congenital abnormalities and a mean birthweight 300 g lower than that of Caucasians.

Black people (Africans and Caribbeans) have an increased PNMR due to sickle cell disease, a higher incidence of pre-eclampsia and eclampsia, a higher rate of twin births, and a mean birth weight 120 g lower than that of Caucasians.

Multiple pregnancy

This predisposes to preterm delivery, pre-eclampsia and low birth weight and so has an increased PNMR. The problems become greater with each extra fetus.

Aetiology

There are three major determinants of perinatal mortality:

1. Congenital abnormalities
2. Low birth weight
3. Asphyxia.

However, it is more useful to look at the causes as below.

Congenital abnormality

This group accounts for 16% of perinatal deaths in the UK. Neural tube defects and chromosomal trisomies can be screened for in the second trimester, and the diagnosis confirmed by ultrasound examination of the fetus or amniocentesis. Termination of affected pregnancies (where the mother wishes) can be performed.

Isoimmunization

Perinatal deaths from haemolytic disease are now rare. The introduction of routine screening of maternal blood for antibodies (in particular anti-D, anti-C, anti-Kell and anti-Duffy) with follow-up by amniocentesis and assessment of the liquor bilirubin level, or by cordocentesis and fetal blood sampling, allows appropriate treatment to be given.

Pre-eclampsia

This excludes essential and renal hypertension which are usually considered a maternal disease, although both increase the risk of developing superimposed pre-eclampsia. Investigations are aimed at detecting fetal asphyxia and growth retardation, as well as ensuring maternal well-being.

Antepartum haemorrhage

Placenta praevia has little effect on PNMR as few babies require early delivery because of it, and those who are delivered early are usually in good condition.

Abruption is more common and accounts for about 20% of perinatal deaths due to asphyxia and prematurity. The risk of abruption increases with smoking and rising parity. It is associated with hypertension and raised maternal serum α-fetoprotein.

Mechanical

These perinatal deaths may be due to uterine rupture and cord accidents (which usually cause asphyxia) or birth trauma (as in breech delivery, forceps delivery or shoulder dystocia).

Maternal disease

Diabetes mellitus is the maternal condition that causes most perinatal deaths. Others of importance are chronic renal disease, SLE or the presence of the lupus anticoagulant alone, and renal transplantation.

Miscellaneous

These are specific causes which cannot be ascribed to prematurity or asphyxia. Examples include the twin to twin transfusion syndrome, milk inhalation and infections.

Unexplained

These are probably due to asphyxia, for which there may or may not be any evidence. Examples include unexplained intrauterine deaths and deaths from unexplained preterm delivery (including respiratory distress syndrome and intraventricular haemorrhage) and are categorized as being:

1. Term or preterm
2. Normal or small for gestational age.

Unclassifiable

These constitute a small group.

Prevention

One of the aims of antenatal care is to detect abnormalities early enough during the pregnancy to allow intervention to improve the likely outcome. This is relatively simple for congenital abnormalities where a careful history coupled with specific investigations, or general screening procedures for the whole population, can identify the abnormal fetus and so allow termination of the pregnancy where desired. It is not possible to cure most abnormalities at present, and it is unlikely that this situation will change for many years.

Isoimmunization with anti-D should be preventable with Rhesus prophylaxis in all pregnant women at risk of sensitization. Care with blood transfusion will reduce the numbers who develop other antibodies.

There is no preventive measure against pre-eclampsia. Early diagnosis and awareness of the risk to the fetus are essential. Treatment of the hypertension is, in itself, of no benefit to the fetus apart from allowing continuation of the pregnancy until the fetus is mature. Cigarette smoking makes the disease less common, but more severe when it does occur, and also increases the incidence of abruption ending in fetal death.

Fatal trauma to the fetus during delivery should be an avoidable event with correct intrapartum care, as should fatal cord accidents. There is no way of preventing antepartum cord accidents.

Ideally, maternal disorders should have been thoroughly assessed and controlled prior to the pregnancy. This is particularly the case with diabetes mellitus, where poor control increases the risk of congenital abnormality as well as increasing the risk of obstetric complications and sudden intrauterine death.

Provision of appropriate neonatal care facilities was emphasized by both the Sheldon Report (1971) and the Short Reports (1980 and 1985). For the high-risk pregnancy, arrangements should be made for delivery in a major obstetric unit with both special and intensive neonatal care units. If appropriate facilities are not available locally, then in-utero transfer is safer for the baby.

Improvement of social and environmental conditions is probably the most important factor in reducing the PNMR, as these are closely linked to both congenital abnormalities and low birth weight babies.

Summary

Perinatal mortality has fallen for a number of reasons and will fall further with improving socioeconomic conditions. Lack of appropriate care is apparent in up to one-third of perinatal deaths and therefore higher standards of obstetric care should result in a further reduction in PNMR. The special problems of the immigrant population must be remembered, and require further investigation. The Confidential Enquiry into Stillbirth and Death in Infancy (CESDI) may help in prevention of these deaths in the future.

MATERNAL MORTALITY RATE

Definition
Number of deaths of women while pregnant, or within 42 days of abortion or delivery, per hundred thousand births.

Interesting facts
In the United Kingdom all maternal deaths are investigated by senior obstetricians, anaesthetists and pathologists and their findings are presented in the Confidential Enquiry into Maternal Deaths which is published triennially. This enquiry has operated since 1952; it details the causes of death and states whether care in each case could be said to be substandard. The rate in the latest

report (1997–1999) is 11.4 per 100 000 maternities. The trend is downward but, as a consequence of better ascertainment of data, appeared to rise in the last triennium. Maternal deaths now comprise only 0.6% of deaths of females aged 15–44 years. (In 1952–54 the figure was 4.0%.)

Substandard care
The main causes of substandard care are:

1. Failure of junior staff or GPs to diagnose or refer the case to a senior colleague or to hospital
2. Failure of consultants to attend, and inappropriate delegation of responsibility
3. In some units, the continuing lack of a clear policy for the prevention or treatment of conditions such as pulmonary embolism, eclampsia or massive haemorrhage
4. Lack of teamwork
5. Failure of the lead professional to identify disease or conditions which do not commonly occur in their own specialty, or to seek early advice.

Classification
The report divides the deaths into four groups:

1. *Direct*. Death due to an obstetric complication arising during pregnancy, labour or the postpartum period, e.g. amniotic fluid embolism.
2. *Indirect*. Death due to a pre-existing disease which was made worse by the pregnancy, e.g. maternal cardiac disease.
3. *Coincidental*. Death due to factors unrelated to, and not influenced by, the pregnancy, e.g. road traffic accident.
4. *Late*. Death between 42 days and 1 year, due to direct or indirect maternal causes.

Demographic features
Age
Direct maternal mortality increases with maternal age. There is a marked increase in the rate in women aged over 35 years.

Parity
Direct mortality is lowest in women having their second baby, and rises with increasing parity.

Race
Maternal mortality in Britain appears to be tripled in black women (ethnic origin Black African, Black Caribbean, Black Mixed and Black Other) when compared to Caucasians and Asians (Indian, Bangladeshi and Pakistani). However, the ethnicity data are only estimates, and future Confidential Enquiries will address this in more detail.

UK area

There are wide variations in the maternal mortality rate in different areas of the UK but they do not correlate with the variations in PNMR.

Direct deaths

These account for 28% of the total, and their relative frequencies are shown in Table 37.1.

Thrombosis and thromboembolism

Approximately half of these deaths occurred during, and half following, the pregnancy. Caesarean section increases the risk of fatal pulmonary embolism 26-fold compared with vaginal delivery but this increase in risk can be reduced by thromboprophylaxis. The risk is also increased by obesity, immobilization, previous thromboembolism and increasing parity. It is markedly higher in women aged over 35 years. There has been little change in the rate over the past 10 years. In many cases the diagnosis of venous thrombosis/embolism was not even considered, despite positive signs on examination.

Hypertensive diseases

These were commonest in the first pregnancy and in older women. The commonest cause of death is again intracranial haemorrhage, with hepatic rupture and acute respiratory distress syndrome (ARDS) being the other major causes. Care was considered to be substandard in over half the cases, with failure to control the blood pressure adequately and to deliver the patient expeditiously being the main points.

Haemorrhage

This had a fatal incidence of 3.3 per million maternities. Three of the seven cases were due to abruption, three to placenta praevia and one to postpartum haemorrhage. Care was deemed to be substandard in two-thirds of the cases. The risk increases with age, particularly after 35 years.

Table 37.1 Causes of direct deaths in the United Kingdom, 1997–1999.

Cause	% of deaths
Thromboembolic disease	33.0
Hypertensive diseases	14.1
Haemorrhage	6.7
Amniotic fluid embolism	7.5
Early pregnancy	16.0
Genital sepsis	13.2
Anaesthesia	2.8
Others	6.7

Amniotic fluid embolism

This had a fatal incidence of 3.8 per million maternities. Two of the eight cases developed symptoms before labour, one dying undelivered, and there were no cases of substandard care. Only one case occurred in a woman under 25 years of age, with the rate increasing with age. Increasing parity was not associated with an increased incidence in this triennium. The mortality rate from histologically confirmed cases has not changed significantly over the past 15 years.

Early pregnancy deaths

The death rate has fallen despite the marked increase in the incidence of ectopic pregnancy. In the ectopic pregnancy cases there was substandard care in two-thirds of cases, usually failure to consider the diagnosis despite clear clinical pointers. Thirteen of the 17 deaths were from ectopic pregnancy and of these care was viewed as substandard in eight. The death rate from ectopic pregnancy is estimated to be 0.4 per hundred thousand ectopic pregnancies and this has not changed over 10 years.

Genital sepsis

There were 14 deaths, in which the commonest causative organism was β-haemolytic streptococcus. The onset of the infection can be insidious and progress rapidly to a fulminating septicaemia.

Anaesthesia

The number of anaesthetic-related deaths has decreased markedly, despite the increase in the number of obstetric anaesthetics given. Despite the improvement, some cases still reflect either poor communication between obstetricians and anaesthetists, or failure to recognize the severity of the patient's condition.

Uterine rupture

There were no maternal deaths from uterine rupture in this triennium. However, stimulation of the uterus, with either prostaglandins or oxytocin, should always be undertaken with extra vigilance in women with a uterine scar.

Indirect deaths

These accounted for 36% of the total, and their relative frequencies are shown in Table 37.2.

Cardiac disease

28% of these deaths were due to congenital defects, comprising either pulmonary hypertension or previous corrective surgery followed by episodes of bacterial endocarditis. Many of these patients had ignored medical advice to avoid pregnancy. 72% were due to acquired disease, of which 20% were the result of ischaemic change.

Table 37.2 Causes of indirect deaths in the United Kingdom, 1997–1999.

Cause	% of deaths
Cardiac disease	25.7
Psychiatric disease	11.0
Malignancy	8.1
Others	55.2

Psychiatric causes

Death from mental illness is the second leading cause of maternal mortality, with psychiatric illness leading to suicide a significant factor in at least 10% of maternal deaths. About 20% of the deaths occurred during the pregnancy, with the others up to nine months after delivery. The standard of documentation made it difficult to assess the standard of care that had been given to these patients. Proper enquiry into previous psychiatric history should be made at the antenatal booking clinic.

Cancer

In most cases it appears that pregnancy has no effect on incidence or prognosis, apart from sometimes delaying treatment. The importance of planned multidisciplinary care is highlighted.

Central nervous system disease

Two-thirds of these deaths were due to intracranial haemorrhage, and most of the remainder to epilepsy. There is a need for specific specialist advice for epileptic women who become pregnant.

Infection

Of the thirteen cases in 1997–1999, the rapidity of overwhelming sepsis was an obvious feature.

Coincidental deaths

These accounted for 8% of maternal deaths covered by the 1997–1999 triennial report. They are excluded from the international definition of maternal mortality.

Late deaths

These occur more than 42 days, but less than 1 year, after a pregnancy or delivery. They are reviewed in the triennial report but excluded from the international definition.

Of the 107 late deaths in 1997–1999, 7 were classified as direct, 39 indirect and 61 as coincidental.

Summary

Maternal mortality should be falling due to the better health of the population and improvements in the obstetric care of the mother. However, as many of the deaths showed evidence of substandard care there is still room for improvement.

38

Neonatal medicine

Ann Duthie

Expectations of the examiners

Candidates should be knowledgeable in the resuscitation and subsequent management of the newborn baby. They should be competent to examine the neonate, recognize abnormalities and deal with feeding difficulties.

ANTICIPATORY CARE

Approximately 70% of infants requiring resuscitation are born following a complicated pregnancy or labour. A paediatrician should be present at delivery in the following situations:

1. Preterm infants < 36 weeks' gestation and other small babies
2. Malpresentations
3. Fetal distress and meconium staining
4. Rhesus incompatibility
5. Instrumental or operative deliveries (excluding Wrigley's forceps lift outs and, in some units, elective repeat caesarean sections)
6. Narcotic analgesia given to the mother within the 4 hours prior to delivery
7. Multiple births
8. Antenatal evidence of malformation
9. Other requests.

The candidate should be competent to resuscitate babies in the event of unforeseen emergencies.

RESUSCITATION

Immediately after birth, the baby should be dried gently but thoroughly and a rapid assessment made of respiratory effort, heart rate, colour, peripheral perfusion, muscle tone and movement. The Apgar scoring system, devised by Dr Virginia Apgar in 1953 (see Table 38.1), is still widely used. It does have limitations, but scores at 1 and 5 minutes give a measure of the need for, and

Table 38.1 The Apgar score (at 1 and 5 minutes).

Score	0	1	2
Heart rate	Absent	< 100/min	> 100/min
Respiratory effort	Absent	Gasping, shallow, weak, irregular	Regular, crying lustily
Muscle tone	Limp	Some flexion	Active, well flexed
Reflex/irritability	None	Grimace	Cough/cry
Colour	Pale/blue	Body pink Extremities blue	Pink

response to, resuscitation. Babies with impaired breathing or apnoea should be resuscitated according to the guidelines of the working party of the Royal College of Paediatrics and Child Health and the Royal College of Obstetricians and Gynaecologists as outlined in Figure 38.1a and b.

If the maternal liquor is heavily meconium-stained, there is a risk of meconium aspiration and subsequent severe respiratory difficulties. At delivery, if the baby is vigorous and pink, gentle suctioning of the nostrils and oropharynx only should be performed. If baby is 'flat', the oropharynx should be gently suctioned and the vocal cords inspected using a laryngoscope. If meconium is seen at the cords, the baby should be intubated and meconium aspirated from the trachea prior to any intermittent positive pressure ventilation being given (see Figure 38.1b).

CARE OF THE NORMAL BABY IN THE DELIVERY ROOM

The umbilical cord
The umbilical cord is usually clamped once the baby is delivered. No advantages/disadvantages to delayed clamping have been proven. The method used should be foolproof to avoid massive haemorrhage, e.g. forceps replaced by a commercial, sterile, disposable cord clamp.

Temperature control
The newborn baby is at risk of hypothermia because of:

1. High heat losses by conduction, convection and radiation
2. Evaporation from a wet skin.
(These losses are exacerbated by the baby's high surface area to volume ratio.)
3. Impaired ability to increase the metabolic rate immediately after birth.

Hypothermia may worsen hypoxia, acidosis and hypoglycaemia (especially in preterm infants) and induce respiratory distress. To prevent this:

1. The delivery room should be warm (20–25°C) and exclude draughts.
2. The baby should be dried and then wrapped with separate dry, warm towels following delivery.
3. Direct physical contact between mother and baby is a means of thermoregulation but, ideally, exposed parts of the baby should be dry and covered.
4. Immediate bathing should be discouraged.
5. The baby should then be nursed in a neutral thermal environment, i.e. where body temperature is normally maintained, heat production is at a minimum and there is no sweating. This is usually achieved by dressing the infant and wrapping him/her in covers in a cot which is situated in a warm room. Energy available for growth is then optimal.

(a)

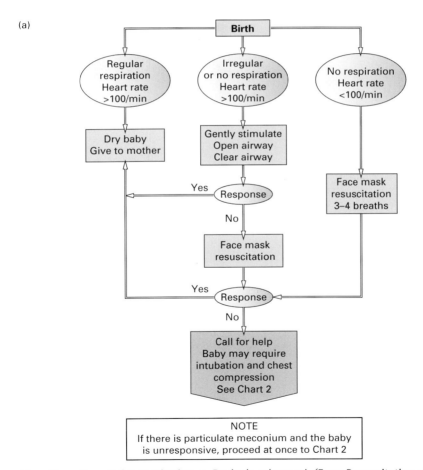

Fig. 38.1 Neonatal resuscitation. a, Basic; b, advanced. (From Resuscitation of babies at birth: A report of the working party of the Royal College of Paediatricians and Child Health and the Royal College of Obstetricians and Gynaecologists 1997, pp57 and 58. BMJ Publishing Group, London, with permission.)

(b)

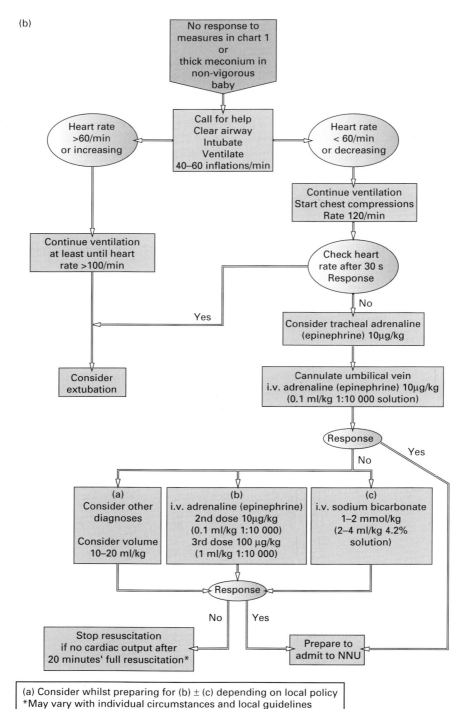

Fig. 38.1 (*cont'd*) Chart 2

Vitamin K₁

Vitamin K₁ is given as prophylaxis against vitamin K deficiency bleeding (haemorrhagic disease of the newborn), a potentially fatal disease which occurs more commonly in wholly breast-fed babies. Other risk factors include prematurity, intrauterine growth retardation, complicated delivery, and babies who are unwell, who are severely bruised, who are unable to feed, who are not absorbing their feeds or who have liver disease. It is also seen more commonly in the babies of mothers who have liver disease, are on anticonvulsant or antituberculous medication, or are misusing drugs. Intramuscular vitamin K₁ given as a single dose at birth, effectively prevents this disease in virtually all babies. A recent report from the UK, although inconclusive, suggested an association between intramuscularly administered vitamin K₁ and childhood cancer. This has been disputed by large studies from the USA, Scandinavia and Denmark. Oral vitamin K₁ regimes can be effective in low-risk babies but doses must be repeated. A suitable regime would be oral vitamin K₁ given at birth and repeated at 7–10 days for all babies, with a further dose at 4 weeks of age in those breast-fed. Currently, only the mixed micelle preparation of injectable vitamin K₁ is licensed for oral administration in babies.

Measurement

The baby's weight and occipitofrontal head circumference should be documented following birth, although the latter is often inaccurate at this early stage because of moulding during labour. Measurement of ankle–crown length by tape measure is useless and may be misleading in follow-up. A stadiometer should be used for complete accuracy.

Labelling

In hospital, name tags are attached to ensure correct identification of all babies.

Bonding

Parent(s) and child should be left alone together as soon as feasible and, if the baby's condition allows, mother and baby should remain together unless the mother requests otherwise. Putting the baby to the breast shortly after delivery may help to promote breast-feeding.

CARE ON THE POSTNATAL WARD

Routine observations

These include recordings of:

1. Temperature
2. Heart rate
3. Respiratory rate
4. Bladder and bowel activity
5. Weight.

Temperature and heart rate

An abnormally high (> 38°C) or low (< 35.5°C) temperature or a tachy-cardia (heart rate > 160/min) which is sustained longer than 1 hour may be indicative of neonatal sepsis. The baby should be examined carefully.

Respiratory rate

In a normal term infant this should not exceed 60 breaths/min. Other signs of respiratory distress include:

1. Expiratory grunting
2. Central cyanosis
3. Subcostal/intercostal/sternal recession
4. Tracheal tug
5. Nasal flaring.

Respiratory distress.　In a term baby this should be treated as neonatal sepsis (likely group B β-haemolytic streptococcal infection) until proven otherwise. Further causes of respiratory distress to then consider are outlined in Table 38.2.

Transient tachypnoea of the newborn.　This diagnosis is based on suspicion when other more dangerous diagnoses, particularly infection, have been excluded. It is attributed to delay in the clearance of fetal lung fluid and is seen more commonly following caesarean section particularly in the absence of labour. Chest X-ray typically shows hyperinflated lung fields, prominent peri-hilar vascular markings and fluid in the horizontal fissure of the right lung.

Bladder activity

Delay in the passage of urine (> 48 hrs after birth) is rare in a healthy baby without obvious physical signs, e.g. enlarged palpable kidneys or bladder. Urine is more likely to have been passed unnoticed during delivery.

A poor, dribbling urinary stream in boys is indicative of congenital post-erior urethral valves and must be further investigated, with urgent ultrasound scan in the first instance.

Urate crystals may be normally precipitated as red streaks on the nappy and should not be mistaken for haematuria.

Bowel activity

Meconium is the viscid, green-black material passed in the first 2–3 days after birth. This changes to 'milk stools', the bright, mustard-yellow, soft and seedy motions of breast-fed babies and the firmer, paler yellow/brown motions of those bottle-fed. Meconium consists of swallowed amniotic fluid, desqu-amated intestinal epithelial cells and intestinal secretions including bile. Delay in its passage beyond 48 hrs of birth is abnormal and may indicate intestinal obstruction or Hirschsprung's disease. A pale, putty-coloured 'milk stool' in a jaundiced baby should raise the suspicion of obstructive jaundice, and extra-hepatic biliary atresia should be excluded.

| **Table 38.2** | Causes of respiratory distress in the term baby. |

1. Infection
Acquired before or during passage down the birth canal. Beware a history of prolonged rupture of membranes > 24 hrs
Organisms: Group B β-haemolytic streptococcus, *Escherichia coli, Staphylococcus aureus, Listeria monocytogenes, Klebsiella, Enterobacter, Streptococcus pneumoniae* and others

2. Meconium aspiration

3. Congenital anomalies
Upper airways obstruction
    e.g. Choanal atresia, Pierre Robin syndrome, laryngeal stenosis or web formation,
        pharyngeal tumours, external compression by vascular rings, neck tumours, e.g.
        goitre etc.
    Tracheo-oesophageal fistula +/– oesophageal atresia
    Diaphragmatic hernia
    Lung defects including
        Congenital lobar emphysema
        Congenital cystic adenomatoid malformation of the lung
        Sequestered lobe
        Pulmonary lymphangiectasia
        Pulmonary agenesis/hypoplasia

4. Spontaneous pneumothorax

5. CNS depression
e.g. Associated with intrapartum asphyxia

6. Intercostal or diaphragmatic paralysis
Associated with:
    Erb's palsy
    Neuromuscular disease, e.g. myasthenia gravis, congenital myopathy

7. Cardiac failure

8. Metabolic disease
With acidosis, e.g. organic acidaemias

9. Transient tachypnoea of newborn

Weight
All normal term babies will lose weight in the first days of life as their energy expenditure and fluid loss are greater than their intake, but this should not exceed 10% of the birth weight. As feeding becomes established, weight should increase and birth weight be regained at 7–10 days of age. Thereafter, babies should gain weight at 20–30 g/day (1 oz/day except on Sundays!) until 6 months of age.

Cord care

Daily cleaning with alcohol-impregnated swabs and the application of hexa-chlorophene-containing powder to prevent colonization by potential pathogenic organisms is advocated by many units; others simply wash the cord with soap and water during baths. The clamp may be removed by the fourth or fifth day.

Skin care

Initial cleaning involves removal of vernix, dried blood and meconium, especially from the flexures. The first full bath can be delayed for one or two days, the baby then being washed with a high-fat baby soap. No special skin care is needed other than the application of a barrier cream, e.g. zinc and castor oil to protect the perineum and baby oil to the dry and cracked skin of post-mature babies.

Parentcraft

This period of postnatal care offers the opportunity to help inexperienced mothers and fathers feed, bathe, change, dress and care for their newborn and so increase their confidence in handling their baby.

Feeding

In 1995 the Department of Health stated that 'of the 64% of women nationally who breast-feed at birth, 12% will have stopped by the time they leave hospital and 20% will have stopped at the end of 2 weeks. By the end of 6 weeks, the proportion of women in England and Wales who breastfeed is only 40%.' Breast-feeding offers the following advantages:

1. There is convincing epidemiological evidence that even in developed countries, where formula feeds can be prepared under sterile conditions, breast-feeding significantly reduces the risk of gastrointestinal and respiratory infections and, in pre-term infants, also of necrotizing enterocolitis. Human milk (especially colostrum) contains factors active against infection which include
   a. Maternal plasma immunoglobulins, e.g. IgG in small quantity.
   b. Secretory IgA specific to antigens in the maternal gastrointestinal and respiratory tracts, including potential pathogens, to which the baby is likely to be exposed.
   c. The bactericidal enzyme, lysozyme.
   d. Lactoferrin, which competes for iron in the gut with certain bacteria, e.g. *E. coli*, and inhibits their growth. Likewise, vitamin B_{12} and folate-binding proteins may deprive bacteria of these free vitamins which are also needed as essential growth factors.
   e. Antiviral agents, e.g. interferon.
   f. Macrophages, lymphocytes, neutrophils, cytokines and complement.

g. Oligonucleotides and glycoconjugates which may act as receptors diverting pathogens away from binding to the baby's pharynx or gut.

 h. Protease inhibitors and antienterotoxin factors.

2. Breast milk contains several hormones in greater concentration than in maternal serum, e.g. calcitonin, epidermal growth factor and prostaglandins E and F. The effect of these hormones on gut mucosal development and activity is unknown.

3. Breast-feeding alone for 6 months lessens the risk of cows' milk protein intolerance. Whether breast-feeding protects against the development of eczema or asthma is still debated but there are grounds to suggest it is important in those genetically at risk.

4. A lower incidence of sudden infant death syndrome has been demonstrated in breast-fed babies in New Zealand. In the UK, published studies have not shown a clear relationship between the two. Despite this, the Chief Medical Officer recommends encouragement of breast-feeding as a preventive measure.

5. The water, fat and protein content of breast milk changes throughout a feed giving a completely balanced diet. The fat and protein are more easily and completely absorbed than those in formula milks.

6. It is cheap and convenient.

7. There is no risk of hypernatraemia as occurs with formula feeds if reconstituted incorrectly.

8. Evidence is accumulating that the long-term benefits of breast-feeding may include a significant advantage in the child's cognitive function and a reduction in risk of juvenile onset diabetes mellitus, lymphoma and maternal breast cancer.

Contraindications to breast-feeding

Maternal factors

1. Severe systemic disease, e.g. cardiac failure, chronic respiratory disease, neoplasia if on chemotherapy or exhausted.

2. Infection, e.g. tuberculosis, septicaemia, bilateral breast abscesses, HIV positivity in this country. There is a small risk of transmission of the HIV virus via milk to the baby. In developing countries, failure to breast-feed carries a higher risk of infection in an immunocompromised baby.

3. inverted nipples which do not respond to local treatment.

4. Treatment with drugs which may be secreted in sufficient quantity to affect the baby seriously (see Table 38.3).

Baby factors

1. Inborn errors of metabolism where milk is harmful, e.g. phenylketonuria (breast-feeding is not contraindicated but is restricted), galactosaemia, alactasia.

In summary There are very few contraindications to breast-feeding and the advantages far outweigh the disadvantages even in our society. Mothers should be encouraged to breast-feed and be supported in their action. Provision of sensible and consistent advice is of paramount importance in this support.

Table 38.3 Drugs which may be secreted in breast milk in sufficient quantity to have the potential to seriously affect the baby. (This list is not exhaustive and further reference should be made to the British National Formulary.)

	Drug	Comments
Anticoagulants	Phenindione	
Antibiotics	Chloramphenicol	Levels could be monitored in baby
	Ethosuximide	
	Isoniazid	
	Metronidazole	Interrupt feeding for 24 hours after an initial single large dose. Then use a daily dosage regime
	Tetracyclines	
Cytotoxics		
Immunosuppressives	Ciclosporin (cyclosporin)	
Radioactive isotopes		Interrupt feeding until radioactivity cleared
Anti-arrhythmics	Amiodorone	
	Atenolol	
Anti-inflammatories	Indometacin (indomethacin)	
	Gold salts	
Antidepressants	Doxepin	
	Lithium	Levels could be monitored in baby
Antimalarials	Dapsone preparations	
Antimigraine	Ergotamine	
Others	High-dose oestrogen	
	High-dose vitamin A+D	

Feeding practice

Healthy term babies exercise autonomous control over feeding and will self-regulate their milk intake if fed 'on demand'. As a guideline, the recommended intake for bottle-fed babies on each day following birth is:

Day 1	60 ml/kg birth weight
Day 2	90 ml/kg birth weight
Day 3	120 ml/kg birth weight
Day 4 and onwards	150 ml/kg body weight (if greater than birth weight)

Examples of formula feed used in the UK are shown in Table 38.4. These milks, particularly those that are whey-based, have a reduced protein content compared to that in breast milk. The proportion of the more digestible lact-albumin to casein is higher in whey-based milks. They also have a lower salt content and are advised for babies up to 6 weeks of age. All are fortified with additional iron and vitamins D and K.

Feeding problems
Maternal (breast-fed babies).

Retracted nipples. Compression of the areola or use of Waller shells may help.

Cracked and sore nipples. Consider the use of a nipple shield or, if it is too painful, rest that nipple from the baby but continue to express milk from that side, allowing breast-feeding to continue on the other side. Application of a bland ointment, e.g. Kamillosan, may be useful.

Acute mastitis. Regular breast-feeding should continue and the baby should start with the affected side to empty that breast.

Breast abscess. Breast-feeding is contraindicated.

Breast engorgement (usually transient). Advise the expression of 20–30 ml milk pre-feed to reduce the tension in the breasts sufficiently to allow baby to fix on.

Incorrect feeding technique. For effective breast-feeding there must be good apposition of the baby's tongue and lower jaw to the breast tissue behind the nipple, where the lactiferous sinuses are located. Poor milk intake will result in a hungry baby who is unsettled and cries incessantly. Frequent, small, green, 'mucous' motions may be passed and there may be pyrexia ('dehydration fever') and hypoglycaemia. Appropriate help and advice should be given. Complementary bottle feeding is not recommended as it has been shown to be a major contributor to failure of breast-feeding.

Baby.

Not interested in feeding, i.e. refusing feeds, feeding for short periods infre-quently or using a weak suck. Examine carefully to ensure the baby is gener-ally well and to exclude:

1. Infection
2. Respiratory distress
3. Congestive cardiac failure

Table 38.4 Examples of formula feed used in the UK.		
Manufacturer	Whey-based	Casein-based
Wyeth	SMA Gold cap	SMA White cap
Farley's	Ostermilk	Ostermilk 2
Cow & Gate	Premium	Plus
Milupa	Aptamil	Milumil

4. Primary neuromuscular problems
5. Dysmorphic syndromes, e.g. Down syndrome
6. Metabolic disorders
7. Congenital adrenal hyperplasia.

A strong suck reflex develops from approximately 35 weeks' gestation, hence premature babies may not suck so effectively.
    A poor suck may follow a history of:

1. Birth asphyxia with poor Apgar scores and need for resuscitation
2. Difficult delivery
3. Sedation from intrapartum or antenatal drug therapy or from drugs excreted in breast milk.

Difficulty sucking.   This implies a mechanical problem and may occur with:

1. Cleft palate, including submucous palatal clefts
2. Micrognathia
3. Nasal obstruction, e.g. choanal atresia, excessive nasal secretions (usually transient in the first few days of life)
4. Maternal breast engorgement
5. Respiratory distress, where the baby has difficulty sucking and breathing at the same time.

'Wind'.   Breast-fed babies may gulp and swallow excessive air if the initial flow of milk is fast. This will similarly occur in bottle-fed babies where the hole in the teat is too large. If it is too small, the baby will have to suck extremely hard to obtain the milk. Bottle-fed babies inevitably swallow more air as they take in the last few drops of milk or if the milk level falls below the level of the hole in the teat. Excessive swallowed air can cause abdominal discomfort with crying and regurgitation, and may be avoided by gently rubbing or patting the baby's back whilst held upright or prone ('winding') during and after feeds.
    Vomiting.   This is common in the first days of life as the baby develops coordination between sucking, swallowing and breathing.
    Persistent vomiting suggests gastro-oesophageal reflux but ensure that feeding technique is correct and that the baby is clinically well as it is also a symptom of:

1. Infection
2. Cerebral disorder—intracranial haemorrhage, hydrocephalus
3. Metabolic disorder, e.g. galactosaemia
4. Congenital adrenal hyperplasia
5. Thyrotoxicosis
6. Cardiac failure
7. Withdrawal from maternal narcotic addiction
8. Intestinal obstruction, e.g. duodenal, jejunal or ileal atresia or stenosis; meconium ileus; volvulus with malrotation of the large gut; necrotizing enterocolitis; Hirschsprung's disease; intestinal duplications or cysts.

Beware vomitus which is:

1. Frothy—indicative of oesophageal atresia with tracheo-oesophageal fistula
2. Bile-stained—suggests bowel obstruction distal to the ampulla of Vater
3. Blood-stained—usually due to ingested maternal blood swallowed during delivery or from a cracked nipple but may, on occasions, be indicative of upper gastrointestinal bleeding secondary to oesophagitis, gastritis, vitamin K deficiency bleeding and, rarely, peptic ulceration, enterogenous duplications and cysts, and haemangiomata.

Examination of the newborn

This enables screening for hidden abnormalities including congenital heart disease or dislocated hips but also allows time for parents to voice any concerns about their baby and to give reassurance about minor abnormalities and normal variants.

A great deal of information can be gained by looking at the infant lying in the cot, e.g. colour (should not be cyanosed or pale), posture (the term infant will lie with hips, knees and elbows strongly flexed, will wriggle spontaneously, stretch and yawn and should be observed to move all limbs), dysmorphic or other obvious abnormal features, and evidence of respiratory distress (see 'Routine observations' above). As the baby is handled and undressed, further information will be gleaned about muscle tone, movement, posture and response to stimuli.

Skin

Minor variants include:

The dry, cracked and peeling skin of postmature infants.

Peripheral cyanosis of hands and feet. This is common in the first 48 hours of life and may become more obvious on exposure.

Traumatic cyanosis. This is the 'blue' discoloration of the face, head and neck produced by masses of petechiae and caused by facial congestion during delivery when the umbilical cord may have tightened around the neck.

Harlequin change. This is flushing of one half of the baby with a clear demarcation from the normal side down the midline.

Mongolian blue spots. Patchy blue-black coloration of the skin over the buttocks and lower back, which should not be mistaken for bruising as it is a normal finding in all babies, particularly non-Caucasians.

Milia. Tiny sebaceous retention cysts produce pinhead-sized white spots scattered mainly over the nose.

Erythema toxicum (urticaria neonatorum). This is a very common, variable, blotchy, erythematous rash which may be associated with yellow pinhead pustules (sterile). It occurs in the first week of life and is harmless and of uncertain cause.

Vascular naevi. These include capillary haemangiomata—small defects of dermal capillaries which produce pale-pink patches on the nape of the neck, forehead and upper eyelids (salmon patches or stork marks). These gradually fade.

Port-wine stains are larger and darker and grow with the child. If they occur in the distribution of the trigeminal nerve and do not cross the midline, there is the possibility of an associated intracranial vascular anomaly with epilepsy and/or hemiplegia (Sturge–Weber syndrome).

Cavernous haemangiomata (strawberry naevi) are rarely present at birth but develop in the first 2 weeks as a bright red spot at any site which then increases rapidly in size over 3–9 months. They do eventually resolve and should not be treated unless in a site which is potentially dangerous, e.g. the eye.

Jaundice.   Onset within 2–4 days after birth is extremely common and likely to be 'physiological' with an increased unconjugated (indirect) bilirubin level due to:

1. A high bilirubin load on the liver from relative polycythaemia in the baby and shortened survival of fetal red cells
2. Decreased hepatic uptake of bilirubin
3. Immaturity of uridine diphosphate glucuronyl transferase which conjugates bilirubin with glucuronic acid
4. Deficiency of hepatic carrier proteins.

The bilirubin level peaks by day 3–4, then falls steadily and is normal by 11–14 days of age.

Beware the following abnormal situations:

Onset of jaundice within the first 24 hours of life.   The most likely causes include:

1. Excessive red cell haemolysis due to Rhesus, ABO or other blood group incompatibility
2. Infection
3. Increased red cell breakdown from
   Extensive bruising
   Cephalhaematoma
   Polycythaemia.

These will result in an unconjugated hyperbilirubinaemia and the baby is at risk of kernicterus which may cause later athetoid cerebral palsy, developmental delay, high-tone deafness or even death. Graphs are available which indicate the level of unconjugated bilirubin at which treatment with phototherapy or exchange transfusion should be commenced, taking into account the baby's age, gestation and health. Levels for intervention are substantially lower if the baby is premature and/or sick.

Investigations at this stage, to elucidate the cause, should include:

1. Full blood count with differential, reticulocyte count and blood film
2. Mother and baby's blood group
3. Coombs test
4. Urine for culture.
5. If baby is unwell, a full infection screen, obtaining blood, cerebrospinal fluid and urine (preferably by suprapubic aspiration) for culture.

If the response to treatment is poor then rare causes of early onset jaundice should be considered and investigated appropriately. They include:

1. Congenital infection with cytomegalovirus, rubella, herpes, toxoplasmosis or hepatitis A, B, C
2. Metabolic causes, e.g. galactosaemia
3. Red cell structural abnormalities, e.g. hereditary spherocytosis
4. Red cell enzyme abnormalities, e.g. pyruvate kinase or glucose-6-phosphate dehydrogenase (G6PD) deficiency
5. Congenitally absent or defective bilirubin uridine diphosphate glucuronyl transferase activity in Crigler–Najjar syndrome.

Note the dangers of phototherapy which include:

1. Retinal damage
2. Dehydration through increased insensible water loss and passage of loose motions
3. Thermal instability
4. Rashes
5. Bronzing if the direct (conjugated) bilirubin level is raised.

Ensure therefore that babies under phototherapy wear eye shields for protection and have a good fluid intake.

Prolonged jaundice > 14 days. Although the most common cause of prolonged jaundice is breast-milk jaundice in breast-fed babies, it is important to consider other causes and extrahepatic biliary atresia should be excluded as a priority. In this condition, surgery to correct obstruction to the flow of bile is more likely to be successful in preventing chronic liver disease with cirrhosis and the need for liver transplantation if performed early (before 8 weeks of age). Babies must have their total and direct (conjugated) bilirubin levels measured. Breast-milk jaundice is characterized by an unconjugated hyperbilirubinaemia. In contrast, in extrahepatic biliary atresia conjugated bilirubin levels will be raised and there may, in addition, be a history of dark urine and pale motions to indicate biliary obstruction.

Other causes of a prolonged, conjugated or mixed conjugated/unconjugated hyperbilirubinaemia include:

1. Infection (congenital or acute as above)
2. Metabolic disease, e.g. galactosaemia, tyrosinaemia, fructosaemia
3. Endocrinopathies, e.g. hypothyroidism, hypopituitarism
4. Genetic disorders, e.g. α_1-antitrypsin deficiency, cystic fibrosis
5. Intrahepatic biliary hypoplasia (may be syndromic, i.e. Alagilles)
6. Increased enteropathic circulation of bile secondary to intestinal obstruction
7. Other obstructive causes including choledochal cyst
8. 'Neonatal hepatitis'—a diagnosis of exclusion after full investigation
9. Rarities, e.g. Zellweger, Wolman, Niemann–Pick type 3.

The first-line investigations for any baby with a prolonged jaundice are therefore:

1. Measure total and direct bilirubin levels
2. Check the colour of the baby's motions!

If there is any suspicion of obstruction then an abdominal ultrasound scan should be performed and referral made (preferably to a specialist centre) for consideration for colloid liver scanning and liver biopsy. Other more specific investigations can be performed as the clinical picture then dictates but initial tests should probably include:

1. Biochemical liver function tests
2. Full blood count and film
3. Urine for culture or, if the baby is unwell, a full infection screen
4. Clinitest and clinistix of urine for reducing substances
5. Thyroid function tests.

Head and neck

Head shape.   This may be markedly affected by moulding during delivery but returns to normal within several days. Caput succedaneum is the oedematous thickening of the scalp over the presenting part. Distinguish from cephal-haematoma where a collection of blood between periosteum and skull bones produces a tense, smooth swelling limited by the suture lines (Fig. 38.2).

An asymmetrical head with flattening of one side of the occiput and the opposite forehead and face (plagiocephaly) may be produced by long-term moulding in utero. Brachycephaly with flattened occiput and reduced AP diameter of the skull is seen in Down syndrome, and a prominent occiput in Edwards syndrome.

Fontanelles and sutures.   The anterior fontanelle is of variable size and eventually closes by about 18 months of age. The posterior fontanelle is small (0.5–1 cm in diameter) and is usually closed by 3 months of age. A third fontanelle, formed by widening of the sagittal suture between the anterior and posterior fontanelles, occurs normally but is more common in Down

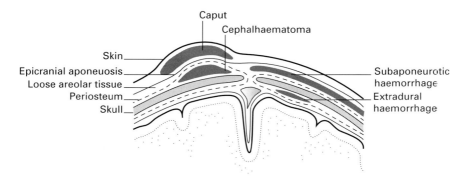

Fig. 38.2   Layers of the fetal skull illustrating possible sites of haemorrhage.

syndrome. A tense, full or bulging fontanelle, suggests raised intracranial pressure, as does undue separation of the sutures. (Up to 1 cm is normal.) The sutures may be overriding (producing a 'step-up' feel) secondary to moulding. This should be distinguished from the rarer 'ridging' of the suture line which occurs with premature fusion of that line (craniosynostosis).
Abrasions or lacerations of the scalp. These may be caused by fetal scalp electrodes or fetal blood sampling during labour.

Facies
This may be typical, for example of Down syndrome, infant of a diabetic mother etc.

Ears
Abnormalities of shape, size or position and the presence of auricular pits, skin tags or accessory auricles may be indicative of dysmorphic syndromes. The ears are low-set if the top of the helix lies below a line drawn at right angles to the facial profile from the outer canthus of the eye.

Nose
Bilateral, complete nasal obstruction as occurs in choanal atresia causes marked respiratory distress as babies are obligate nose breathers. Transient increased nasal secretions blocking the small neonatal nose may cause mild distress. Nasal flaring may be a sign of respiratory distress (see above).

Eyes
These may be abnormal in:

1. Size (small in microphthalmia; prominent in congenital glaucoma)
2. Slant (e.g. mongoloid in Down syndrome)
3. General appearance (e.g. sunsetting of the iris in raised intracranial pressure).

Conjunctival haemorrhages are common following birth as are mildly 'sticky' eyes with a mucopurulent discharge. If this worsens, swabs should be taken to exclude pathogenic infection, particularly with *Gonococcus* or *Chlamydia*.

Pupils may be irregular if there is a defect in the iris (coloboma). This may be associated with a retinal defect. Congenital cataracts are usually excluded when the normal red, retinal reflex is obtained on direct ophthalmoscopy. This method is not foolproof, however, as cataracts may develop after birth. For more detailed examination of the lens a +20 dioptre ophthalmoscope lens should be used. Cataracts may be:

1. Familial (usually autosomal dominant)
2. Part of a syndrome, e.g. Down
3. Of metabolic cause, e.g. galactosaemia
4. Associated with congenital infection, e.g. rubella, toxoplasmosis.

Immediate referral to the ophthalmologist is indicated.

Mouth and tongue

Obvious abnormalities include macroglossia (e.g. in hypothyroidism, Beckwith–Wiedemann syndrome) and micrognathia. Facial palsy, caused by direct pressure on the nerve by forceps or by compression on the maternal sacrum during delivery, may only be evident when the baby cries or grimaces.

A cleft lip (unilateral, bilateral or of more complex deformity) will be obvious but small soft palate clefts and submucous palatal clefts can easily be missed unless the palate is both directly viewed and palpated.

Other minor abnormalities include:

1. Sucking blisters on the lips
2. Epithelial (Epstein's) pearls—tiny white spots on the hard palate
3. High arched palate, e.g. in Marfan syndrome
4. Ranula—mucus retention cyst on the floor of the mouth
5. Neonatal teeth—should be removed if loose lest they be inhaled.

Neck

This may be webbed in Turner syndrome or swollen with a:

1. Cystic hygroma
2. Congenital goitre
3. Sternomastoid tumour—a firm swelling anywhere along the length of this muscle, usually with an associated torticollis with the head turned away from the side of the lesion. It represents a small haematoma or fibrous malformation.

Loss of continuity, swelling or crepitus of the clavicles may indicate a fracture.

Chest

Shape and movement may be abnormal, e.g. bell-shaped in pulmonary hypoplasia, tachypnoea with intercostal recession in respiratory distress. Palpation of the precordium will reveal thrills and ventricular heave and will locate the apex beat (displaced in dextrocardia, diaphragmatic hernia and pneumothorax). Auscultation will reveal abnormal heart sounds and heart rate and will exclude any heart murmur. Breath sounds should be vesicular and air entry equal over both lung fields. Very occasionally, bowel sounds may be audible with a diaphragmatic hernia.

The breasts may be engorged and lactation may occur in both males and females. This is normal unless there is associated erythema indicative of mastitis.

Abdomen

Major defects, e.g. gastroschisis or omphalocele, will be evident at birth. A distended abdomen will be evident on inspection, as will visible peristalsis and erythema at the base of the umbilical cord ('umbilical flare').

The cut end of the cord. This should show two arteries and one vein. (A single artery is only very occasionally associated with renal abnormalities.)

An umbilical hernia.   This may be large and unsightly but rarely causes complications. Surgery is rarely indicated before 2 years of age as the majority will close without intervention.

Urine discharging from the umbilicus.   This indicates a persistent patent urachus and requires surgical treatment.

Abnormal masses.   These may be palpated. A soft liver edge is often palpable 1–2 cm below the costal margin and the spleen is often 'tippable'. It is abnormally large if palpable more than 1 cm below the costal margin. In a well-relaxed baby, the kidneys are usually palpable.

The inguinal region.   Indirect herniae may be visible. (Surgical referral is needed.) Both femoral pulses should be palpable and, if not, it is important to determine the blood pressure in all four limbs to exclude coarctation of the aorta.

The anus.   This should be directly visualized to determine position and patency so as to exclude an imperforate anus. Examination should not be deterred by the presence of meconium as a fistula will allow the passage of meconium whilst the anus remains imperforate.

Genitalia

In males.   True micropenis associated with hypopituitarism is rare. More commonly, it may appear deceptively short when buried in suprapubic fat. The position of the urethral meatus will be abnormal in hypospadias, which may or may not be associated with chordee (curvature of the shaft of the penis). These babies should not be circumcised as the foreskin will be required for later surgical correction. At full term, both testes should be palpable. Hydroceles usually resolve spontaneously.

In term females.   The labia minora should be covered by the labia majora. Virilization, e.g. in congenital adrenal hyperplasia, produces an enlarged, prominent clitoris. A white (occasionally blood-stained), mucoid vaginal discharge is normal as are small skin tags and mucoid cysts around the vaginal opening.

Ambiguous genitalia.   Chromosome analysis should be requested urgently and these results awaited before the sex of the baby is given to the parents.

Spine

Major spina bifida will be obvious at birth. Swellings, sinuses, 'birthmarks' or hairy patches over the vertebral column may indicate an underlying vertebral or spinal cord abnormality. An ultrasound scan of the spine should be requested. Sacrococcygeal pits are common. Their bases should be intact to distinguish them from dermal sinuses which communicate through to the theca (risk of meningitis unless dealt with surgically). The spine should be straight.

Limbs

Ensure movement is symmetrical and posture and shape are normal.

Birth injuries.

1. A fractured humerus or clavicle will result in paucity of movement of that arm, the former often with obvious deformity.

2. Brachial plexus injury with contusion of
   a. The upper roots from downward traction of the arm or shoulder will produce paralysis of the muscles supplied by the cervical nerves, C5 and C6, i.e. Erb's palsy (Fig. 38.3) with lack of arm movement and characteristic 'waiter's tip' posture *or*
   b. The lower roots by upward traction on the arm will produce paralysis of muscles supplied by C8 and T1, i.e. the intrinsic muscles of the hand and flexors of the wrist and fingers with Klumpke's palsy.
3. Wrist drop may result from pressure or traction on the radial nerve as it spirals around the upper humerus.

Excessive moulding in utero (especially with oligohydramnios). This may produce abnormal posturing of the feet and ankles, e.g. talipes calcaneovalgus or equinovarus (postural or true type). A calcaneovalgus foot will usually correct spontaneously. In postural talipes equinovarus, the foot can always be straightened passively. (Gentle abduction and dorsiflexion of the foot should result in the little toe touching the outside of the leg.) Referral to an orthopaedic surgeon is needed for true talipes equinovarus.

Hands and feet
Dysmorphic features include polydactyly, syndactyly, brachydactyly, clinodactyly, hypoplastic nails, single palmar creases, the characteristic clenched hand and position of the thumb with 'rocker bottom' feet in Edwards syndrome, oedematous dorsum of the feet in Turner syndrome etc.

Fig. 38.3 Erb's palsy.

Hips

Congenital dislocation of the hip is more common in girls than in boys, in those delivered in the breech position and if there is a family history. There is an association with oligohydramnios, myelomeningocele and other neuro-muscular abnormalities. It is important to detect this at birth as early inter-vention will usually be curative. The following tests are used:

Ortolani's test. This will detect a dislocated hip. The hips and knees are flexed. With the examiner's middle fingers over the outer aspect of the thighs, their tips on the greater trochanters and the thumbs over the inner aspects of the thighs, the baby's legs are gently pulled away from the pelvis, abducted and externally rotated. Gentle pressure is applied anteriorly and medially on the greater trochanter and if the hip is dislocated, a definite 'clunk' is felt as the femoral head slips forward into the acetabulum.

Barlow's test. This will detect a dislocatable hip. The pelvis on one side is sta-bilized. The other leg is held as above. The hip is brought into an adducted position and then pushed posteriorly and laterally with the thumb. A dislo-catable femoral head will 'clunk' out of the acetabulum.

If there is any doubt about hip stability then ultrasound examination is indi-cated and referral to an orthopaedic surgeon, who has a specialist interest in such problems, should be made.

Neurology

Muscle tone. This can be assessed by traction response and recoil in the limbs and by measuring the tightness of the popliteal angle.

At term, as the baby is pulled to sit by gentle traction on both upper arms, the head should lift in line with the body with minimal head lag.

In ventral suspension, the head should come up in line with the body for a few seconds and the limbs should flex against gravity.

Primitive reflexes. Assessment is usually limited to obtaining the Moro reflex; the baby's head is lifted from the supine position and supported in the exam-iner's hand. It is then allowed to drop suddenly backwards a short way. There should be rapid outward flinging of the arms, opening of the hands and exten-sion of the legs followed by a slower return to the normal position. If a neu-rological problem is suspected, then other primitive reflexes, e.g. the palmar reflex, plantar reflex, asymmetric tonic neck response, and stepping and walking reflexes, should be elicited.

Biochemical screening tests

All babies born in the UK are currently screened for phenylketonuria (PKU) and hypothyroidism. A small blood sample is obtained by heel prick on days 5–9 of life and is allowed to dry as blood spots on blotting paper as provided in the standard 'Guthrie cards'. The baby should have been on a normal milk intake prior to testing.

Screening for cystic fibrosis is performed in some health regions by mea-surement of immunoreactive trypsin levels from one of the blood spots.

Any positive result obtained on a screening test must be checked by more sophisticated laboratory investigation.

Immunizations

Tuberculosis (TB).   It is recommended that in communities where TB is of high prevalence, BCG (Bacillus Calmette–Guérin) vaccination be given to all babies following birth.

Hepatitis B.   The following immunization regime is recommended for all infants of mothers who are hepatitis B surface antigen positive. If the mother is hepatitis B 'e' antigen negative and hepatitis B 'e' antibody positive, then only (2) is needed:

1. Hepatitis B specific immunoglobulin 200 IU intramuscularly within 12 hours of birth *and*
2. Hepatitis B vaccine 10 μg intramuscularly at birth (on the contralateral side), and at 1 month and 6 months of age. The baby's antibody status should be checked at 1 year of age and a booster dose of hepatitis B vaccine given if antibodies are undetectable at this stage.

SPECIAL PROBLEMS

Potential neonatal problems may be anticipated before delivery in certain situations and the paediatrician should then be alerted. Consider the following:

Pre-existing maternal disease

Selected examples include:

Diabetes mellitus

During pregnancy the fetus is subjected to an excessive carbohydrate load with resultant pancreatic islet cell hyperplasia and hyperinsulinaemia. Insulin is an anabolic hormone which stimulates growth and, together with altered release of insulin-like growth factors, produces a baby who is large for gestational age. This macrosomic baby may have an enlarged heart (risk of hypertrophic cardiomyopathy) and liver and typical facies with bulging cheeks, plethora and hirsutism. Although this is most commonly seen if maternal diabetic control is poor during pregnancy, it can still occur when control has been good. The main hazards to be anticipated in the baby are:

1. A difficult vaginal delivery with an increased risk of shoulder dystocia and birth injury.
2. An increased risk of hyaline membrane disease because of delayed maturation of the pulmonary surfactant system.
3. Severe hypoglycaemia with jitteriness and fits when the rich source of maternal glucose stops at birth and there is still a circulating hyperinsulinaemia. High levels of glucose supplementation may be required.

4. Increased risk of congenital anomaly (particularly anencephaly, meningomyelocele, congenital heart disease and sacral agenesis with or without agenesis/hypoplasia of the femora) in infants of diabetic mothers.

Thyroid disease

Transplacental passage of thyroid stimulating autoantibodies may cause overt neonatal thyrotoxicosis in 1 in 100 infants of mothers with Graves' disease. Most affected infants have a palpable goitre, and proptosis and lid retraction may be evident at birth. Symptoms of irritability, hyperactivity or jitteriness, tachycardia and occasionally cardiac arrhythmias with cardiac failure, excessive appetite with diarrhoea, weight loss or poor weight gain, excessive sweating or flushing, hepatosplenomegaly with thrombocytopenia, bruising or petechiae may develop soon after birth or some days or weeks later.

Antithyroid medication given to the mother during pregnancy may inhibit the fetus's own thyroid hormone synthesis and cause a goitre if the baby responds with increased secretion of thyroid stimulating hormone (TSH). Breast-fed babies of mothers on antithyroid treatment should have their thyroid function monitored fortnightly for the first 2 months and monthly thereafter if all is well.

Narcotic analgesic addiction

Infants of narcotic analgesic drug addicts are at risk of being small for gestational age, of delivering prematurely and of developing withdrawal symptoms with jitteriness (occasionally with generalized, clonic convulsions), irritability, sweating, sneezing, a high-pitched cry, diarrhoea, vomiting and poor feeding usually starting 24–48 hours following birth. Babies may require treatment with oral methadone to control these symptoms and intravenous methadone or morphine should fits occur.

Human immunodeficiency virus (HIV)

Vertical (maternal–infant) transmission of HIV infection occurs during late pregnancy, around the time of labour and delivery and through breast-feeding. In the developed world, the risk of transmission when no interventions are made ranges from 15 to 25%. Breast-feeding increases mother-to-child transmission of HIV by 14%, i.e. it approximately doubles the rate of transmission.

In the Health Service Circular HSC 1999/183, the NHS Executive recommended that 'all pregnant women should be offered and recommended an HIV test along with other ante-natal screening tests, as an integral part of their ante-natal care'. By 31 December 2002, an uptake of 90% was to be achieved, with 80% of HIV-infected pregnant women identified and offered appropriate advice for their antenatal and postnatal care. This should include advice not to breast-feed. In addition, it is usually advised that zidovudine (AZT) be given to the baby within 6–8 hours of birth and be continued for 4 weeks. There are only two situations when combination therapy for neonates should be considered:

1. When an unplanned delivery occurs either prematurely prior to the mother starting antiretroviral therapy, or after a late presentation when details of maternal HIV parameters may not be available
2. When the mother is found to be HIV-positive after delivery.

Babies should not be given BCG vaccine until their HIV status is established; otherwise their immunization schedule should proceed as normal.

Babies are usually followed up by a designated paediatrician and will require diagnostic tests to establish their HIV status at 2–3 days, 3–4 weeks, and 2 and 6 months of age.

Carriage of group B streptococcus (GBS)

Group B streptococcal disease is the most common cause of serious bacterial infection—in UK infants with a minimal incidence of 0.6/1000 live births and a mortality of 11%. Early onset disease (EOGBSD) occurs before 7 days of age (usually within the first 24 hours of life) as pneumonia or septicaemia, is vertically transmitted and is more common (66%) than late onset disease (34%). Late onset disease occurs between 7 and 90 days of age, is more likely to be horizontally acquired, and tends to present as meningitis or focal infection. Several risk factors for the development of EOGBSD have been identified:

1. Previous sibling with GBS infection
2. Known maternal carriage of GBS
3. Prematurity
4. Prolonged rupture of membranes
5. Maternal pyrexia > 37.8°C during labour.

It is recognized that EOGBSD can be prevented by intrapartum or postpartum antibiotic prophylaxis. Various preventive strategies have been proposed, but at present these tend to be ad hoc within different UK units.

The postnatal management of a term infant born to a mother known to be a GBS carrier or who is at high risk for GBS infection depends on whether the mother received intravenous antibiotics at least 4 hours prior to delivery. If this is the case, then the baby can be discharged home at 24 hours if, after careful monitoring and assessment, he/she remains completely healthy. If antibiotics were not given, the baby requires investigation (partial infection screen) and treatment with intravenous antibiotics for at least 48 hours until he/she is proven not infected.

Problems in the baby recognized antenatally

Congenital abnormalities

Abnormalities such as diaphragmatic hernia and gastroschisis may necessitate antenatal transfer of the mother to a unit where specialist neonatal advice, including surgical treatment, is immediately available.

Abnormal antenatal renal ultrasound scan

The most common abnormal finding on antenatal renal ultrasound scan is hydronephrosis, i.e. dilatation of the renal pelvis with an anteroposterior diameter persistently greater than 7 mm at 28 weeks' gestation and 10 mm at term. Postnatal investigations will clarify whether this is due to obstruction, e.g. pelviureteric obstruction, vesicoureteric reflux or duplex kidney.

Babies with bilateral hydronephroses require follow-up ultrasound within 48 hours of birth and early referral to a paediatric urologist to exclude bladder outflow tract obstruction, e.g. posterior urethral valves in boys. Otherwise, the initial ultrasound scan should be delayed until at least 48 hours after birth. Paediatric follow-up is needed. It is usually advised that a prophylactic antibiotic be commenced, e.g. trimethoprim, until subsequent investigations to establish the cause of the renal abnormality are completed. Such investigations may include a micturating cystourethrogram (MCUG) and radionuclide scans.

Small for gestational age baby
The definition varies: a baby whose birth weight is either more than two standard deviations below the mean or below the 10th centile for that gestational age.

Dysmorphic features may suggest a chromosomal abnormality. Hepatosplenomegaly with thrombocytopenic purpura suggests congenital infection.

Potential neonatal problems include:
Increased risk of birth asphyxia. This is particularly true if there have been adverse intrauterine conditions such as placental insufficiency.
Hypoglycaemia. This occurs because of lack of adequate glycogen stores and relative hyperinsulinaemia. Early, regular feeding should be instituted and blood sugar levels monitored. Nasogastric tube feeding may be needed.
Hypothermia. See 'Temperature control' above. This is potentially a greater problem in these babies because of the lack of subcutaneous fat.
Polycythaemia. This carries an increased risk of:

1. Cerebral vein thrombosis
2. Cardiac failure with pulmonary hypertension
3. Pulmonary haemorrhage
4. Jaundice requiring phototherapy
5. Necrotizing enterocolitis
6. Renal vein thrombosis.

Hypocalcaemia. This may result in jitteriness and fits.

Preterm baby
A preterm baby is defined as a baby born before 37 completed weeks' gestation irrespective of birth weight.

Potential neonatal problems include:
Respiratory distress syndrome (hyaline membrane disease). This is due to deficiency of pulmonary surfactant, which acts to reduce surface tension within the alveolar sacs and prevents their complete collapse during expiration. Exudation of plasma and other blood constituents from the congested pulmonary capillaries produces an amorphous 'hyaline' membrane which lines the terminal bronchioles and alveoli, preventing gas exchange. Signs of respiratory

distress (see above) develop within 3–4 hours of birth (sooner in very preterm infants). The natural history depends on the disease severity and gestational age but, in general, the condition improves from 36–48 hours of age as the proteinaceous material and cellular debris in the alveoli are removed by macrophages and surfactant is produced. Supportive therapy including oxygen, ventilatory support, artificial surfactant and inotropic support may be needed in the interim. Long-term ventilation and oxygen therapy increase susceptibility to chronic lung disease of prematurity (bronchopulmonary dysplasia).

Intraventricular haemorrhage (IVH).   This is the most common cerebral complication. Haemorrhage may be limited to the subependymal layer or germinal matrix of the cerebrum, or may extend into the ventricles with subsequent dilatation if the reabsorption or flow of cerebrospinal fluid is impaired. Venous infarction, usually secondary to a severe IVH, will result in haemorrhagic necrosis of periventricular white matter with a high risk of subsequent neurological impairment. Pathogenesis is complex and involves the following factors:

1. Intravascular—impaired autoregulation of cerebral blood flow in preterm infants and episodes of increased cerebral venous pressure, both affecting cerebral perfusion
2. Extravascular—poor vascular support in the germinal matrix in premature infants
3. Vascular—fragility of the germinal matrix vasculature
4. Platelet and coagulation factors.

If preterm labour and delivery cannot be avoided, prevention of IVH involves avoiding prolonged labour, difficult or traumatic delivery and birth asphyxia. It also involves careful neonatal care and handling post-delivery to prevent hypothermia, respiratory distress and systemic hypo- or hypertension, with provision of appropriate ventilatory support (with early paralysis if necessary) to prevent episodes of hypoxia, hypo- or hypercapnia. The arterial partial pressure of carbon dioxide, Pa_{CO_2} is normally a major regulator of intracranial vascular resistance and hence cerebral blood flow.

Infection.   There is increased susceptibility in preterm infants.

Jaundice.   Comparatively low levels of unconjugated hyperbilirubinaemia will produce kernicterus in the preterm baby with an increased risk of later athetoid cerebral palsy. Intervention with phototherapy and exchange transfusion is required at progressively lower levels of bilirubin with increasing immaturity.

Hypothermia.   See above.

Fluid and electrolyte imbalance.   This is due to immaturely functioning kidneys.

Feeding difficulties.   These involve functional intestinal obstruction and increased risk of necrotizing enterocolitis.

Apnoeas and bradycardias.

Persistent patent ductus arteriosus.   This may require surgical ligation.

Retinopathy of prematurity.   This is a vasoproliferative retinopathy which may result in total retinal detachment and blindness. Excessive oxygen administration has been implicated in its pathogenesis.

39 Sexually transmitted infections in women

Simon Barton

Expectations of the examiners

The candidate will be expected to understand the general principles of the diagnosis and management of sexually transmitted infections (STI). These include the following:

1. Appropriate history-taking and clinical examination.
2. Where possible, the relevant tests that should be performed to obtain an accurate diagnosis prior to commencing therapy.
3. The finding of one STI suggests that others may also have been acquired. As several conditions may be totally asymptomatic (e.g. cervical gonorrhoea or chlamydial infection, latent syphilis, vaginal condylomata acuminata), it is essential that both clinical examination and laboratory investigations screen for a wide range of infectious diseases.
4. The management of STI should include advice and education of the patient as well as contact tracing of partners. This will help to prevent reinfection after treatment, as well as reduce the reservoir of infection within the community. Often the presentation of a woman with a suspected STI will provide a valuable opportunity for her to receive advice about contraception.

It is essential that the candidate has a clear understanding of which clinical conditions can be managed by general practitioners, and which should be referred to departments of genitourinary medicine or gynaecology for specialist assessment and therapy.

Definition

A major problem with producing a satisfactory definition of an STI is that certain organisms produce an entirely local genital condition (e.g. trichomoniasis, genital warts), whereas others may cause severe systemic disease (e.g. *Treponema pallidum* and secondary syphilis, HIV and AIDS). Moreover, not all STI are *always* transmitted by sexual contact (e.g. vertical transmission of congenital syphilis or HIV infection). The question of whether to include conditions which are associated with sexual activity but not necessarily transmitted by, such as bacterial vaginosis, is a vexed one.

Interesting facts

Women with STI can present with four manifestations:

1. Vaginal discharge
2. Pelvic inflammatory disease
3. Genital lesions (ulceration or condylomata)
4. Systemic infections.

Individual infectious agents can cause disease in more than one of these categories and most can also be asymptomatic.

This chapter will consider each of these broad clinical categories in turn, describing the common causes of each and their management.

VAGINAL DISCHARGE

Pathophysiology

The normal vaginal secretions of a premenopausal adult woman consist of desquamated vaginal epithelial cells, vaginal wall transudate, cervical mucus, a variable volume of fluid from the upper genital tract, and microorganisms (mainly Döderlein's lactobacilli). There is an individual and often cyclical variation in the amount of these secretions, as well as considerable variation in different women's perceptions of what constitutes a 'normal discharge'.

Aetiology

The causes of an alteration in vaginal discharge are summarized in Table 39.1. Several of these may coexist; for instance a woman who has recently commenced sexual activity may also have begun to take the pill, have vaginal

Table 39.1 Aetiology of altered vaginal discharge.

Non-infectious	Infectious
Physiological	Vaginal
Puberty	*Candida albicans*
Menstrual cycle	*Trichomonas vaginalis*
Sexual activity	Bacterial vaginosis
Pregnancy	Others
Menopause	Human papillomavirus
Pathological	β-haemolytic streptococcus
Foreign body	Cervical
Chemical vaginitis	*Neisseria gonorrhoeae*
Drug-related	*Chlamydia trachomatis*
Gynaecological	Herpes simplex virus

candidiasis and have tried douching with antiseptics to treat this. Such cases mean that accurate history-taking, careful clinical examination and obtaining suitable specimens for laboratory tests are essential to make a correct diagnosis.

Non-infectious causes of alterations in vaginal discharge include the hormonal changes which occur at puberty and the menopause, as well as changes during the menstrual cycle. Retained foreign objects usually present with an offensive vaginal discharge, the cause often being a piece of tampon. Chemical vaginitis usually occurs with the use of antiseptic douches, but also as a reaction to the use of perfumed or disinfectant bath additives. Non-infectious, gynaecological causes are less common and include genital tract neoplasms, uterine prolapse and vaginal fistulae.

The commonest infectious cause of a symptomatic vaginal discharge is the yeast *Candida albicans*. More than 50 000 cases of vaginal candidiasis are treated in STI clinics annually in the UK and many more are self-treated or treated by GPs. In a small percentage of cases, other candidal species such as *Candida glabrata* may be the yeast involved, but the clinical picture is similar. Another frequently identified cause is *Trichomonas vaginalis*, a flagellated protozoon, which accounts for 25% of cases of vaginal discharge in the USA.

In the considerable number of women who present with vaginal discharge but have no evidence of either of these infections, a diagnosis of bacterial vaginosis is often made; however, a specific aetiological agent has not been identified for this condition (see below). Rarer causes of vaginal discharge include streptococcal infection or that associated with extensive vulvovaginal warts (although this is often due to secondary infection).

Infection of the columnar epithelium of the endocervix by *Neisseria gonorrhoeae* or *Chlamydia trachomatis* (serotypes D–K) can result in vaginal discharge alone, be complicated by pelvic pain and systemic symptoms, or be completely asymptomatic (see 'Pelvic inflammatory disease' below). Herpes simplex virus (HSV) infection may produce a vaginal discharge secondary to cervical lesions during a primary or recurrent episode; indeed, it is important to note that cervical and vaginal HSV lesions can occur in the absence of any externally visible vulval lesions (see 'Genital lesions' below).

Assessment

Points in the history and examination which may suggest particular infectious causes of an increased vaginal discharge include the following:

1. Pregnancy, diabetes mellitus, immunosuppression (including that due to HIV infection), recent antibiotic treatment, itchy vulval irritation or superficial dyspareunia suggest candidiasis.
2. New sexual partner, copious irritant discharge and malodour suggest trichomoniasis.
3. Presence of an IUD, malodorous vaginal discharge and dyspareunia suggest bacterial vaginosis. However, as no specific historical features are pathognomonic for any particular infection, clinical examination is essential.

4. Vulvovaginal erythema and oedema, vulval excoriation and the presence of curdy discharge with white/yellow plaques suggest candidiasis.
5. Excessive, often frothy yellow/green malodorous discharge suggests trichomoniasis.
6. Thin, adherent, homogenous, grey/white, offensive-smelling discharge suggests bacterial vaginosis.

Despite these typical appearances, reliance on clinical diagnosis will often be misleading or miss the presence of multiple infections.

Investigations

A vaginal smear on a microscope slide can be Gram-stained to demonstrate typical Gram-positive ovoid spores or tubular pseudohyphae of *Candida albicans*. Sabouraud's media can be inoculated to provide culture confirmation.

A drop of discharge on a slide, suspended in saline under a coverslip, can be examined as a wet mount preparation. This may reveal the presence of motile, flagellated trichomonads. Although this is a very reliable method of diagnosing trichomoniasis, it can be confirmed by using Whittington–Feinberg culture medium.

The diagnosis of bacterial vaginosis is based on the Amsel criteria which include: finding of typical 'clue cells' in a Gram-stained vaginal smear. These are characteristically granular epithelial cells, with coccobacillary organisms attached to their surface giving a 'salt and pepper appearance', a pH > 4.5 of vaginal fluid, release of a fishy odour on adding 10% potassium hydroxide and a thin, white homogeneous discharge. No microbiological test has been shown to be diagnostic of bacterial vaginosis and women without symptomatic bacterial vaginosis can have *Gardnerella*, *Mobiluncus* and anaerobes detected. The pH of vaginal discharge is also raised in trichomoniasis, but is usually < 4.5 in cases of candidal infection; this can be a quick and helpful guide to diagnosis. Ideally, though, all women with vaginal discharge should have a full range of microbiological tests performed on vaginal and cervical samples (to exclude gonococcal and chlamydial infection).

Treatment

Vaginal candidiasis may be treated topically using an imidazole derivative, such as clotrimazole (500 mg × 1 or 200 mg × 3 nocte) or econazole (150 mg × 1 or × 3 nocte). These may be administered as vaginal creams or pessaries and will produce a cure in over 90% of cases. The availability of these treatments 'over the counter', without prescription, means that many women will have tried these remedies before they present to a doctor.

In these cases, or in women with recurrent infection or a history of sensitivity to topical antifungals orally administered, triazoles such as fluconazole 150 mg stat or itraconazole 200 mg b.d. for 1 day are valuable options. It is essential that women complaining of recurrent symptoms are assessed to exclude the presence of a concomitant infection such as genital herpes or a dermatological cause such as vulval psoriasis or eczema.

Metronidazole 400 mg b.d. for 5 days is the treatment of choice for trichomoniasis. The same dose has proven efficacy against bacterial vaginosis, although avoidance of systemic side-effects and equivalent efficacy by the use of metronidazole gel (Zidoval) intravaginally for 7 days is becoming increasingly popular amongst patients, especially those with recurrent bacterial vaginosis. Unfortunately, such relapses are described in a significant minority of women. Confirmation of the diagnosis, followed by the use of either prophylactic antibiotic therapy or agents such as Aci-Jel to encourage an acidic environment in the vagina to support lactobacilli proliferation, is anecdotally reported as being helpful.

As *T. vaginalis* has been found to infect the male urethra and cause some cases of non-specific urethritis (NSU), it is important that the male partners of infected women are treated to prevent reinfection. However, there is less evidence to support such contact tracing for cases of candidiasis and bacterial vaginosis. This is only usually performed in cases of recurrent infection. Indeed, a further problem lies in the high prevalence of apparently asymptomatic women with laboratory evidence of these two conditions. Whilst further research is awaited on the local immune responses to candidal carriage and the role of *Gardnerella vaginalis* and anaerobes in bacterial vaginosis, most authorities do not advocate treating asymptomatic women.

All women with vaginal discharge should also be given simple advice on wearing looser cotton underwear, avoiding irritant soaps or bath additives and general health information.

Summary

Vaginal discharge is a common presenting complaint which merits a proper clinical assessment and accurate diagnosis to ensure the correct management. In women with atypical or recurrent symptoms or those who do not respond to therapy, referral to the genitourinary medicine specialist for further investigation and management is advised.

PELVIC INFLAMMATORY DISEASE

Definition

Pelvic inflammatory disease (PID) is an infection of the endometrium, fallopian tubes and/or contiguous structures which is usually attributed to the ascent of microorganisms via the vagina and cervix.

Interesting facts

It is estimated that nearly 100 000 women in the UK develop PID each year. After one episode of infection, 12.8% of women will suffer from tubal infertility; after three episodes, this figure rises to 75%. In addition, chronic pelvic pain, dyspareunia, pelvic adhesions and an increased subsequent risk of ectopic pregnancy add to the morbidity associated with this condition.

Pathophysiology

It is unknown why only 10% of women with gonococcal or chlamydial cervical infection will develop PID. The barriers to the ascent of microorganisms include cervical mucus, which forms a mechanical barrier in the narrow endocervical canal and contains lysozyme and immunoglobulins (especially IgA), and cyclical menstrual shedding of the endometrium may also contribute to preventing the establishment of uterine infection. In addition, the uterotubal junction and the downward flow of tubal mucus appear to act as further mechanical barriers to ascending infection.

Except in the few cases where infection is spread intra-abdominally (e.g. from an infected appendix), all of these barriers have to be passed by an ascending pathogen. This is often precipitated by trauma to the cervix and uterus as occurs in spontaneous and induced abortions, childbirth or surgical procedures, especially the insertion of an IUD.

There is some evidence that spermatozoa and the motile protozoon, *T. vaginalis,* may play a role in carrying *N. gonorrhoeae, C. trachomatis* or other microorganisms into the upper genital tract. Once there is infection by one organism, the local damage to the fallopian tubes may result in an increased susceptibility to infection by other microorganisms, such as anaerobes and coliforms.

Aetiology

The question of whether PID is caused by a single or multiple infectious agents is unanswered. The current consensus view is that most commonly *N. gonorrhoeae* or *C. trachomatis* (types D–K) initiate an attack, but are often replaced later by opportunistic bacterial invaders, such as the anaerobic species *Peptococcus* and *Bacteroides.* The detection of *Mycoplasma hominis, Ureaplasma urealyticum* and even herpes simplex virus from the fallopian tubes of women with PID has implicated these agents as pathogens, but further evidence is awaited. Finally, it is important that pelvic tuberculosis is not forgotten as an occasional cause of PID. It rarely presents as an acute infection nowadays, but it is essential to exclude it as a cause of infertility and pelvic pain, especially in women from higher-risk groups.

Assessment

The spectrum of symptoms and signs present in cases of PID is very wide, and although bilateral low abdominal pain and an increased vaginal discharge are common presentations, no clinical picture is reliable. Because of this, gynaecologists will only make an accurate clinical diagnosis of PID in two-thirds of cases. This may be partly improved by using strict diagnostic criteria:

1. Abdominal tenderness, with or without rebound tenderness
2. Cervical motion tenderness ('excitation')
3. Adnexal tenderness.

All three must be present with at least one of the following:

1. Gram-negative intracellular diplococci seen on microscopy of endocervical secretions
2. Fever > 38°C
3. Leuckocytosis > 10 000/mm^3
4. Purulent material in peritoneum on laparoscopy or culdocentesis
5. Pelvic abscess on clinical examination or ultrasound or at laparoscopy.

The inaccuracy in clinical diagnosis of PID, as well as the potentially fatal error of missing important differential conditions such as ectopic pregnancy, has led some authors to recommend that all women with pelvic pain should have a diagnostic laparoscopy performed. However, few centres have facilities for this and most will only perform laparoscopy on the most severe cases or those who do not respond after 48–72 hours of antibiotic therapy. Early laparoscopy allows the microbiological sampling of the peritoneum and tubal fimbriae, which may give a more accurate guide to the causative organisms than samples from the vagina or cervix.

Investigations

In all cases of suspected PID, endocervical swabs should be taken for culture of *N. gonorrhoeae* and the detection of *C. trachomatis* (by culture, or EIA or, preferably, PCR tests). The addition of a urethral swab will increase the sensitivity of detecting *N. gonorrhoeae*. High vaginal swabs are only useful for the detection of associated candidiasis, trichomoniasis or other vaginal infections. A full blood count and differential white cell count should be performed.

As part of the investigations to exclude other differential diagnoses in women with acute pelvic pain, a midstream specimen of urine for microscopy and culture, a pregnancy test and an ultrasound examination are often indicated.

Treatment

As no single agent is suitable for this purpose, combinations of antibiotics are essential. Recommended regimes must be tailored to whether the patient has been admitted to hospital or is being managed as an outpatient. These include:

1. Intravenous cefoxitin 2 g t.d.s., plus intravenous doxycycline 100 mg b.d. (or oral doxycycline) followed by oral doxycycline 100 mg b.d. plus oral metronidazole 400 mg b.d. for a total of 14 days
2. Oral ofloxacin 400 mg b.d. plus oral metronidazole 400 mg b.d. for 14 days
3. Intramuscular ceftriaxone 250 mg immediately, or intramuscular cefoxitin 2 g immediately with oral probenecid 1 g followed by oral doxycycline 100 mg b.d. plus metronidazole 400 mg b.d. for 14 days.

The most important component of outpatient therapy is the need for regular reassessment every 2–3 days to assess the clinical response to treatment.

In women who are managed on an outpatient basis, it is essential that if there is a failure to respond to therapy judged by a reduction in symptoms, a reduction in fever and abdominal tenderness, they are immediately reassessed or hospitalized for laparoscopy. As PID lacks a specific diagnostic test, it is essential that the diagnosis is constantly reviewed in patients who do not respond adequately to treatment. Failure to do so may result in major adverse consequences for women with a misdiagnosis of torted ovarian cysts, appendicitis or ectopic pregnancy.

In addition to treatment of the patient herself, it is essential to undertake partner notification for those in primary care or gynaecological services. However, this may be impractical. Liaison with local genitourinary medicine services, particularly the health advisers, would enable this to be undertaken. Only in exceptional circumstances, often involving a partner living abroad or entirely unwilling to attend the health service, should treatment for the women ever be prescribed without seeing the partner/s and screening him/them for other STIs.

Summary

The clinical diagnosis of PID is often inaccurate, especially if a diagnostic laparoscopy is not performed. It is essential that endocervical specimens for *N. gonorrhoeae* and *C. trachomatis* are taken prior to commencing appropriate antibiotic therapy. There is overwhelming evidence that the introduction of a screening programme for asymptomatic cervical infection by *C. trachomatis* will result in a reduction in the incidence of PID and the complications of tubal infertility and ectopic pregnancy. The Department of Health has recently announced the results of pilot projects which are expected to lead to the national introduction of screening to be coordinated across primary care, including family planning and sexual health clinics, in the future. Whatever the success of this programme, it is important that clinicians aim for earlier and more accurate diagnoses of PID, provide frequent clinical reassessment, and carry out contact tracing of sexual partners such that the severe morbidity and even mortality (via ectopic pregnancy) of PID may be reduced completely.

GENITAL LESIONS

GENITAL ULCERATION

Interesting facts

Our understanding of the natural history of genital herpes has resulted in a major change. Instead of it being seen as a relatively rare condition, transmitted from individuals during recurrent lesional episodes, it is clear that prevalence of serological evidence of HSV II infection (presumed to be almost exclusively genital herpes) is as high as 20% in some populations. The major mechanism of transmission is from an asymptomatic individual without symptomatic lesions. The discovery that individuals with no clinical history of genital herpes but serological evidence of HSV II infection are as likely to shed the virus asymptomatically as those that have been diagnosed because of a florid primary or recurrent episode, is a most unsettling fact for patients and their doctors alike. This has caused considerable anxiety and emphasized the need for specialist information and supportive counselling of newly diagnosed individuals.

Pathophysiology/aetiology (see Table 39.2)

Primary infections of the genitals by HSV infection can be a severe condition associated with a mixture of symptoms including fever and meningism, as well as florid and extensive anogenital ulceration. Although most new infections are due to HSV type II, which almost exclusively affects the genital area, some clinics have reported that up to 50% of new acquisitions are due to HSV type I.

It is important to differentiate between these two viral subtypes because of the difference in median recurrence rates after initial infection. There are 0.3–0.4 recurrences per month for those infected by HSV type II and 0.08 recurrences per month for those with HSV type I infection. Furthermore, patients with immunosuppression, including that caused by HIV, are more likely to suffer frequent, more severe, recurrences. However, the major cause of clinical concern in those with recurrent symptomatic HSV is a psychosexual disturbance, particularly regarding anxiety about transmission to a sexual partner.

Assessment

Careful history-taking of any previous episodes, a typical prodrome of itching, dysuria, painful groins and legs and blistering prior to ulceration strongly suggest recurrent HSV infection. The use of new soaps or antiseptics, recent drug ingestion, previous dermatological problems and recent foreign travel, as well as a full sexual history, are all also important.

Table 39.2 Differential diagnosis of genital ulceration.

Non-infectious	Infectious
Physical or chemical trauma	Herpes simplex virus
Erythema multiforme	Primary or secondary syphilis
Stevens–Johnson syndrome	Lymphogranuloma venereum
Behçet's disease	Granuloma inguinale
Lichen planus	Varicella zoster
Crohn's disease	Scabies/pediculosis pubis
Vulval malignancy	

Clinical examination must include thorough inspection of the lower genital tract and perianal region, as well as a general physical examination with a diligent search for lymphadenopathy or coexistent oropharyngeal lesions or other skin rashes.

In the UK, painful genital ulceration is usually herpetic in origin whereas painless ulcers are syphilitic; solitary ulceration suggests a primary chancre and multiple ulcers secondary syphilis. However, as these infections can and do coexist, it is essential that tests for both are performed on women with genital ulceration.

Investigations

All new cases of genital ulcers should have samples taken for viral culture of HSV. If facilities exist, a specimen of serum expressed from the ulcer should be obtained and examined by dark ground microscopy to search for the live organisms of *T. pallidum*. Whether this is done or not, it is mandatory to obtain a venous blood sample for syphilis serology, which should be repeated 6 weeks later in cases of a suspected primary chancre. The times of appearance of positive serological tests for syphilis are shown in Table 39.3.

The Venereal Disease Research Laboratory (VDRL) test is a non-specific test which is often used in conjunction with the *Treponema pallidum* haemagglutination assay (TPHA) in screening antenatal patients for syphilis. It can be complicated by a biological false positive reaction following acute viral infections, typhoid or yellow fever immunizations and autoimmune conditions such as disseminated lupus erythematosus and rheumatoid arthritis. Thus it is essential that any positive test is repeated and combined with clinical examination before any treatment is commenced. In patients with a history of overseas travel or sexual contacts from the developing world, it may be indicated to take cultures for *Haemophilus ducreyi*, a Gram-negative facultative anaerobe which causes chancroid, and blood for serological diagnosis of lymphogranuloma venereum, which is caused by *C. trachomatis* serotypes L_1, L_2, and L_3. Recent outbreaks of syphilis across the UK are the subject of much public health concern. It is essential that all primary care physicians understand that serological screening for syphilis ('the great mimicker'), contact tracing and follow-up in genitourinary medicine clinics are of continued importance.

A diagnosis of genital herpes infection can be confirmed by viral culture antigen detection or PCR. However, in patients who present with a history of but no current lesions, the use of type-specific serology can be helpful in supporting or refuting the diagnosis. As yet, there is no consensus to advocate generalized type-specific serology testing in the UK.

Table 39.3 Syphilis serology: time from exposure to positivity.

Fluorescent treponemal antibody test (FTA)	3–4 weeks
Venereal Diseases Research Laboratory (VDRL) test	3–5 weeks
Treponema pallidum haemagglutination assay (TPHA)	8–10 weeks

It is essential that a full screen for other STIs is obtained from all patients who present with genital ulceration, which is usually best performed in departments of genitourinary medicine.

Treatment

Primary and first episode cases of genital HSV infection should be treated with systemic antiviral therapy. There is no difference in efficacy, but a variety of oral dose frequencies are available, e.g. aciclovir 200 mg five times daily, valaciclovir 500 mg b.d., and famciclovir 250 mg t.d.s. These will diminish the symptoms and new ulcer formation as well as reduce the risk of complications such as urinary retention occurring. This latter complication should be managed by analgesia, urinating into a warm bath, local anaesthesia and, only if all else fails, suprapubic catheterization. Counselling and advice are important to provide in these patients.

In recurrent HSV infection, most patients will be able to tolerate two to three annual episodes of slight genital discomfort with simple measures, such as saline bathing, wearing loose underwear and avoiding sexual contact until the lesions have healed. However, in cases where the attacks are very frequent (more than one per month) or severely painful, or in those patients suffering psychosexual problems because of their HSV recurrences, continual antiviral therapy is indicated. Integral dosages include: aciclovir 400 mg b.d. or 200 mg t.d.s.; valaciclovir 500 mg once or twice daily, or famciclovir 250 mg b.d. which have been evaluated and shown to significantly reduce herpetic recurrences, viral shedding and psychological morbidity.

Some women will describe very clearly how they experience typical prodromal symptoms before a recurrence. Such women may benefit from being prescribed an episodic antiviral course for them to self-initiate treatment. Suitable dosages would include aciclovir 200 mg five times daily for 5 days, valaciclovir 500 mg b.d. for 5 days or famciclovir 125 mg b.d. for 5 days. Although there are data to suggest that asymptomatic shedding is significantly reduced by the use of antiviral therapy, it is important that women receiving antiviral treatment are informed that such therapy does not eliminate this phenomenon completely and that barrier methods, designed to further reduce the risk of transmission to a sexual partner, should be recommended.

HSV in pregnancy

The major risk of transmission of genital HSV to a neonate occurs in a situation where a mother acquires primary genital herpes during her pregnancy. It is now considered that the repeated viral swabbing of pregnant women for the detection of HSV if they have reported a past history of genital herpes is an ineffectual measure in reducing neonatal transmission. Although no antiviral agent is licensed for use during pregnancy, a number of studies have reported the use of aciclovir to suppress both lesional and asymptomatic shedding during pregnancy in women with recurrent genital herpes and to reduce the need for caesarean section. In women who have first acquired genital herpes in pregnancy, the use of antiviral treatment along with recommendations that delivery should be by caesarean section is the recommended protocol. Collaborative management between specialist genitourinary physicians, obstetricians and midwives is essential for women who acquire genital HSV during pregnancy.

Syphilis should be treated by aqueous procaine penicillin 600 000 units/day i.m. for 15–20 days, or in patients allergic to penicillin, by a 30-day course of erythromycin or oxytetracycline (500 mg q.d.s. orally). Patients with primary and secondary syphilis should be warned of the Jarisch–Herxheimer reaction, a self-limiting febrile illness (thought to be related to the release of treponemal toxins and immune complex formation) which may be lessened by oral aspirin therapy. However, as more serious complications of therapy can occur in patients with later stages of cardiovascular or neurosyphilis, such cases should only be treated as inpatients under medical supervision.

Although contact tracing is desirable in new cases of genital HSV infection, for syphilis this is mandatory and patients should be referred to the health adviser at the local genitourinary medicine clinic to facilitate this, as well as for the appropriate serological follow-up of the index patient.

Summary

Genital ulceration is an increasingly common problem in the UK. The range of disease extends from microscopic, solitary painless ulcers to multiple, severely painful systemic disease. Whatever the presentation, the correct diagnosis will only be obtained by careful clinical investigation and appropriate follow-up. Much of the morbidity of genital herpes relates to psychosexual problems which need to be addressed by the availability of clear information, supportive counselling and the use of antiviral treatment.

GENITAL WARTS

Pathophysiology/aetiology

Genital warts are caused by human papillomavirus (HPV). The lesions produced range from large exophytic warts (often HPV types 6 and 11) to flat subclinical lesions (often types 16 and 18) which are only visible on colposcopic examination. All epithelia in the lower genital tract may be infected by HPV, often by multiple types. Infection of the cervical epithelium with HPV types 16 and 18 has been strongly implicated in the aetiology of cervical neoplasia. A less convincing association has also been proposed between vaginal and vulval HPV infection and premalignant conditions at these sites (VAIN— vaginal intraepithelial neoplasia—and VIN). In view of the association of HPV with CIN, it has been recommended that women with a history of genital warts should have more frequent cervical cytology performed (i.e. annually); however, evidence suggests that the prevalence of CIN in women with a history of external genital warts is no different to that found in women with any other STI.

The main differential diagnoses of genital warts are from molluscum contagiosum, caused by a pox virus, and condylomata lata, the classic lesions of secondary syphilis. Occasionally benign skin tags, sebaceous cysts or pigmented naevi can also confuse the diagnosis.

Assessment

A history of slow-growing, painless, vulvovaginal lumps is highly suggestive of genital warts. This is one of the few STIs to be diagnosed solely from their clinical appearance. However, a third of women who present with genital warts will have another STI present on more detailed investigation.

The lesions of molluscum contagiosum are also characteristic, being pearly white, umbilicated papules which may also be found on other parts of the body; they are transmitted by close, but not always sexual, contact.

Condylomata lata are coalescent, large fleshy masses of the papular lesions of secondary syphilis found in moist body areas. Other signs of secondary syphilis are usually present.

Investigations

A thorough examination of the lower genital tract is essential. If there is any suspicion of cervical or high vaginal lesions then the use of a colposcope is recommended. A cervical cytology smear does not need to be performed more frequently in women because of a diagnosis of genital warts. However, a screen for other STI should be undertaken. In cases of secondary syphilis, a dark ground examination of a smear from the condylomata lata will reveal spirochaetes and serological tests will be positive.

If the examining clinician is not 100% certain of the diagnosis being genital warts, then a biopsy must be discussed. Cases where condylomata acuminata have been confused with intraepithelial neoplasia or even squamous cell carcinoma have been described.

Treatment

Over the past decade a major shift towards patients treating their own external genital warts by self-application medication has occurred. Use of topical podophyllotoxin (Warticon) three times weekly has reduced the need for patients to reattend to have their warts painted by nurses in genitourinary medicine clinics. Treatment is only applicable to external lesions. It is essential that internal lesions are treated by physical methods due to the increased risk of side-effects, both local and systemic, with chemical agents. The use of cryosurgery, hyfrecation or laser treatment did have equivalent efficacy. All the above treatment methods appear to have comparable cure rates initially of between 70% and 90%. However, long-term recurrence rates have been shown to approach 50%. This leads to considerable despondency amongst patients, hence also amongst clinicians. To address this problem, an approach of using immune response modifiers has been developed. The use of imiquimod (Aldara) as a topical treatment to be applied by the patient thrice weekly gives a comparable initial cure rate and anecdotal reports suggest that sustained long-term clearance can be achieved in the majority of cases.

Contact tracing to find the male partners of women with genital warts serves to screen them from HPV and other STI. The value of condom use by the male partner during, and for some time after, treatment has been suggested, but there is little evidence for this. Molluscum contagiosum is treated either by applying neat phenol on a wooden stick into the centre of each lesion, or by using cryotherapy or electrocautery.

Summary
Genital warts often serve as a marker for other STI. As no systemic anti-HPV agent exists, the treatment is local. Long-term cure rates are often poor. Genital HPV infection, like other STI, acts as a risk factor for the development of cervical neoplasia; hence regular cervical cytological sampling of all women with warts, or any other STI, must be recommended.

INFESTATIONS

Unless there is a high level of clinical awareness and a good light in the examination room, the detection of the ectoparasites which cause pediculosis pubis or scabies will be missed. In the former, *Phthirus pubis* ('crabs') itself or its eggs ('nits') is visibly attached to the base of pubic hairs. In the latter, if the typical burrows of the scabies mite are lifted with a needle and the contents placed in 10% KOH on a slide, *Sarcoptes scabiei* may be visualized on microscopy.

Scabies and pediculosis pubis should be treated by 25% benzyl benzoate or 1% γ-benzene hexachloride applications from the neck downwards. Sexual partners and close family contacts should be seen and also treated.

SYSTEMIC INFECTIONS

Aetiology
The three most important systemic infections which may be sexually transmitted are syphilis, hepatitis B and HIV infection. All of these have asymptomatic phases in their natural history, all may be transmitted vertically by a pregnant woman, and all may be fatal.

Currently, despite large and continuing research efforts, only one vaccination effective to protect against a sexually transmitted systemic infection exists—hepatitis B. Recently, the sexual transmission of infectious agents such as hepatitis C and human T-lymphotrophic virus-1 (HTLV1) has been described. Serological testing of populations for these latter agents, accompanied by an increase in understanding of their natural history and mode of transmission, is currently being evaluated before any decision on routine screening can be made.

Assessment

Although each of these infections does produce well-described clinical syndromes, the initial infection and subsequent carriage may be completely asymptomatic. Thus, the diagnosis will often be missed unless serological screening is performed in patients presenting with another STI. It is important that the patient understands the nature of any screening test performed and is counselled before the result is known.

Investigations

Hepatitis B may only be diagnosed by serology. Within 4–12 weeks of infection, hepatitis B surface (HBsAg) and e antigens (HBeAg) appear in the serum. HBsAg is usually cleared by 4 months from the onset of the infection and this usually precedes the appearance of HBsAb, the antibody which confers long-term immunity. During this serological window, hepatitis B core antibody may be the only positive indication of infection. HBeAg is usually cleared rapidly unless a chronic carrier state develops. Liver enzymes must be checked at regular intervals, but no pattern is pathognomonic of hepatitis B virus infection.

Seroconversion for HIV antibodies typically occurs 4–12 weeks after the initial exposure. However, longer delays have been described. The earlier detection of infection by the presence of HIV P24 antigen or PCR RNA testing can be useful following a specific exposure (e.g. a needle stick injury or sexual assault) or in certain circumstances where time is of the essence such as during pregnancy. All positive HIV antibody tests must be repeated, along with a full screen for other STI before proceeding to specialist investigations of immunosuppression and viral load which are used to manage HIV infection in specialist centres.

Treatment

Acute viral hepatitis B is usually self-limiting and management is usually supportive. Advice on a low-fat, high-energy diet, the avoidance of alcohol and bed rest is given and the patient's liver enzymes are regularly checked until normal. In chronic hepatitis, advances in antivirals (e.g. ribavirin or lamivudine) and immunological (pegylated α-interferon) therapy will require specialist referral for management and follow-up. The contacts of patients who are infectious for hepatitis B must be identified and tested under the auspices of the local communicable diseases specialist. Information should be offered to the non-immune contacts of known hepatitis B patients, as well as those in higher-risk groups (e.g. female sex workers and those who regularly travel to high endemicity areas). It is essential that all medical, nursing and laboratory staff who come into contact with potentially infected patients or their blood are vaccinated against hepatitis B.

The management of HIV infection has been transformed over the past 5 years by the use of highly active antiretroviral therapy (HAART). Essentially, this means the use of combinations of antiretroviral medicines, usually containing two classes of drug (e.g. nucleoside analogues and either protease inhibitors or non-nucleoside reverse transcriptase inhibitors), in order to reduce the HIV concentration in the plasma to undetectable levels to allow immune reconstitution. The success of such approaches greatly reduces the prevalence of immune suppressed individuals because HIV has led to new problems of side-effects of medication such as metabolic abnormalities, including lipodystrophy, as well as the need to find strategies to cope with the spectre of transmissible viral resistance. The consequence of improvement in treatment and in prognosis of individuals infected by HIV has been a decreasing incidence and, therefore, a decreasing familiarity of physicians with opportunistic infections. It is essential that primary care physicians in the UK are aware that at least 40% of individuals infected by HIV remain undiagnosed. Advancing, untreated immune suppression in such individuals involves a high proportion of women who present with evidence of opportunistic infections such as *Pneumocystis carinii* pneumonia (PCP), CMV retinitis, recurrent candidal infection or opportunistic neoplasia, including squamous cell carcinoma of the cervix. A low threshold of recommending HIV testing as part of the investigation of patients who present with respiratory, gastroenterological or neurological symptoms, is essential so that patients receive the appropriate and earlier management of HIV infection.

SYSTEMIC STI AND PREGNANCY

For many years, women attending antenatal clinics have been screened for syphilis and often hepatitis B infection on serum samples obtained at their booking visits. In the UK it is now the policy advocated by the Department of Health that women are also recommended to have an HIV antibody test. This is strongly influenced by the clear evidence that the use of antiretroviral therapy during pregnancy reduces the viral load to undetectable levels, and elective caesarean section and the avoidance of breast-feeding have been shown to reduce significantly the risk of transmission of HIV to neonates. Women diagnosed as HIV-seropositive in pregnancy require specialist support, information and management to ensure that they receive optimal advice on how to maintain their own health, as well as significantly reducing the risk of transmission to their infants.

Ideally, however, the time to diagnose asymptomatic infections, which may be transmitted vertically, is prior to the pregnancy, as part of comprehensive preconceptual care. This service is increasingly being facilitated, particularly in relation to HIV infection, by the development and improvement in facilities of sexual health clinics, and an increase in the number of sites where women may be tested for HIV and other infections.

Syphilis
Vertical transmission via the placenta is almost inevitable if the mother is suffering from secondary syphilis; it is likely if she has a primary chancre, but

becomes more unlikely with increasing duration of latent disease. In 30% of women with untreated early syphilis, the pregnancy will end in a second trimester spontaneous abortion or stillbirth. If a live infant results, it may rarely be born showing signs of early congenital syphilis, or more usually be born well, developing signs within the first few weeks, months or even years of life. With successive pregnancies, the outcome tends to improve.

Adequate treatment of maternal syphilis prior to a pregnancy will prevent any transmission to the fetus or infant. It should be remembered that infection of the mother may also occur during pregnancy and therefore screening at 14–16 weeks' gestation will not prevent all cases of congenital infection. Furthermore, if reinfection is considered a possibility during a pregnancy, then retreatment is essential.

Hepatitis B

Infection of a pregnant woman carries a maternal mortality risk of 1.8% and a 2% increase in preterm delivery, although there is no specific association with congenital abnormalities. These figures relate to Europe and North America, but in India and the Far East fulminant hepatitis is more common, with a reported maternal mortality of 72% for cases of third trimester infection. The reason for this geographical variation is thought to include ethnic differences in host immunity. There is also a geographical difference in the risk of vertical transmission by a mother who is a chronic carrier of HBsAg throughout her pregnancy. This varies from a 7% risk of vertical transmission in Greece, compared to 73% in Japan. These differences seem to be directly related to the titre of HBsAg and also the presence of e antigen in maternal serum.

For infections acquired during pregnancy, the risk of vertical transmission to the fetus is determined by the gestational age at the time of maternal infection. A third trimester infection carries a 66% risk of transmission, compared to less than 10% if the virus is acquired earlier.

There is no evidence that any therapy given during pregnancy alters the risk of transmission or the maternal or perinatal morbidity. However, to prevent the risk of neonatal transmission, infants born of HBsAg-positive mothers should receive hepatitis B immunoglobulin and a dose of hepatitis B vaccine, at separate sites, within a few hours of birth.

SUMMARY

An increasing number of cases of syphilis in the UK and the advances in anti-viral treatment of hepatitis B and HIV have led to a clear consensus that women must be recommended to undergo serological testing for these infections during pregnancy. It is essential that screening is undertaken by trained staff using verbal as well as written information to back up the recommendation for screening. It is important that all units undertaking screening have a clear policy of how to manage positive test results. The initial management should acknowledge the importance of psychological and counselling support, of including the woman's partner, and the repeating of the specimen and taking of blood for evaluation of immune suppression, viral load and other HIV-related investigations, as well as a clearly determined referral pattern to specialists working alongside an obstetrician with experience and training in managing such infections in pregnancy.

40

Family planning

Valerie Price and Helen Massil

Expectations of the examiners

The candidate will be expected to have the following theoretical knowledge:

1. The factors influencing motivation for contraception and emotional/psychological factors related to fertility control
2. The acceptability and choice of contraceptive method
3. Safety and effectiveness of all available methods
4. How to provide counselling and advice about contraception
5. Methods of contraception including advantages/disadvantages and risks/benefits
6. The management of associated complications (including resuscitation if required at IUD insertion and in the case of anaphylactic reaction to medication)
7. The organization of family planning services.

MOTIVATION

The following factors are known to influence whether an individual or a couple will seek contraception:

1. The personal/cultural ideal family size and norms for child rearing
2. The sex of the existing children in the family
3. Religious beliefs
4. Socioeconomic conditions
5. Expected dependency or assistance from children
6. Opportunities and education for women
7. The stage in family building
8. Age and marital status
9. The stability of the male/female relationship
10. The perceived risk of pregnancy
11. The availability of information about contraceptive services
12. Expectations about the confidentiality of services.

ACCEPTABILITY OF CONTRACEPTIVE METHODS

Even when a couple are motivated to use contraception, they may find their choice of method difficult and may finally opt for a method which is seen simply as the least of several evils. They will be influenced by the following factors:

1. Effectiveness of the method
2. Perceived safety of the method
3. Whether the method is used by the man or the woman
4. Convenience and simplicity of use
5. Whether action is required at the time of coitus
6. Freedom from forethought
7. Whether the method is well known or novel
8. Whether or not the method has religious or ethical approval
9. Availability of the method.

CHOICE OF METHOD

To cater for as many needs and preferences as possible, it is important that couples and individuals are free to choose where they obtain their advice and their method of contraception. Confidentiality is very often important particularly to groups such as young people. The role of the professional is to give information, and after taking a thorough history (and examining the patient if this is indicated), to advise the individual or couple. Any factors which might influence the effectiveness or the safety of the method(s) being considered should be discussed. The final choice is for the individual or couple to make. It is likely to be most successful when they are in agreement.

Commonly, partners will opt to use more than one method during their reproductive life, changing their method to suit changing circumstances. An example of this could be the following:

1. First using the combined pill to delay the onset of childbearing
2. Then using an IUD or other long-acting method such as Implanon to space their children
3. Finally using sterilization when the family is complete.

SAFETY

Contraceptive safety should be assessed in comparison with the morbidity and mortality associated with pregnancy. Evaluations of absolute risk are dependent upon personal medical history (including age and smoking status), and also on the availability of high-quality maternity services and safe, legal abortion. Where maternal mortality and morbidity are high, e.g. Latin America and Africa, the relative safety of contraceptive methods is very great. In developed countries where maternal mortality and morbidity rates are substantially lower, the risks of contraceptive use assume a relatively greater importance, but when the additional non-contraceptive health benefits of birth control methods are taken into account, most contraceptive practices will still yield a positive health benefit for most women. The careful selection of methods for women who may have particular risk factors can further improve the safety of fertility control and underlines the importance of having access to a full range of contraceptive methods. The simultaneous use of more than one contraceptive method may also benefit health, e.g. the use of male or female condoms as an additional protection may substantially reduce the risk of STI including HIV.

WHO has recently reviewed the contraindications for all the main methods of contraception and created a system of medical eligibility criteria for classifying these. This classification is helpful, as it is evidence-based and clarifies the absolute and relative contraindications for the different methods of contraception. Also, it separates relative contraindications into two categories:

WHO classification system: medical eligibility criteria for initiating and continuing selected family planning methods

WHO 1   A condition with no restriction for the use of contraceptive method.

WHO 2   A condition where the benefits of using the method generally outweigh the theoretical or proven risks.

WHO 3   A condition where the theoretical or proven risks generally outweigh the advantages of using the method. The method should only be used with caution if no other method is acceptable.

WHO 4   A condition which would represent unacceptable health risks if the method were used.

The WHO medical eligibility criteria tables can be found in the WHO publication 'Improving Access to Quality Care in Family Planning', in specialist contraceptive textbooks and on the Internet.

EFFECTIVENESS

Definitions

Theoretical effectiveness is defined as what might be achieved under ideal circumstances but in practice is never achieved.

User-effectiveness is defined as that actually achieved in practice.

Method failure is defined as failure inherent to the method itself.

User failure is defined as failure due to using a method inadequately or not at all.

Some methods of contraception are particularly vulnerable to 'user failure', e.g. oral contraceptives and condoms, while others are almost entirely vulnerable to 'method failure', e.g. IUDs and sterilization.

Measurements of effectiveness

Pearl index

This method takes into account the length of time the woman has been exposed to the risk of pregnancy. It is expressed in terms of a rate per 100 woman-years (HWY) and is calculated as follows:

$$\text{Failure rate per HWY} = \frac{\text{Total no. of pregnancies} \times 1200}{\text{Total months of use for all those using method}}$$

Life-table analysis

This method takes into account the changing probability of pregnancy over a period of time and is therefore more accurate. Calculations are expressed in terms of a rate per 100 women after 'n' months or years of use.

The effectiveness of any method varies in practice with differences due to personal, social and cultural factors in the user, the provider and the user–provider relationship. When user failure is important, failure rates are highest in couples who are young or inexperienced. Fertility diminishes with age, particularly sharply in women after the age of 35 with a consequent lowering of failure rates. For example, the progestogen-only pill has a failure rate of 3 per HWY in motivated users in the 25–30 age group and only 0.3 per HWY in women over 40.

COUNSELLING

For the purposes of counselling patients, methods may be usefully classified into three groups according to the best results that can be obtained in practice with near-perfect use. However, note that oral contraceptives, barrier methods and 'natural methods' have a much wider range of failure when used incorrectly or inconsistently.

Very highly effective methods

(Failures less than 1 per HWY)

1. Sterilization (male or female)
2. Combined oestrogen/progestogen pills (COC)
3. Depot progestogen injections
4. Subdermal contraceptive implants
5. Intrauterine devices (high-dose copper)
6. Intrauterine systems (high-dose progestogen).

Highly effective methods

(Failures 2–5 per HWY)

1. Progestogen-only pills (POP)
2. Diaphragm with spermicide
3. Male condom with spermicide
4. Periodic abstinence (symptothermal method)
5. Lactational amenorrhoea method
6. Female condom
7. Low copper-containing IUDs.

Less effective methods

(Failures may sometimes be as high as 10 per HWY or more.)

1. Spermicide alone
2. Cervical caps
3. Periodic abstinence (calendar method)
4. Coitus interruptus
5. Home-made barriers and spermicides.

Further research is required into the effectiveness of the disposable polyurethane cervical cap before it can be assigned to the above classification.

METHODS OF CONTRACEPTION

HORMONAL CONTRACEPTION

COMBINED OESTROGEN-PROGESTOGEN PILLS (COMBINED ORAL CONTRACEPTIVE OR COC)

Mechanism of action

The sex steroids (oestrogens and progestogens) used in available hormonal contraceptive preparations have the following actions:

1. Hypothalamus and pituitary inhibition of GnRH, FSH and LH by oestrogen via 'feedback' system.
2. Ovary—consequent inhibition of follicular activity, ovulation and luteal function.
3. Endometrium—inadequate secretory phase prejudices implantation. The endometrium becomes atrophic.
4. Cervical mucus—progestogens render it thick and scanty, making it resistant to sperm penetration.
5. Fallopian tubes—impaired function interferes with sperm migration and sperm transport.

Note: These actions are dose-dependent and vary from one woman to another.

Popularity

Currently used by 65–70 million women worldwide, this is the most popular reversible method of contraception in the UK. Since it was first marketed in the early 1960s, the dose of oestrogen and then the dose of progestogen have been greatly reduced. In the early 1980s newer progestogens (third generation, claimed to produce more beneficial lipid profiles) were introduced. In 1995 several published studies reported evidence of an increased risk of venous thromboembolism, associated with the use of several of these third generation pills containing desogestrel and gestodene, when compared with second generation levonorgestrel- and norethisterone-containing pills.

Advantages

Contraceptive benefits

1. Very highly effective—failure rate 0.2–3/HWY
2. Convenient—no action required at time of coitus
3. Reversible—do not cause subsequent infertility.

Non-contraceptive benefits

1. Improvements in the menstrual cycle
   a. Reduced blood loss and less iron deficiency anaemia
   b. Reduced dysmenorrhoea
   c. Reduced premenstrual problems
   d. Prevention of 'mittelschmerz' (ovulation pain/bleeding)
   e. Increased regularity of bleeding (withdrawal bleeds)
   f. Ability to manipulate the cycle, e.g. tri-cycle regime
2. Reduction in gynaecological disease
   a. Reduction in functional ovarian cysts, and possibly fibroids and endometriosis
   b. Reduction in pelvic inflammatory disease, and therefore a reduction in tubal infertility and ectopic pregnancy
   c. Prevention of ectopic pregnancy in women with a history of the condition
   d. Reduction in ovarian and endometrial cancers (both duration of use and ex-use effects)
3. Reduction in benign breast disease
   a. Fibroadenoma and fibrocystic disease without atypia
4. Other possible benefits
   a. Reduction in seborrhoeic conditions
   b. Reduction in thyroid disease, peptic ulcer and possibly severe forms of rheumatoid arthritis.

Disadvantages

1. Minor side-effects may be experienced, especially in the early months of use. These may include nausea, breast discomfort, acne, weight gain, headache (unusual with modern low-dose pills), 'break-through bleeding', mood changes, hirsutism and chloasma.

2. There may be serious health hazards for a minority of women. The taking of a thorough history, with an appropriate examination and investigations, if indicated, is essential to exclude contraindications.
3. No protection against sexually transmitted infections.
4. Requires continuous motivation to take the pill correctly.
5. Requires medical supervision.
6. Not immediately effective unless started on the first or second day of the menstrual cycle.

Cardiovascular disease

An observed increase in venous thromboembolic disease (VTE) in current users has been attributed to oestrogen-induced changes in clotting factors. It now seems likely that progestogens may also modify this effect, although they do not cause it. The risk of VTE, with both second- and third-generation pills, is still less than that associated with pregnancy.

An observed increase in arterial disease (ischaemic heart disease and cerebrovascular disease) in current users has been attributed to oestrogen-induced changes in clotting factors plus progestogen-induced changes in serum lipids (mainly HDL reduction). Recent epidemiological studies have confirmed that the absolute risk of myocardial infarction in women taking low-dose combined oral contraceptives is extremely small but significantly increased in smokers of cigarettes and those with hypertension. The risk is greater in current users who smoke than in smokers who do not take the COC. The risk is also greater in women with hypertension who use the COC, than in those with hypertension who are not current users. The estimated excess risk of all types of stroke attributable to low-dose oral contraceptive use is also extremely low but greater for ischaemic than for haemorrhagic stroke. Smoking and hypertension increase these risks significantly and several studies point to a further association with migraine.

Both arterial and venous clotting do not appear to be influenced by duration of use and there is no ex-use effect after the pill is discontinued.

Mean blood pressure rises slightly in COC users but remains within normal limits for most women. Asymptomatic, progressive and reversible hypertension develops occasionally, necessitating cessation of pill-taking. Epidemiological studies have demonstrated some lowering of risks with lower-dose pills.

Excess mortality and morbidity from arterial disease appears to be confined almost completely to women over the age of 35 who smoke.

Neoplasia

Carcinoma of the breast. Reanalysis of numerous studies suggests that women who are current users of combined oral contraceptives or who have used them in the past 10 years are at a slightly increased risk of having breast carcinoma diagnosed, although the additional cancers diagnosed tend to be localized to the breast. There is no evidence of an increase in the risk of having breast cancer diagnosed 10 or more years after cessation of use, and the cancers diagnosed then are still less advanced clinically than the cancers diagnosed in never-users. There is no evidence that COC use increases mortality from breast cancers (confirmed in the 1999 RCGP study by Beral et al.) and the excess risk of diagnosis is very slight, compared with the effect of other risk factors, e.g. positive family history.

Carcinoma of the cervix. There is some evidence of an association between COC use and an increased risk of CIN/invasive cancer with a duration-of-use effect. This has not been confirmed by all studies and confounding factors such as sexual behaviour, exposure to HPV and smoking need to be taken into account. A causal relationship is not reliably established. Combined oral contraceptive users should be encouraged to have regular smears, in line with the NHS cervical screening programme.

Liver tumours. Benign and malignant tumours may be increased by long-term use of high-dose pills but are extremely rare in British women.

Contraindications to COC use

Absolute (WHO 4)

1. Hormone-dependent tumours—breast, endometrial, trophoblastic.
2. Cardiovascular disease
    a. Venous—thromboembolism (DVT/ pelvic vein thrombosis/pulmonary embolism) or thrombophlebitis.
    b. Arterial—thrombosis, ischaemic heart disease including angina, cerebrovascular disease, transient ischaemic attacks, peripheral vascular disease, Raynaud's disease, cardiomyopathies.
    c. Valvular heart disease, with risk of embolization or pulmonary hypertension.
    d. Hypertension—systolic blood pressure > 160, diastolic > 100 (untreated).
    e. Migraine with aura, migraine which commences during COC therapy or migraine that needs treating with ergot preparations.
    f. Conditions predisposing to clotting, e.g. thrombophilias (inherited or acquired), immobility, elective major surgery, during treatment of varicose veins (sclerosant therapy or surgery), autoimmune disorders such as SLE, polyarteritis nodosa and scleroderma.
3. Impaired liver or renal function including active hepatitis, cholestatic jaundice of pregnancy, acute hepatic porphyrias, certain rare inherited disorders, e.g. Dubin–Johnson and Rotor syndromes, hepatic tumours, severe decompensated cirrhosis and gallstones.
4. Breast-feeding if the infant is less than six weeks old.
5. Diabetes with nephropathy/retinopathy or neuropathy.
6. Serious conditions known to have been made worse by previous pregnancy or sex steroids, e.g. herpes gestationis, otosclerosis, chorea, porphyria, haemolytic-uraemic syndrome. WHO category 3 or 4 contraindications to COC use are listed in the British National Formulary and in the product characteristics for some of these very rare diseases. However, for many there is no direct research evidence of the effects of the COC on the condition. Nevertheless, it would be wise to exercise great

caution as the conditions are serious and often irreversible. In the rare situation of the COC being the only acceptable contraceptive for a woman with such a medical history, the advice of a specialist should be sought.

Relative (WHO 2 and 3)
(More than one in combination may be a very strong contraindication, e.g. a smoker over 35.)

1. Age over 35 years.
2. Current smoker.
3. Hypertension—systolic blood pressure 140–159, diastolic 90–99.
4. History of subarachnoid haemorrhage.
5. Hyperlipidaemia.
6. Diabetes without complications.
7. Migraine without aura and without the need for treatment with ergot preparations.
8. Obesity—BMI > 30.
9. History of premature cardiovascular disease in first-degree relative (stroke under the age of 60, coronary artery disease under the age of 50).
10. Lactation if the infant is less than six months old. The COC may diminish the supply of milk.
11. Puerperal psychosis/severe mood disorder.
12. Homozygous sickle cell disease (not the trait).
13. Some diseases may be made worse by the COC, e.g. inflammatory bowel disease.
14. Oligomenorrhoea/amenorrhoea or irregular vaginal bleeding should be investigated before prescribing the COC. Specialist advice may be required depending on the outcome.

Prescribing principles
Choose:

1. Low oestrogen dose (20–35 µg ethinylestradiol)
2. Low progestogen dose (e.g. 500 µg norethisterone or 150 µg levonorgestrel)
3. Monophasic regimen which is simple for the patient
4. Low-cost preparation.

Note: Newer progestogens (desogestrel, gestodene and norgestimate) have been developed to reduce the depressant effect on HDL cholesterol. Claims for the superiority of these more expensive preparations can only be substantiated by long-term epidemiological studies or randomized controlled trials, and at present must remain speculative. Women who wish to use desogestrel- or gestodene-containing combined pills (e.g. when the concomitant increase in sex hormone binding globulin may improve a tendency to acne) should be advised about the possibly small increased risk of VTE compared with other preparations.

Practical prescribing

Drug interactions

The most important which may affect contraceptive efficacy are:

Broad-spectrum antibiotics. These may impair oestrogen reabsorption in the enterohepatic circulation (affects oestrogen only). In short-term antibiotic use, extra precautions should be used during treatment and for 7 additional days. In long-term antibiotic use, the large bowel flora responsible for the recycling of oestrogens are replaced with resistant organisms within about 2 weeks. Therefore, if a woman is started on long-term antibiotics when she is on the COC, she needs to use extra precautions for about 3–4 weeks. If she is already on long-term antibiotics when she starts the COC, she does not need to take extra precautions.

Enzyme-inducing drugs (rifampicin, griseofulvin, some anticonvulsants, protease inhibitors used in the treatment of HIV). These interfere with oestrogen and progestogen metabolism in the liver (affecting COC and progestogen-only methods). Patients wishing to use the COC and enzyme inducers should be prescribed a COC with a high dose of oestrogen (at least 50 μg) and progestogen. Even then, great care should be taken when the patient is using a very powerful enzyme inducer such as rifampicin.

Elective major surgery

The combined oral contraceptive should be stopped 6 weeks in advance of major surgery with immobilization, to allow clotting factors to normalize. It should not be restarted until at least 2 weeks after full mobilization.

The lowest dose monophasic levonorgestrel or norethisterone preparation

This should be prescribed first and the patient warned to expect spotting or break-through bleeding for up to the fourth month of use. If cycle control is not attained by then, the dose of progestogen may be increased. (An increase in oestrogen is not usually practicable or desirable but some women may be helped by a triphasic preparation.)

The simplest regime

This is to advise the patient to take her first pill on the first or second day of menstrual bleeding and to take 21 consecutive pills (one per day) followed by a 7-day break. The COC is then immediately effective, and a regular 28-day cycle is the norm. The COC may be commenced immediately after therapeutic abortion or 3 weeks after childbirth, if not breast-feeding.

Contraceptive efficacy

This may be lost if a pill is taken more than 12 hours late, malabsorbed or subjected to drug interaction. An alternative contraceptive method should be advised during the lapse and for 7 days after resuming COC use. If the 7 days extend into the pill-free interval, two packs of pills should be taken consecutively. When an enzyme-inducing drug is used, contraceptive efficacy may not be regained until 8 weeks after stopping the therapy.

Teaching
All patients need careful instructions about how to take their pills and counselling as to any side-effects they may experience. This information also should be given in writing. Leaflets should be available for this purpose.

PROGESTOGEN-ONLY CONTRACEPTION

Progestogens have effects on the cervical mucus (making it impenetrable to sperm), on the endometrium (preventing implantation) and on tubal function with secondary effects on ovulation. These effects are variable, are probably dose-related and depend on the potency of the progestogen.

PROGESTOGEN-ONLY PILL (POP)

Mechanism of action
The effects on the cervical mucus and on the endometrium are the most important ones in this low-dose preparation. To maximize the effect on cervical mucus, the POP may be more effective if taken regularly about 4–6 hours before the likely time of intercourse. This only applies if intercourse usually occurs at the same time of day. To ensure effectiveness, the most important thing is for the pills to be taken regularly at the same time every day.

Advantages
1. There are no significant metabolic effects. The POP can therefore be used in older women, in women who smoke and in women with medical conditions such as diabetes mellitus, migraine and mild hypertension.
2. In lactating mothers there is no adverse effect on lactation or on the infant and no decrease in the milk volume.
3. Where oestrogen is contraindicated the POP may be a useful alternative to the combined pill.
4. The continuous daily regimen may be simpler for some patients to remember.

Disadvantages
1. Like the COC it requires continuous motivation and medical supervision.
2. Not immediately effective unless started on the first day of the menstrual period.
3. Less effective than COCs. The failure rate is age-related (0–4%).
4. Possible menstrual irregularity (spotting, short cycles or amenorrhoea) which may prove unacceptable to the patient.

5. Probably offers less protection against ectopic pregnancy than COCs because the POP does not prevent ovulation.
6. Increased risk of developing functional ovarian cysts due to partial suppression of follicular development. This may cause diagnostic confusion with suspected ectopic pregnancy.
7. Need for very regular pill-taking with only a 3-hour window for late pills.

Contraindications to POP use (WHO 3 or 4)

1. Hormone-dependent tumours (unless agreed with oncologist).
2. A history of functional ovarian cysts.
3. Enzyme-inducing drugs may reduce its efficacy.
4. A past history of ectopic pregnancy is a relative contraindication, as methods which consistently prevent ovulation offer more protection against a recurrence.
5. Acute porphyria.
6. Current VTE (consult with physician).
7. Current breast cancer (discuss with oncologist).
8. Severe liver disease.

Prescribing principles

There is no convincing evidence that any preparation is superior to another; therefore the cheapest should be prescribed.

Practical prescribing

1. Start the first pill on the first day of menstrual bleeding.
2. Continue with one pill daily at the same time each day. After pregnancy, the POP may be started immediately (regardless of gestation) but bleeding patterns may be more acceptable if the first pill is postponed until 3 weeks postpartum.
3. Contraceptive efficacy may be lost. This may happen if pills are forgotten (more than 3 hours late), malabsorbed or subjected to drug interaction from enzyme-inducing drugs, which may have an effect for up to 8 weeks from discontinuation. An alternative contraceptive method should be advised during the period at risk and for 7 days thereafter.

Teaching and counselling

The patient should be carefully taught how to take the POP and the instructions reinforced by written information (CES leaflets).

DEPOT PROGESTOGEN INJECTIONS

Mechanism of action

The dose of progestogen is sufficiently large to inhibit ovulation. The endometrium tends to become atrophic with no secretory activity, and cervical mucus thickens.

Advantages

1. Very highly effective, and immediately so if given during the first 5 days of the menstrual cycle.
2. No user-failure between injections—needs no continuous motivation or action at the time of coitus.
3. Safe—no mortality reported.
4. Reversible—does not cause permanent infertility.
5. Lactation not suppressed—may be enhanced.
6. Can be used when oestrogens contraindicated.
7. Erythropoiesis stimulated and red cell membrane stabilized—reduces crises in homozygous sickle cell disease.
8. Probable reduction in menstrual disorders—as with the COC. (Irregular bleeding may occur initially, but amenorrhoea usually supervenes with continuing use.)
9. Protection from endometrial cancer.

Disadvantages

1. Bleeding irregularities may be unacceptable to the patient.
2. May be some delay in return to fertility (up to 2 years but usually about 6 months).
3. Early postpartum period—because of the risk of heavy and prolonged bleeding it is preferable to wait until 5–6 weeks after delivery to give the first Depo-Provera injection.
4. Cannot 'stop' in an emergency.
5. Some women dislike injections.
6. Requires medical supervision.
7. Weight gain affects some patients. (This is usually secondary to an increase in appetite.)
8. Metabolic effects on glucose tolerance (reduced) and HDL-cholesterol (reduced) but significance unknown.
9. Theoretical risk of fetal masculinization if given in pregnancy but unlikely in the dose used.

Contraindications (WHO 3 and 4)

1. Pregnancy.
2. Pregnancy desired in near future.
3. Anxiety about possible menstrual disturbance.
4. In breast-feeding mothers of premature infants it probably should be avoided as it is excreted in small quantities in breast milk.
5. Acute or chronic liver disease (as for the COC).
6. Porphyria.
7. In view of the metabolic effects, caution should be exercised before use in women with impaired glucose tolerance.
8. Current breast cancer (discuss with an oncologist).
9. Current cardiovascular disease.

10. Hypertension greater than 160/100.
11. Enzyme-inducing drugs.

Practical prescribing

Depo-Provera (DMPA—depot medroxyprogesterone acetate) and Noristerat (NET-OEN—norethisterone enantate) are both marketed in the UK and may be offered to suitable patients after giving information and counselling. Manufacturer's information leaflets and audiotapes are available for Depo-Provera in English and a number of ethnic minority languages. Noristerat has a product licence for short-term use as a contraceptive, but doctors may assume responsibility for long-term prescribing. The usual doses are Depo-Provera 150 mg 12-weekly or Noristerat 200 mg 8-weekly. Both should be given by deep intramuscular injection into the gluteal muscle. In obese patients the deltoid may be a preferable site, to avoid subcutaneous injection. The injection site should not be massaged as this may result in higher initial blood levels and possible shortening of the duration of action. The DMPA should be shaken before injection. In the case of Noristerat this needs to be warmed to body temperature before injection, as it is thick and oily.

Patients should have their blood pressure, weight and BMI measured initially. Pelvic examination and breast examination should only be carried out if clinically indicated. In the case of a cervical smear, this should be taken if it is due. Counselling patients about possible changes in their menstrual bleeding pattern is very important. Excessive bleeding (defined as more than 7 days out of 21) should be actively managed after excluding other causes of bleeding. Unfortunately the efficacy of regimens of 'add-back oestrogen' or shortening the intervals between injections has not been compared in randomized controlled trials and this treatment remains empirical.

When women are on enzyme-inducing drugs and no method other than the injectable is suitable, the interval between injections can be shortened (Depo-Provera to be given 8–10-weekly).

SUSTAINED RELEASE SYSTEMS

Long-acting sustained steroid-releasing contraceptive methods are currently available and others are being developed. These methods all depend on the capacity of a non-biodegradable polymer to release lipophilic drugs at a relatively constant rate.

Effectiveness is proportional to the daily dose of steroid released. Currently only the subdermal implant (Implanon) and the levonorgestrel-releasing intrauterine system (Mirena) are marketed in the UK. They are both highly effective methods with no user failure.

The acceptability of all progestogen-only methods is mainly limited by the frequency of unpredictable menstrual bleeding patterns, but their safety, effectiveness and convenience assure them a place in overall contraceptive provision.

Implanon subdermal implant

Implanon is a newly marketed subdermal implant system which gives highly effective, reversible, low-dose contraception for 3 years. It consists of a single flexible polymer rod containing 68 mg of the progestogen, etonogestrel. The most important mode of action is the suppression of ovulation. The etonogestrel also acts by thickening the cervical mucus and by suppression of the endometrium. The hormone is released at a rate of 60–70 μg per day by week 5–6. This rate decreases to 35–45 μg at the end of the first year, 30–40 μg at the end of the second year and 25–30 μg by the end the third and final year. The implant is inserted subdermally into the inner aspect of the upper non-dominant arm, using local anaesthetic. It is a simple procedure but clinicians must have appropriate training in the insertion and removal techniques before prescribing Implanon. Patients should be counselled prior to insertion particularly about the possibility of irregular bleeding and/or amenorrhoea.

Advantages
1. Very highly effective—no pregnancies at all in the phase 3 trials
2. No user failure
3. Long-term contraception
4. Safe
5. Reversible
6. Immediate return to fertility when implant removed
7. Acne may improve.

Disadvantages
1. Expensive.
2. Irregular bleeding may occur, particularly in the first few months. It can sometimes be prolonged.
3. Requires fitting by a trained clinician.
4. Progestogenic side-effects such as acne, weight gain and breast tenderness may occur.
5. Headaches may occur.
6. Enzyme—inducing drugs may reduce the effectiveness.
7. Lactation—the manufacturers suggest that this is a relative contraindication, although there is no evidence to support or refute this. Etonogestrel has been detected in breast milk.

Contraindications (WHO 3 and 4)
1. Active venous thromboembolism
2. Progestogen-dependent tumours
3. Severe hepatic disease
4. Pregnancy
5. Undiagnosed vaginal bleeding
6. Hypersensitivity to any of the components of Implanon
7. Acute porphyria.

Practical prescribing
1. Implanon should be inserted on day 1–5 of the menstrual period.
2. Following childbirth or second trimester abortion, it should be fitted on day 21–28. If it is fitted later condoms should be used for a week.
3. It can be fitted immediately following first trimester abortion.
4. If changing from another progestogen method: Implanon may be inserted on any day when switching from the minipill, the day the next injection is due when changing from Depo-Provera, and the same day when replacing an implant.
5. When changing from the COC Implanon should be inserted the day after the last active pill.

Norplant—subdermal implant
This was first marketed in the UK in 1993 but is no longer being marketed in this country. However, there are women who are still using Norplant who may attend their GP or family planning clinic for advice or removal of the system. Six silastic rubber capsules, each containing levonorgestrel, are placed subdermally on the medial aspect of the upper non-dominant arm. The capsules are not biodegradable and should be removed. Removal (which can be difficult) requires local anaesthesia and aseptic technique and should only be undertaken by accredited practitioners.

Mirena—intrauterine system
This intrauterine system was first marketed in the UK in 1995. It is a modified Nova T/ Novagard device with a silastic capsule fixed to the vertical stem containing 52 mg of levonorgestrel which is released into the uterine cavity at the rate of 20 μg/24 hours. The system is licensed for 5 years' use in Europe.

Mechanism of action
1. The progestogen released by the IUS produces an endometrium unsuitable for implantation. This suppression of the endometrium is the main mode of action.
2. Modification of ovarian function with some anovulatory cycles particularly in the first 12 months of use.
3. Foreign body reaction of the endometrium with infiltration with macrophages, leukocytes and plasma cells.
4. Thickening of the cervical mucus.

Advantages
1. Highly effective.
2. Safe.
3. Menorrhagia treatment—the device can benefit women with this condition. The effect on the menstrual bleeding pattern is mainly due to the local effect of the levonorgestrel on the endometrium. The system was originally marketed as a treatment for menorrhagia and is licensed for this use.

4. Oligo-amenorrhoea may occur and is often seen as an advantage.
5. The effect of levonorgestrel on cervical mucus is likely to give some protection against PID.
6. High continuation rates.
7. Immediately reversible.
8. No sustained motivation needed.
9. Long-term contraception.

Disadvantages
1. The device is expensive.
2. Irregular bleeding often occurs in the early months of use and can be troublesome.
3. Amenorrhoea may occur and be unacceptable.
4. The IUS is not suitable for emergency contraception.
5. Progestogenic side-effects (breast discomfort, abdominal bloating, headaches, acne) may occur.
6. Functional ovarian cysts.

Contraindications
These are the same as those for the IUD (see next section) with the exceptions of menorrhagia, copper allergy and anticoagulant therapy. Current VTE, current or history of ischaemic heart disease and severe liver disease appear as WHO 3 categories for the IUS.

Practical prescribing
Irregular bleeding or amenorrhoea will lead some women to request removal. The IUS can be expected to reduce or eliminate menstrual blood loss after the first few months of use. It is important to give careful counselling about the possible changes in the menstrual bleeding pattern before the system is fitted. Careful preinsertion assessment and counselling should maximize continuation rates.

The method of insertion of Mirena is quite specific and different from that of the Nova T. The diameter of the introducer is 4.8 mm (compared with 3.7 mm for the standard Nova T). Local anaesthesia and dilatation of the cervix to Hegar 5 are sometimes required for successful insertion. Lack of attention to this factor may lead to failed insertions.

INTRAUTERINE DEVICES (IUD)

Popularity
Worldwide popularity exceeds that of oral contraceptives. An estimated 100 million women are current users of IUDs.

Mechanisms of action

The main mode of action is believed to be alteration/inhibition of sperm migration, fertilization and ovum transport, all of which lower the fertilization rate. In addition there is the production of a sterile inflammatory response in the endometrium which inhibits implantation of the blastocyst. IUDs may therefore be used as an emergency method of contraception and should not be removed from the uterus within 7 days of coitus if pregnancy is not desired. The IUD is not abortifacient.

Advantages

1. Safe — mortality is very rare and there are no metabolic effects.
2. Highly effective.
3. Effective immediately or postcoitally.
4. Continuation rates are high. The method proves to be acceptable to the majority of users.
5. Reversible.
6. Requires no sustained motivation or action at the time of coitus.
7. Can provide long-term contraception cheaply.

Disadvantages

1. Need for specially trained personnel to fit IUDs and give follow-up care.
2. Possible complications at the time of insertion of the device include pain, bleeding, vagal inhibition and perforation of the uterus (rare).
3. Infection is most likely to occur in the first 3 weeks following the fitting and is related to STI risk.
4. Menstruation is often heavier and more prolonged than is normal for the woman.
5. Complications include pain, intermenstrual bleeding, expulsion, displacement, lost threads or male dyspareunia. There is an increased relative risk of ectopic pregnancy.
6. The method provides no protection from STI or PID.

Contraindications

Absolute (WHO 4)

1. Pregnancy
2. Malignancy of the genital tract
3. Acute or chronic pelvic infection
4. Certain congenital abnormalities of the uterus
5. Large fibroids which distort the uterine cavity
6. Wilson's disease or copper allergy (only for copper-bearing devices)
7. Trophoblastic disease.

Relative (WHO 2 and 3)

1. STI risk—a sexual lifestyle which increases this risk. This is especially important in young people with the current high incidence of STI, particularly chlamydia.

2. Undiagnosed abnormal vaginal bleeding. (If pathology has been excluded an IUD may be fitted.)
3. Menorrhagia.
4. Malignant disease of the genital tract.
5. Fixed retroversion of the uterus.
6. Past history of ectopic pregnancy.
7. History of PID.
8. Nulliparity.
9. Recent uterine wall surgery.
10. Congenital or rheumatic valvular heart disease (may require antibiotic cover for insertion).
11. Compromised immune system particularly if there is an increased risk of STI.
12. Anticoagulant therapy—this may lead to very heavy periods with copper-containing IUDs. An intrauterine system would be more suitable.

Prevention and management of complications

Patients should be carefully assessed for contraindications to the method. The taking of an in-depth history, a pelvic examination and investigations, if indicated, are essential. Patients who have risk factors for STIs, where no other method is appropriate or acceptable, should have high vaginal and endocervical swabs taken and a test for chlamydia. It is important to remember that the method is relatively contraindicated for this group of patients. If the fitting is absolutely necessary—for instance, in the case of emergency contraception —prophylactic antibiotics such as doxycycline should be given prior to the swab results being available.

Before fitting the IUD, counselling about the device, including possible complications and side-effects, is essential. Also, it is important to explain what the fitting will involve, the use of analgesia, and the possibility of pain.

Insertion of the device should be carried out in a calm, relaxed manner with due attention to aseptic technique, analgesia for the patient if necessary, and precise adherence to the recommended fitting procedure, which differs for each device.

Women with epilepsy should have their IUD fitted by an experienced clinician and facilities should be available for treatment of an epileptic seizure.

Women who experience vagal inhibition resulting in bradycardia may be treated with i.v. atropine 0.6 mg. It may be necessary to remove the device if the patient does not recover quickly. Facilities for basic cardiopulmonary resuscitation should be available whenever IUDs are fitted.

The device may have to be removed if menstrual pain and bleeding are unacceptable. Intermenstrual pain/bleeding may be due to infection or partial expulsion/displacement of the device. Suspected infection should be investigated and treated promptly in a department of genitourinary medicine, with follow-up of the partner.

Ectopic pregnancy should always be considered if there is unexplained lower abdominal pain or irregular vaginal bleeding, particularly if there is a history of a scanty or late period.

Perforation of the uterus may be suspected when threads are absent and should be investigated by pelvic ultrasound. A follow-up abdominal X-ray should be performed if the device is not seen in the uterine cavity. If its presence in the abdominal cavity is confirmed, laparoscopic removal of the device should be arranged without delay.

If pregnancy occurs with the device in situ, the patient should be advised to have the device removed immediately while the threads are accessible. Previous expulsion is not a contraindication to the insertion of another device.

Practical prescribing

The devices currently recommended for use in Britain are:

1. T-Safe Cu380A (The OrthoGyne-T 380 Slimline which was the gold standard is no longer being manufactured)
2. Multiload Cu375 and Multiload Cu250 (short and standard)
3. Nova-T 380
4. GyneFix
5. Flexi-T 300.

The choice of device may be made on the basis of its relative effectiveness and on uterine size and tightness of the cervix, determined by sounding the uterus. The choice of device is probably less important than the selection of the patient and the skill of the operator. IUDs may be fitted at any time in the menstrual cycle if contraception has been used effectively. After delivery, it has been customary to insert the IUD 6 weeks postpartum, when the uterus is usually fully involuted. Devices may be fitted with caution at the time of delivery, if this is in the best interest of the woman. Postplacental insertion is associated with high expulsion rates and possibly an increased risk of perforation. IUDs may be fitted at the time of termination of pregnancy.

Devices releasing the highest amounts of copper (the Cu380A and the Multiload 375) are the most effective but if the cervical canal is narrow it may be easier to fit a Nova-T device. When loaded, the Cu380A is wider than the Mirena. Therefore, local anaesthesia and dilatation may be needed for the fitting.

Despite the varying recommendations of the manufacturers it is likely that all devices can be left in utero for 5 years without loss of efficacy. Studies continue to define the optimal life of the more effective modern devices with data indicating the continued effectiveness of the Cu380A and Multiload 375 devices for at least 8 years. IUDs inserted in women over the age of 40 may be left in situ until after the menopause. It is probably advisable to remove them a year after the menopause, before cervical/uterine atrophy makes the procedure difficult.

BARRIER METHODS OF CONTRACEPTION

Popularity
There has been renewed interest in barrier contraceptives in response to concern about the increase in STIs and HIV infection. Theory and clinical experience suggest that maximum contraceptive efficacy can only be obtained by using a barrier and spermicide together. The commonly used spermicide nonoxinol '9' has been shown to be active against HIV in vitro.

Advantages
1. Protection from sexually transmitted infection.
2. Protection from carcinoma of the cervix.
3. Instantly effective (after initial learning).
4. No systemic side-effects.
5. Cervical caps do not interfere with the sensation of either partner (although condoms and possibly diaphragms are reputed to do so).
6. Most types of barrier method are available from non-medical sources.

Disadvantages
1. Need trained personnel to fit cap initially and check periodically.
2. Require continuous motivation and supplies.
3. Action required at time of coitus (for condom use).
4. User-failure can be high, e.g. the young/inexperienced.
5. Couples may find barrier methods messy or distasteful.
6. Small increase in cystitis/vaginal infections in cap users.

PRACTICAL PRESCRIBING

Caps
Mechanism of action
This method works by acting as a barrier between the sperm and the ovum and also as a vehicle for spermicide.

   There are three types of cap, as described below.
Diaphragm (flat-spring, coil-spring and arcing types).   These can be successful when the pelvic floor has good muscle tone. An arcing diaphragm is particularly useful when the cervix is difficult to cover. A coil-spring diaphragm is often found to be comfortable when a flat-spring one is not.
Suction cap (cervical, vault and vimule types).   These can be used when there is prolapse of the vaginal walls. They may sometimes be useful when a diaphragm is uncomfortable.

Oves cap.   This cervical cap has recently been marketed. It is made from a medical-grade silicone elastomer and is hypoallergenic. It is said to adhere to the surface of the cervix, not by suction but by surface tension. An initial study has shown good efficacy but this study was very small. The results of a larger trial are awaited. The oves cap is available over the counter.

The patient should be fitted with a suitable cap and then taught how to remove and reinsert the device several times under supervision before she relies on the method. She should also be instructed in the correct use of spermicide and be given written instructions on the use of the method (see CES leaflet). Periodic checks of the fitting and correct placement of the cap should take place during use.

Sponges
Contraceptive sponges are no longer marketed in the UK.

Condoms
Male and female condoms are available. These may be dispensed free of charge in hospitals, community health family planning clinics, some general practices and genitourinary medicine clinics, as well as some clubs and youth projects. Male condoms vary in shape, thickness and lubrication. They may have features, e.g. texture, colour or taste, designed to enhance their attractiveness to the user. Some brands have a spermicide incorporated in the lubricant. There is a British standard for condoms and those without the 'kite mark' should not be used. There is also now a European standard for condoms which runs concurrently. Condoms are available over the counter.

Most male condoms are made of latex rubber. Avanti is a polyurethane male condom. One type of female condom is marketed in the UK, the Femidom. It is made of polyurethane rather than latex rubber and has an inner flexible ring to aid insertion and an outer ring to aid retention around the vulva. Efficacy studies suggest that the female condom is as effective as the diaphragm.

For clients who are allergic to latex, polyurethane male or female condoms may be used. Unfortunately these are expensive.

Clients should be given detailed instructions in the use of condoms and should also be made aware of the availability of emergency contraceptive methods (see CES leaflets.)

Spermicides
These are available as tubed creams, jellies or pastes, aerosol foam, soluble pessaries, foaming tablets and water-soluble plastic film. High failure rates are to be expected if they are used without a barrier. The active ingredient is usually nonoxinol '9'. Note: Oil-based spermicides or other products should not be used with latex caps/condoms as they can damage the tensile strength of the rubber.

STERILIZATION

Popularity
In the UK almost 30% of couples and 50% of those over 40 use either male or female sterilization for contraception.

Methods
Bilateral vasectomy in the male, and tubal procedures performed at laparoscopy or minilaparotomy in the female, are the preferred methods. Clips or rings are preferred to diathermy for female sterilization. Nowadays, however the ring is rarely used. Interval sterilization has a better prognosis than sterilization carried out in association with pregnancy.

Advantages
1. Very highly effective.
2. Needs no continuing motivation.
3. One-off procedure with no ongoing cost.
4. Safe—side-effects and health hazards are rare.

Disadvantages
1. Regret is possible. Reversal is expensive and cannot be guaranteed.
2. Needs a surgical procedure and therefore involves a relatively large capital outlay. This tends to restrict availability.
3. Higher failure rate of female sterilization than previously thought.

Importance of counselling the couple
From the medicolegal point of view it is important to stress both the irreversibility of the procedure and the very small failure rate. Alternative

Table 40.1 Implications of the male and female sterilization options.

	Male	Female
Immediacy	Not immediately effective	Immediately effective
Failure	Very small: 1 in 2000	Small: 1 in 200
Mortality	1 in 100 000	1 in 10 000
	(mostly under local anaesthetic)	(mostly under general anaesthetic)
Morbidity		
Early	Below 5% (bleeding, infection)	Below 5% (bleeding, infection, trauma)
Late	Sperm granuloma	Ectopic pregnancy
Reversibility	Chances dependent on extent of original procedure	
Availability	Marked regional/district variations	

contraception should be discussed as well as the implications of the male and female sterilization options (see Table 40.1). Suggestions that tubal procedures in the woman predispose to later menorrhagia have not been substantiated. Recent suggestions that vasectomy has a causal relationship with an increased risk of prostatic and testicular cancers or renal calculi remain unproven and do not currently justify avoidance of the operation.

PERIODIC ABSTINENCE

This method is also referred to as natural family planning, the rhythm method or the safe period. It is based on the principle of avoidance of coitus during the 'fertile days' of a woman's menstrual cycle but in practice this is difficult to determine because:

1. Sperm may survive in the female genital tract for several days (up to 7) post-coitus.
2. Ovulation cannot be predicted accurately in advance.

High effectiveness can therefore only be achieved by restricting coitus to the postovulatory phase of the cycle after the ovum is presumed to be incapable of being fertilized. The most accurate way of determining the 'infertile' days is to use various methods in combination—the 'symptothermal' method:

1. Observation from a menstrual calendar of the longest cycle length and calculation of the last fertile day by subtracting 10.
2. Observation of basal body temperature and reckoning on the infertile phase beginning on the third morning of elevated temperature readings following mid-cycle release of the ovum.
3. Observations of cervical elevation and softening at the time of ovulation; ovulatory pain, bleeding or breast discomfort; and serial observations of cervical mucus. The infertile phase is reckoned to begin on the fourth evening after peak mucus production.

Since 1996 a small device, incorporating a microcomputer and hormone assay system to measure LH and oestradiol from urinary dipsticks, has been marketed in Britain under the trade name Persona. This provides an alternative method of determining the 'fertile' days of a woman's cycle by signalling 'safe' and 'unsafe' days with green and red lights. It has a higher failure rate than the symptothermal method and is expensive.

The successful use of periodic abstinence is dependent on the couple's motivation to avoid intercourse on the 'fertile' days.

Advantages
1. Free of any known physical side-effects.
2. May be acceptable to couples whose religion or culture debars them from other methods.
3. Always available and cheap (after teaching). However, Persona is expensive.

4. The knowledge gained by couples practisng the method may also assist them when planning conception.

Disadvantages
1. High user failure rates which vary between 6 and 25 pregnancies per HWY.
2. The infertile period may be difficult to identify, e.g. during fever.
3. The couple have to accept considerable limitations on the days available for coitus. Sustained motivation and cooperation are essential to success.

Practical prescribing
Temperature charts and fertility thermometers are available on prescription in Great Britain. The couple should be counselled and taught effectively and offered ongoing support. A CES leaflet is available.

LACTATIONAL AMENORRHOEA METHOD

Women who have delivered a baby in the preceding 6 months, who are breast-feeding fully (without giving any supplemental feeds) and who are amenor-rhoeic have only a 1–2% chance of becoming pregnant. If these three conditions are fulfilled, it may be reasonable to rely on them alone for con-traceptive protection. It is important to counsel the woman, so that she under-stands that ovulation will precede menstruation and she will have no warning that fertility has returned.

POSTCOITAL CONTRACEPTION (EMERGENCY CONTRACEPTION)

A request for emergency contraception should lead to a review of the couple's ongoing contraceptive strategy. In order that the method can be used at all, the population needs to be educated about its existence and availability. The method should be accessible on every day of the week. There are two methods: hormonal and IUD insertion.

HORMONAL

Levonelle
This is a progestogen-only postcoital contraceptive. It was approved by the Committee on the Safety of Medicines for use in the UK in 1999. It is pres-ented in a two tablet pack. Each tablet contains 750 mg of levonorgestrel. The first tablet must be taken within 72 hours of unprotected sexual intercourse and the second 12 hours later. The 1998 WHO trial showed that Levonelle

prevented 86% of expected pregnancies. The sooner the pills are taken after unprotected sexual intercourse, the more effective the product. If levonelle is taken in the first 24 hours after unprotected sexual intercourse 95% of expected pregnancies are prevented, at 25–48 hours 85%, and at 49–72 hours 58%. The only contraindication is established pregnancy. Some women may experience nausea as a side-effect but vomiting is rare. It is available over the counter but is expensive.

PC4-Yuzpe method

This is no longer available in the UK. It may still be valuable in developing countries where financial constraints prevail.

IUD INSERTION

This is effective if fitted within 5 days of exposure to unprotected coitus. It can be fitted in good faith up to day 19 of a 28-day cycle, or within 5 days of the earliest estimated ovulation, where the patient has come for treatment more than 5 days after unprotected intercourse. Nulliparity and rape are relative contraindications because of the greater susceptibility to STI. However, if infection is suspected the fitting can be covered with a course of antibiotics such as doxycycline in an emergency. A past history of ectopic pregnancy is a relatively strong contraindication. The method is virtually 100% effective and may be retained by the woman as her ongoing method or removed with the next period if so desired.

ORGANIZATION OF FAMILY PLANNING SERVICES

Family planning services in the UK used to be provided, mainly, by the Family Planning Association (a charitable body) until they were transferred to the National Health Service during the 1974 reorganization. The intention was that all who needed advice and help with family planning (regardless of sex or marital status) should be able to choose a free service from the following sources (DHSS Circular HSC(l S) 32 May 1974):

1. Community health services.
2. Hospital services.
3. Family practioner services.
4. Pharmacists—More recently, pharmacists have been providing services in some areas.

These services should be seen as complementary to each other and liaison should be encouraged.

Community health services
Family planning advice and supplies may be delivered by:

1. Sexual and reproductive healthcare clinics (family planning clinics)
2. Young people's clinics (youth advisory centres)
3. Community youth projects
4. Domiciliary and outreach family planning services
5. Community midwives and health visitors.

Hospital services
Family planning advice and supplies may be delivered by:

1. Hospital outpatient sexual and reproductive healthcare clinics (family planning clinics).
2. Hospital family planning 'visitors' who see patients in postnatal and postabortion wards.
3. Hospital midwives working in antenatal/postnatal clinics and parentcraft classes.
4. Genitourinary medicine clinics.
5. Hospital gynaecology clinics, especially termination of pregnancy (TOP) request clinics.
6. Hospital staff in any department may find it appropriate to advise or refer patients as part of their regular clinical care. They should be aware of the possible interactions of various medications and the effects of surgery on the safety or effectiveness of different contraceptive methods.

Family practitioner services
General practitioners and practice nurses often provide family planning services within normal surgery hours and/or in special 'sessions'.

Future services
Primary Care Trusts
Since April 2002 most community services have been in Primary Care Trusts (PCTs) instead of community trusts. This gives the opportunity for close working of all those providing family planning services.

The recently published National Sexual Health Strategy leads the way to the development of integrated sexual health services, both in community family planning clinics and in general practice. This will extend the role of these primary care services and should provide more holistic care for patients.

41

Psychosexual counselling

Helen Massil

Expectations of the examiners

The candidate will be expected to have an understanding of the principles involved in counselling patients with psychosexual problems.

Introduction

This chapter will outline the principles of psychosexual counselling and is not intended to provide a comprehensive account of this therapeutic work. It should be noted that the chapter is mainly related to individuals and couples within a heterosexual relationship, although the general principles apply to all individuals and relationships.

Human sexuality encompasses gender identity (maleness/femaleness), sexual object choice (partner/other object of desire), sexual drive and sexual function. Individuals display wide variations in their sexuality and therefore it is a general principle that it is the client who decides whether any particular state is a 'problem'. Professionals should be sensitive to this issue and should not make assumptions about their patient's wishes. However, confidentiality cannot always be maintained if others are at risk (paedophilia, sexual abuse).

Classification

In 1999 a new classification was developed for female sexual dysfunctions (International Consensus Development Conference) which included a new category of 'other sexual pain disorders'. The new category includes vulvodynia (vulval pain) and pelvic pain, both of which can be non-coital in origin.

The classification of sexual problems can be related to the human sexual response cycle (see Fig. 41.1 and Table 41.1). The components of the human sexual response include the underlying sexual drive, desire (initiation), arousal (sexual excitement), orgasm and resolution. The differentiation between sexual drive and desire is important; the former may be defined as an omnipotent force that can lead to all forms of sexual outlet, while sexual desire is

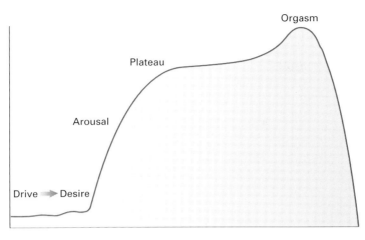

Fig. 41.1 The human sexual response and sexual dysfunction.

an object-focused drive. Thus a patient may be able to masturbate and experience sexual fantasies, but have no sexual desire for his or her partner. Problems in sexual drive suggest an organic aetiology, while low sexual desire is more likely to be psychological in origin.

Statistics

The true incidence of sexual problems is not known but complaints are common and most relate to sexual dysfunction, i.e. problems of sexual

Table 41.1 Classification of sexual dysfunction related to the human sexual response.

Stage	Female	Male
Initiation	Low sexual drive or desire	
	Incompatible sex drive or desire	
	Excessive sexual interest	
	Fear of painful intercourse	
	Phobia of sex	
Arousal	Unresponsiveness	Erectile dysfunction
	Lack of lubrication	
Penetration	Vaginismus	Erectile dysfunction
	Dyspareunia	
Response	Orgasmic dysfunction	Premature ejaculation
		Failure to ejaculate

function or interest. There is ample evidence, none the less, that many patients find it difficult to ask for professional help in this area and that of those who do, the sexual dysfunction may be associated with other more fundamental problems in the relationship or the personality. It is also likely that many patients experience sexual dysfunction but do not regard it as a problem.

Presenting problems

Sexual dysfunctions that impede or prevent a couple from having or enjoying sexual intercourse include the conditions listed in Table 41.2.

Some sexual problems are gender-specific, while there are many conditions common to both men and women. Problems in one partner almost always affect the other and an individual or couple may have more than one coexisting difficulty, be it sexual or within the general relationship. It is not uncommon for a cyclical pattern to develop (e.g. initial dyspareunia leading to low sexual desire and arousal, thus maintaining a vicious cycle). Sexual dysfunction may also be classified according to whether it is primary (life-long), or secondary (acquired) to a period of normal function.

Table 41.2 Presenting problems.

Sexual and relationship problems for men and women	Female-specific sexual problems
Relationship problems	Painful or difficult intercourse
Non-consummation	Dyspareunia
Loss or lack of sexual desire	Vaginismus
Loss or lack of arousal	Inability to achieve orgasm
Gender orientation	Physiological events
Major events	Childbirth
Sexual or physical abuse	Menopause
Bereavement	Other sexual pain disorders (unrelated to intercourse)
Illness	Vulvodynia
Medication	
Antidepressants	**Male-specific sexual problems**
Antipsychotics	Inability to achieve or maintain an erection
Antihypertensives	Premature ejaculation
Drugs and alcohol	Inability to ejaculate
	Dyspareunia

Aetiology

Psychological factors play a part in sexual dysfunction, even when physical factors are mainly responsible. Counselling the individual or couple is therefore an important element of management.

Physical causes of sexual dysfunction

Illness. Any physical or mental illness may interfere with sexual life. Chronic illnesses, stress, fatigue and depression may be associated with loss of sexual interest. Vascular disease and neuropathy, e.g. in diabetics, may prevent erection. Endocrine disorders that reduce free testosterone may be associated with lack of sexual drive. It is common for women to experience a loss of sexual interest after childbirth which may be attributed to a complex interaction of stressful life events, changing relationship roles, fatigue, physical and hormonal changes (particularly in the lactating mother), and possible dyspareunia from an episiotomy scar.

Age. Although many individuals/couples enjoy sexual expression well into old age, most will have to adjust to changes in their sexual responsiveness as they become older. Erectile difficulties are a common complaint in men over 50 which may simply reflect a general reduction in sexual responsiveness and the need for more foreplay, but organic factors (as yet imperfectly understood) may also be important.

Drugs. Many drugs (both therapeutic and recreational) can affect sexual functioning. Alcohol may inhibit sexual response through central nervous system effects. It may lessen inhibitions to good effect (e.g. override vaginismus). When assessing the possible role of therapeutic drugs in patients with sexual dysfunctions, it is often difficult to determine to what extent the drug therapy, e.g. antihypertensives or antidepressants, might be responsible for symptoms which could also be attributed to the disease being treated, e.g. hypertension or depression. In addition there may be a secondary effect on the relationship.

Psychological causes of sexual dysfunction

Immediate causes.

Lack of knowledge. Sexual ignorance continues to play a part in sexual problems. Unrealistic expectations may also contribute to sexual dissatisfaction (e.g. if 'vaginal orgasm' is believed to be the 'norm' for women). Couples sometimes do not relate their socioeconomic difficulties, e.g. living virtually without privacy, to the sexual problems they are experiencing.

Sexual anxiety. Sexual anxiety can prevent the physiological changes of sexual arousal for women and contribute to premature ejaculation in men. Fear of failure contributes to erectile failure in men who may feel that they are expected to 'perform'. Other men who experience premature ejaculation may have an excessive need to please their partner and may be so over-concerned about this that they are unable to focus on their own sexual pleasure.

Lack of communication between the sexual partners. Some couples find it difficult to talk about sexual matters and may therefore give less pleasure to each other than they could if they knew more about each other's preferences. Feelings of rejection and guilt may develop due to lack of understanding and can cause unnecessary distress.

Relationship difficulties between sexual partners. Serious conflict, general communication difficulties, lack of commitment, lack of trust and disappointment in the partner may be associated with sexual problems that are unlikely to improve unless the basic relationship difficulties can be resolved.

Personal factors. Each partner may have difficulties related to their upbringing, past experience and attitudes towards sexuality. They may experience conflict with the idea that sexual behaviour should be pleasurable and feel consequent guilt and shame. Negative sexual experiences such as childhood sexual abuse or rape are increasingly recognized as contributors to these difficulties.

Sociocultural context. It is becoming increasingly important to take into account the impact of cultural norms and values and of the media (e.g. body image, the emphasis on youth, isolation/integration within society), and to realize the interconnection of this context with physical and psychological factors (see Table 41.3).

Assessment
The professionals' attitude
As most people still find it difficult to present their sexual problems, the attitude of the professional to whom they first unburden themselves is extremely important. The attitude of the doctor is probably more important than any specific knowledge or skill in treating sexual problems. Many individuals/

Table 41.3 Taking a sexual history.

Medical model	Model of sexuality
Total or situational	Biological
Primary or secondary	Childbirth
Technical problems	Menopause
Medical problems	Ageing
Medication	Psychological
Drugs	Thoughts, beliefs, anxiety, depression
Alcohol	Body image, self-esteem, guilt
Motivational	Sociocultural
Fear and phobias	Relationship with people
Loss of interest	Major life events
Mismatched sexual drive	

couples will be helped at a 'primary' level by the following features in the therapist:

1. Listening skills and the use of open-ended questions
2. Genuine concern about the patient
3. Lack of embarrassment—being at ease with sexual matters
4. A non-judgmental attitude and avoidance of 'standard-setting'
5. The use of ordinary language and avoiding medical jargon.

As the problem unfolds it may become apparent that 'secondary' or specialist help is needed but it is important not to refer patients on too quickly in case they feel rejected and unable to contemplate the process of unburdening themselves a second time to another professional.

As a quick check, exclude the sexual problem from the narrative and consider what is left: a stable or problematic relationship, rigidity or flexibility, an optimistic or pessimistic personality? Also consider the impact of losses or changes on the homeostasis of the relationship and lifestyle (e.g. hysterectomy, children leaving home). These may have positive or negative longer-term effects. It is also useful to identify why patients have presented now and whether their expectations of treatment are realistic before referral.

How sexual problems present

For some patients there may be little hesitation in presenting the sexual nature of their problem to the clinician. This may be because the patient knows the professional well and finds him or her trustworthy or because the consultation has indicated that the professional is open to discuss issues of a sensitive nature. However, many patients will find it difficult to express their feelings and present covertly either consciously with a so-called 'visiting card' or unconsciously with a variety of presenting problems. In these situations the clinician may feel that the interview is not going well; there may appear to be a conflict between what the patient is saying and how he or she responds to questions, or body language may hint at other underlying issues. It is always worthwhile stopping at this point and asking if there are any other issues that the patient wishes to talk about (see Table 41.4).

Table 41.4 How sexual problems present.

Overt

Covert

Conscious: the 'visiting card'	Unconscious
Request for contraception	Psychosomatic symptoms
Request for health check	Difficulty with contraception
Refusal to be examined	Accidental pregnancy

Doctors working in gynaecological situations need to be alert to these covert presentations. Common examples include dyspareunia, persistent vaginal discharge without any infectious or physical causation (the 'worried well'), difficulty in using contraception, pelvic pain and early presentation for a cervical smear.

Taking a sexual history

The factors that need to be considered are outlined in Table 41.3. The first column is familiar to doctors as it follows the normal medical assessment model. The model of sexuality runs in parallel with the medical factors and together they provide a more holistic view and a clearer perspective of the patient's world.

Examination

Clinical examination may be an important part in the assessment of sexual problems. The main purpose will be to assess the part played by organic disease in any complaint but the examination may also serve to educate the patient or to increase his/her sexual confidence (e.g. in vaginismus). However, it may not be either possible or desirable to examine a patient with vaginismus—such patients are often phobic in many aspects of their life and these issues may need to be addressed in the first instance.

The timing of a vaginal examination needs to be considered carefully if there has been a history of previous sexual abuse. It is essential to engage the patient before attempting examination, which otherwise could be experienced as a perpetuation of the abuse.

Investigations

The urine should be tested for glucose in all men presenting with secondary impotence or late-onset ejaculatory problems. Superficial or deep dyspareunia in women may indicate the need for a variety of tests such as a vaginal swab or full genitourinary screening. Pelvic ultrasound or laparoscopy may be needed in the further assessment of deep dyspareunia. In men, measurements of erectile function such as nocturnal tumescence studies, measurement of penile blood pressure and blood flow, and more invasive procedures such as arteriography, intracavernosal injections of smooth muscle relaxants and peripheral nerve conduction tests are also specialist techniques.

It is customary to measure serum testosterone, FSH, LH and prolactin levels in men complaining of loss of sexual interest (low drive). For men presenting with erectile or ejaculatory difficulties, with or without secondary low desire, it is usually unnecessary to check hormone levels as they are rarely outside normal limits. However, it is important to check their cardiovascular and diabetic status.

Formulation

Once the history and appropriate examination and investigations have been completed it is important to pull together the history and feed your understanding back to the patients. This is known as the formulation. This process allows patients to agree or disagree with your formulation and helps them to understand the often multifactorial nature of their problem. A useful working model is outlined in Table 41.5.

Treatment

The general principles of treating sexual dysfunctions include:

1. Consider treating the couple irrespective of which partner presents.
2. Define the problem and what the couple would like to change.
3. Aim to reduce sexual anxiety by education and 'permission giving', which may modify unhelpful attitudes. Fear of unwanted pregnancy may be a source of anxiety and contraceptive counselling may prove to be therapeutic.
4. Facilitate communication between the partners.
5. Encourage new behaviour that will give mutual pleasure to the couple.
6. Specific problems may need specific treatment programmes, e.g. vaginismus.
7. Tackle more difficult interpersonal or intrapersonal problems if they appear to be 'blocking' progress.
8. The presenting diagnosis may therefore change during the subsequent counselling.

Management of specific problems

Low sexual drive or desire

The management should be directed to the underlying cause. Low sexual drive is more likely to have an organic origin. Endocrine abnormalities are rare and more often the problem is lack of sexual desire secondary to stress, fatigue, depression, physical illness, drugs (e.g. alcohol), other sexual dysfunctions or relationship difficulties. There is often a circular pattern to this problem, both

Table 41.5 Formulation.	
1. Brief statement of what the problem appears to be	Random failure, e.g. erectile failure Anxiety/depression/stress
2. Predisposing factors Parental attitudes Poor sex education Early trauma, e.g. sexual or physical abuse	**4. Maintaining factors** Performance anxiety Poor communication Partner demands/mismatched desire Lack of knowledge
3. Precipitating factors Discord in general relationship Childbirth	**5. Positive prognostic factors** **6. Diagnosis/hypothesis**

intra- and interpersonally. It may be helpful to depict this diagrammatically to illustrate the complexity, especially when one partner has been presented as the 'problem'.

Failure of sexual arousal

Failure of the lubrication/swelling response in women may result in dyspareunia, lack of enjoyment, resentment and withdrawal from sexual encounters. It may be treated as outlined in the general principles. It may be particularly beneficial to ban sexual intercourse for a limited time and to encourage graded pleasuring exercises as a substitute. Once sexual arousal and enjoyment have been re-established the couple may regain the confidence to enjoy intercourse again.

Erectile difficulties may be treated successfully by the same means, provided there is no major organic deficit. When organic factors predominate or where the couple are not motivated towards a psychological approach, then sildenafil may be the treatment of choice. The alternative mechanical aids to erection include intracavernosal injections of vasoactive drugs, e.g. prostaglandin E, vacuum devices, penile bands, vascular surgery (if appropriate), or a penile prosthesis as a last resort.

Vaginismus

This is an involuntary spasm of the pelvic floor muscles surrounding the lower third of the vagina, which may prevent penetration or render it painful. It appears to be a learned response triggered by fear of penetration and although it is usually primary (occasionally associated with childhood sexual abuse), it may occur secondary to a traumatic experience such as childbirth or rape. If found at routine examination it may be iatrogenic; time to relax should be offered and a sensitive enquiry made to elicit whether it is present in other situations.

Treatment should aim to help the couple understand the nature of the problem. (Pictures and models are helpful.) The woman should be helped to understand the avoidance tactics often exhibited in any phobic condition and how this is often mirrored in other aspects of her life. In parallel she can embark on a programme of relaxation and deep breathing exercises before starting a system of graded exercises (using fingers or Amielle vaginal trainers) while learning progressively to gain control and relax the pelvic floor muscles (Kegel exercises). It may be more relevant to deal with the phobic issues (specific and general) within the session and encourage the exercises to take place within the home setting, especially if the partner is motivated to become involved in treatment. Operative treatment should not be considered before an expert psychosexual assessment indicates that surgical intervention is appropriate.

Dyspareunia

The management of dyspareunia (pain during intercourse) involves treating the underlying cause, whether psychological or physical. Physical conditions include the following:

Male dyspareunia. This is rare but may be caused by lacerations from over-sharp IUD threads or from candidal or other infections which may also affect the female partner.

Female dyspareunia. It is important to distinguish, from the clinical history, between superficial (vulval and vaginal) and deep dyspareunia (pelvic pain) and the timing and type of pain in relation to intercourse. The causes of female dyspareunia that may require treatment (in addition to failure of sexual arousal or vaginismus) include:

1. Vulval conditions: candidal vulvitis, herpes genitalis, urethral caruncle, urethral diverticulum, bartholinitis, vestibulitis, female genital mutilation
2. Vaginal conditions: atrophic vaginitis, infective vaginitis (candidal or trichomonal), chemical vaginitis, vaginal scars, congenital abnormalities, foreign body
3. Pelvic conditions: cystitis, PID, pelvic pain syndrome, endometriosis, fibroids, ovarian tumours, constipation, inflammatory bowel disease.

Orgasmic dysfunction

It is first important to establish whether the woman has ever experienced orgasm and in what situation. Many women do not experience orgasm during sexual intercourse although they are orgasmic during clitoral stimulation. This knowledge may be therapeutic to women who regard themselves as 'inadequate' because they require additional clitoral stimulation to reach orgasm. The capacity to experience orgasm may be helped by encouraging a couple to increase their sexual arousal (by increased sexual foreplay and fantasy) and by learning to relax and 'lose control' when high levels of sexual arousal are reached. Many men do not understand the different level of sexual stimulation required by women and further discussions on what is 'normal' can be extremely therapeutic. It is important to address both partners' needs, rather attributing any individual blame. A useful self-help book is *Becoming Orgasmic* by J. Heiman and J. LoPiccolo which addresses both personal and couple aspects of orgasmic dysfunction.

Premature ejaculation

The complaint of premature orgasm appears to be limited to men. After orgasm an erection is lost rapidly and the man remains refractory to sexual arousal for a variable period. His orgasm therefore usually terminates sexual intercourse, whereas a woman is capable of multiple orgasms without a refractory period. Anxiety reduction and re-education to control the ejaculatory reflex are the basis for most therapeutic approaches for men who are distressed by premature ejaculation. After a psychosexual assessment, treatment with topical preparations or paroxetine may be considered in conjunction with a programme of exercises.

SUMMARY

Sexual problems are common and may be presented to doctors overtly or covertly. The patient will choose to present the problem because she/he believes the doctor has some expert interest, knowledge or skill and therefore problems are frequently aired in discussions about contraception, obstetrics or gynaecology.

Concerned attention by the doctor at the first presentation may need to be followed by referral to a specialist but this should not be the initial response. The management of some conditions described in this chapter will be within the scope of the primary care doctor.

Section III

Appendices

Appendix I

Obstetric terms and definitions

Amniotomy. Surgical rupture of the membranes to induce or enhance labour.

Android pelvis. A funnel-shaped male-type pelvis with diameters which decrease from above downwards.

Antepartum haemorrhage. Bleeding from the birth canal in the period from the 24th week of gestation to the birth of the baby.

Asynclitism. Tilting of the fetal head in labour so that the anterior or posterior parietal bone presents.

Attitude of the fetus. Relationship of the fetal head and limbs to the fetal trunk, usually flexion.

Bregma. Anterior fontanelle.

Brow. The part of the fetal head between the root of the nose and the anterior fontanelle.

Caput succedaneum. Oedema from obstructed venous return in the fetal scalp caused by pressure of the head against the rim of the cervix or birth canal.

Cephalhaematoma. Collection of blood beneath the periosteum of a skull bone, limited to that bone by periosteal attachments.

Cervical dystocia. Difficult labour due to failure of the cervix to dilate, in spite of adequate uterine contractions.

Chloasma. The brown pigmented facial mask of pregnancy.

Couvelaire uterus. The uterus appears purple due to haemorrhage within its musculature, and occurs with severe placental abruption.

Crowning of the head. Phase in the second stage of labour when a large segment of the fetal scalp is visible at the vaginal orifice, the perineum being distended and the anus dilated.

Engagement. Engagement occurs when the widest diameters of the presenting part have passed through the pelvic inlet.

Erythroblastosis fetalis. Haemolytic disease of the newborn usually due to Rhesus antibodies.

Fontanelle. Space at the junction of three or more skull bones, covered only by a membrane and skin.

Fourchette. The fold of skin formed by merging of the labia minora and labia majora posteriorly.

Funnel pelvis. (See Android pelvis.)

Hyaline membrane. A homogeneous membrane lining the alveoli, alveolar ducts and respiratory bronchioles, and an important cause of death in premature infants.

Hydrops fetalis. Gross oedema of fetal subcutaneous tissues together with ascites and pericardial and pleural effusions, usually due to erythroblastosis.

Kernicterus. Yellow staining of the baby's brain due to high blood levels of unconjugated bilirubin causing severe neurological damage or death.

Lie of the fetus. Relationship of the long axis of fetus to the long axis of the uterus, usually longitudinal but can be transverse or oblique.

Linea nigra. Brown or black pigmented line in the middle of the abdominal wall during pregnancy.

Lochia. The discharge from the uterus during the puerperium, initially red, then yellow, then white.

Lower uterine segment. The thin expanded lower portion of the uterus which forms in the last trimester of pregnancy.

Moulding. Alteration in shape and diameter of the fetal head during labour (the fontanelles and sutures permit the force of contractions to compress the head against the bony pelvis and adapt its shape to that of the birth canal).

Naegele's rule. To estimate the probable date of confinement add 9 months and 7 days to the first day of the menstrual cycle (correction required if cycle not 28 days).

Neonatal death. A liveborn infant who dies within 28 days of birth.

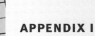

Obstructed labour. There is no descent of the presenting part in the presence of good contractions.

Operculum. The plug of mucus that occludes the cervical canal during pregnancy.

Pawlik's grip. Suprapubic palpation with the outstretched hand to identify the presenting part of the fetus, its position, flexion and engagement.

Pelvic brim or inlet. The plane of division between the true and false pelvis. The plane passes from the upper border of the symphysis pubis, along the pubic crest to the iliopectineal eminence, then to the sacroiliac joint, along the wings of the sacrum to the centre of the sacral promontory.

Pelvic outlet. Runs from beneath the symphysis pubis along the ischiopubic ramus to the ischial tuberosity along the sacrotuberous ligament to the fifth sacral vertebra.

Pelvimetry. Measurement of the size of the pelvis.

Perinatal mortality. Stillbirths plus first week deaths expressed per 1000 total births.

Placenta accreta. Absence of decidua basalis, so that the chorionic villi are attached to uterine muscle.

Placenta circumvallata. Placenta with a double fold of amnion forming a ring on the fetal surface some distance in from the edge of the placenta.

Placenta increta. Chorionic villi are in the uterine muscle.

Placenta percreta. The villi are through the uterine muscle.

Placenta succenturiata. There is one or more accessory lobe of the placenta.

Position of the fetus. The relationship of a defined area on the presenting part (called the denominator) to the quadrants of the maternal pelvis.

Presenting part. That part of the fetus felt on vaginal examination.

Prolonged pregnancy. A pregnancy that lasts longer than term (37–42 completed weeks).

Puerperium. The period during which the reproductive organs return to their prepregnant condition (usually regarded as an interval of 6 weeks after delivery).

Show. A discharge of mucus and blood at the onset of labour when the cervix dilates and the operculum (cervical mucus plug) falls out.

Sinciput. That part of the fetal head in front of the anterior fontanelle.

Spalding's sign. Overlapping of the fetal skull bones, seen radiographically after fetal death.

Station. The level of the presenting part within the mother's pelvis (the ischial spines are the reference points on vaginal examination).

Symphysiotomy. Division of the pubic symphysis to enlarge the diameters of the bony pelvis.

Third degree tear. A perineal laceration passing through the anal sphincter.

Vasa praevia. Fetal vessels lying in the membranes in front of the presenting part (there must be an associated velamentous insertion of the cord, succenturiate lobe or bipartite placenta).

Velamentous insertion. The umbilical cord inserts onto the membranes over which the vessels course to reach the fetal surface of the placenta.

Vernix caseosa. Produced by sebaceous glands and prevents waterlogging and maceration of the fetal skin by the amniotic fluid.

Vertex. The area between the anterior and posterior fontanelles and the parietal eminences.

Wharton's jelly. The mucoid connective tissue supporting the umbilical cord vessels.

Appendix II

Risk factors in obstetrics

General factors

Age less than 18 years
Age more than 36 years
Nullipara of 35 or more
Parity greater than 4

Menstrual history uncertain

Last period more than 2 weeks
Pill stopped within 3 months of last period
Cycle length before last period more than 30 days
Intrauterine device in situ
Vaginal bleeding since last period

Previous obstetric history

Stillbirth or neonatal death
Small baby, less than 2.5 kg
Large baby, more than 4.0 kg
Fetal congenital abnormality
Significant antibodies (defined by haematologist)
Hypertension or proteinuria
Eclampsia
Two or more legal abortions (less than 13 weeks)
Two or more miscarriages (less than 13 weeks)
Late miscarriage or legal abortion (13 weeks or more)
Preterm delivery (less than 37 weeks)
Cervical suture
Caesarean section, hysterotomy or myomectomy
Postpartum haemorrhage or manual removal of placenta
Labour less than 2 hours
Labour more than 12 hours
Operative vaginal delivery
Postnatal depression

Maternal health

Relevant medical condition
Pelvic abnormality (including fibroids)
Smoking more than 10 per day at booking
Social factors
Problems with housing
Family history of diabetes
Family history of congenital abnormality
Haemoglobinopathy
Risk of transmissible viral factors
Drinking more than 10 units of alcohol per week at booking
Current drug abuse by woman or partner
Not fluent in English

Booking examination	Blood pressure more than 140/90
	Proteinuria
	Weight more than 90 kg
	Weight less than 45 kg
	Height less than 1.52 m
	Cardiac murmur
	Uterus large or small for dates
	Other pelvic or abdominal mass
	Blood group Rhesus negative

City and Hackney District Health Authority system (from Carroll et al. 1988 Journal of Obstetrics and Gynaecology 8: 222–227).

Appendix III

The fetal skull

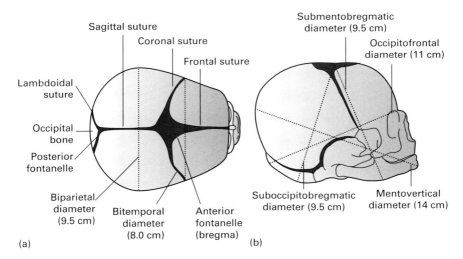

Fig. III
Frontal suture—between the two frontal bones
Coronal suture—between the frontal and parietal bones
Sagittal suture—between the two parietal bones
Lambdoidal suture—between the occipital bone and the parietal and temporal bones.

Anterior fontanelle (bregma)—large diamond-shaped depression where the frontal coronal and sagittal sutures meet. Closes at 18 months of age.
Posterior fontanelle—smaller triangular-shaped depression where the sagittal suture meets the lambdoidal sutures.

Diameters of the fetal skull
Biparietal diameter: 9.5 cm (vertex presentation)
Submentobregmatic: 9.5 cm (face presentation)
Occipitofrontal: 11 cm (deflexed head, usually occipitoposterior)
Mentovertical: 14 cm (brow presentation)
Suboccipitobregmatic: 9.5 cm (vertex presentation).

Appendix IV

Diameters of the normal female pelvis

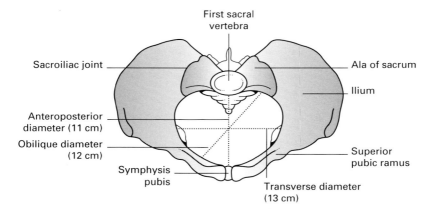

Fig. IVA. The pelvic brim. The outline of the brim follows the upper border of the first sacral vertebra, the alae, the sacroiliac joint, the ilium, the superior pubic ramus and the symphysis pubis.

Anteroposterior diameter: 11 cm
Oblique diameter: 12 cm
Transverse diameter: 13 cm.

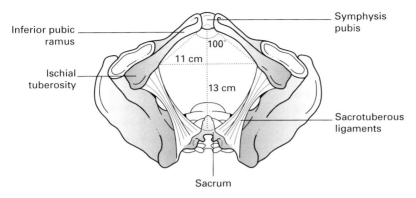

Fig. IVB. The pelvic outlet. The boundary of the outlet passes from the symphysis pubis, down the inferior rami of the pubic bones to the ischial tuberosities, and then obliquely upwards and posterior along the sacrotuberous ligaments to the tip of the fifth sacral vertebra.

Anteroposterior: 13 cm
Transverse: 11 cm
Oblique diameter: 12 cm.

Appendix V

Normal values in pregnancy

Haemoglobin concentration	12 weeks	12.0 g/dL
	36 weeks	11.1 g/dL
White cell count	12 weeks	8.1×10^9 L
	36 weeks	10.2×10^9 L
Packed cell volume		< 0.35
Platelets		$150{-}400 \times 10^9$ L
ESR	32 weeks	44–114
Serum urate	32 weeks	< 0.35 mmol/L
	36 weeks	< 0.40 mmol/L
Serum glucose (fasting)		< 5.5 mmol/L
Serum glucose (random)		< 8.7 mmol/L
Glomerular filtration rate		170 mL/min
24-hour urinary protein		< 0.3 g/24 h

Appendix VI

Partograms—the graphic description of labour

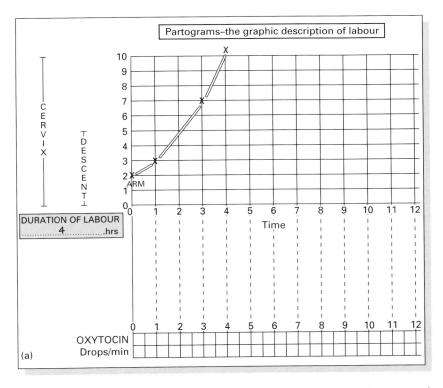

Fig. VI. Partograms showing (a) normal labour and (b) inefficient uterine action corrected with oxytocin.

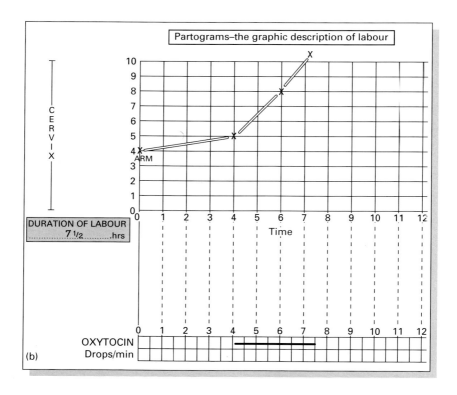

Partograms–the graphic description of labour

DURATION OF LABOUR
.... 7 ½ ....hrs

Time

OXYTOCIN
Drops/min

(b)

Appendix VII

The obstetric flying squad

Obstetric flying squads were pioneered by E. F. Murray in Newcastle in the 1930s and comprised an obstetrician, midwife and anaesthetist with the necessary equipment to resuscitate a woman prior to her transfer to hospital.

Nowadays some 30% of calls are for intrapartum problems and 50% for PPH or retained placenta. Removal of a retained placenta is one of the few operative procedures now performed at home. On occasion a paediatrician may accompany the flying squad where the problem relates to the neonate.

With the introduction of paramedics into the ambulance service the role of, and necessity for, the flying squad is being re-examined.

Indications to summon the flying squad are:

1. Intrapartum haemorrhage
2. Eclampsia or severe pre-eclampsia
3. Postpartum haemorrhage
4. Retained placenta
5. Neonatal apnoea.

Suggested reading

Janice Rymer

OBSTETRICS

Beischer N, Mackay E 1997 Obstetrics and the newborn, 2nd edn. W B Saunders, London
McDonald M 1996 Loss in pregnancy—guidelines for midwives. Baillière–Tindall, London
Magowan B 1996 Churchill's pocketbook of obstetrics and gynaecology. Churchill Livingstone, Edinburgh
Why mothers die—the confidential enquiries into maternal deaths in the United Kingdom 1997–1999. HMSO, London
Studd J (ed) 1981–2001 Progress in obstetrics and gynaecology, vols 1–15. Churchill Livingstone, Edinburgh

GYNAECOLOGY

Loudon N (ed) 2000 Handbook of family planning and reproductive healthcare, 4th edn. Churchill Livingstone, Edinburgh
Magowan B 1996 Churchill's pocketbook of obstetrics and gynaecology. Churchill Livingstone, Edinburgh
Shaw R W, Soulter W P, Stanton S L 1997 Gynaecology, 2nd edn. Churchill Livingstone, New York
Studd J (ed) 1981–2001 Progress in obstetrics and gynaecology, vols 1–15. Churchill Livingstone, Edinburgh
Whitfield C R (ed) 1995 Dewhurst's textbook of obstetrics and gynaecology for postgraduates, 5th edn. Blackwell Scientific, Oxford (for reference)

SEXUALLY TRANSMITTED DISEASES

Clinical Effectiveness Group August 1999 UK national guidelines on sexually transmitted infections in closely related infections. Sexually Transmitted Infections. Vol 75, Suppl 1. Available via web site: www.mssvd.org.uk
Hermione H, Lyall M, Blott A et al October 2001. Guidelines for the management of HIV infection in pregnant women and the prevention of mother to child transmission. HIV Medicine. Vol 2, No. 4, pp. 314–335. Available via website: www.bhiva.org.uk
Holmes K, King K 1990 Sexually transmitted diseases, 2nd edn. McGraw–Hill, London (for reference)
Willcox R, Willcox J 1982 Venereological medicine. Blackwell Scientific, Oxford

PSYCHOSEXUAL MEDICINE

Heiman J, LoPiccolo, J Becoming orgasmic. Piatkus, London
Mini symposium of psychosexual disorders in The Diplomate (Dec 1997, RCOG)
Spence S H 1991 Psychosexual therapy. Chapman & Hall, London

NEONATAL MEDICINE

Rennie J M, Roberton N R C 1997 Textbook of neonatology, 3rd edn. Churchill Livingstone,
    Edinburgh

EXAMINATION REVISION

Dooley M, Reid M 1997. DRCOG practice exams—MCQ and OSCEs. PasTest
James D K, Pillai M, Rymer J et al. 2001. Interactive CD-ROM in obstetrics, gynaecology and
    neonatalology. Churchill Livingstone, Edinburgh
Rymer J, Ahmed H 1999 OSCEs in obstetrics and gynaecology. Churchill Livingstone,
    Edinburgh

Index

INDEX

INDEX